The Residential Psychiatric Treatment of Children

The Residential Psychiatric Treatment of Children

Edited by

PHILIP BARKER, MB, MRCPEd, MRCPsych, DPM, DCH

Crosby Lockwood Staples London

Granada Publishing Limited
First published in Great Britain 1974 by Crosby Lockwood Staples
Frogmore St Albans Herts and 3 Upper James Street London W1R 4BP

ISBN 0 258 96891 5

Printed in Great Britain by
Richard Clay (The Chaucer Press) Ltd, Bungay, Suffolk

Foreword

The first children's psychiatric hospital outpatient and inpatient unit was built at The Maudsley Hospital, London, in 1938, although the admission of inpatients did not start until 1946. The late Dr Kenneth Cameron then developed the psychiatric inpatient care of children there and so was the leader in this field in the United Kingdom. Thus he should have been the writer of this Foreword; my excuse is that I worked for him in this unit in 1947 and remember well its early days.

This book describes the working of a number of hospital inpatient units for children that have since opened up. Each had to start from scratch and so was a pioneer in its own area, and each has developed its own expertise. Some have a special slant, but their functioning overlaps and together they give a composite picture of inpatient child psychiatry as practised today – taking its place with the other kinds of residential care of disturbed children. If the various accounts given sometimes appear to recur, they emphasise that each separately has had to undertake a similar task. The reader will incidentally gain new insights into some of the well-known syndromes to be met in child psychiatry, while the continuity of psychiatric practice as between children and younger adolescents is underlined.

The need to provide for the psychiatric inpatient care in special hospital units for both children and adolescents has been assured for at least a decade. The point has now been reached when moves to develop further hospital care have to be considered so that experiences described in this book are opportune. Should similar children's hospital units be further multiplied, and if so where should they be placed? Or, because of more and better alternative facilities now available, for instance in schools for the maladjusted, community homes and so on, will the demand for hospital beds become less urgent? In any case, should not the experience of psychiatric care gained in these hospital units be spread more widely to influence other kinds of residential care of disturbed children and adolescents?

Hospital units have been set up in a variety of settings and this has to some extent determined the kinds of patient admitted; for instance, very disturbed children cannot be placed in hospital near the physically sick. However, a psychiatric inpatient unit should not be isolated and, with the spread of district general hospitals, it is clear that any child psychiatric department for both outpatients and inpatients should be linked with the general psychiatric department; for disturbed children are apt to have psychiatrically disturbed parents. Still more does the children's unit need to be linked with the paediatric department.

There are other hospital developments to be kept in mind. How far should day-hospital care of psychiatrically disturbed children be developed? Again, there are some children with chronic conditions that require long-term hospital care. What can be developed for them? Finally, the whole matter of the hospital care of handicapped children, including the mentally handicapped, is now an open question. What should be arranged for them?

The Maudsley Hospital
London
August 1973

W. WARREN
MA, MD, FRCP, FRCPsych

List of Contributors

PHILIP BARKER, MB, MRCPEd, MRCPsych, DPM, DCH
Consultant in Clinical Charge, Charles Burns Clinic, Birmingham B13 8QD
Part-time Lecturer and Post-graduate Clinical Tutor in Child Psychiatry, University of Birmingham

S. BROWN, SRN, SCM, Certificate of Child Psychiatry Nursing
Nursing Officer, Nuffield Child Psychiatry Unit, Newcastle

L. A. HERSOV, MD, MRCP, FRCPsych, DPM
Physician, The Bethlem Royal Hospital and The Maudsley Hospital, London
Senior Lecturer and Hon. Consultant in Psychological Medicine, The Royal Postgraduate Medical School and Hammersmith Hospital, London

I. KOLVIN, BA, MD, FRCPsych, DipPsych
Physician in Psychological Medicine, Nuffield Child Psychiatry Unit, Newcastle
Research Director, Human Development Unit, University of Newcastle

PHILIP PINKERTON, MD, FRCPsych, DPM
Senior Consultant and Lecturer in Paediatric Psychiatry, University of Liverpool
Physician-in-Charge, The Unit for Psychosomatic Disorders, Royal Liverpool Children's Hospital, Heswall, Wirral, Cheshire

D. A. Pond, MA, MD, FRCP, FRCPsych
Professor of Psychiatry, The London Hospital, E.1
H. M. N. Rees, MB, MRCP, MRCPsych, DPM
Consultant Children's Psychiatrist, Charles Burns Clinic, Birmingham B13 8QD
Part-time Lecturer in Child Psychiatry, University of Birmingham
Co-Director of the Child Treatment Research Unit, University of Leicester
D. McI. Scott, BA, DipPsych, DipEd, ABPsS
Principal Psychologist, Nuffield Child Psychiatry Unit, Newcastle
George Stroh, MB, BS, MRCPsych, DPM
Psychiatrist-in-Charge, High Wick Hospital, St Albans, Herts
Consultant Psychiatrist, The Child Guidance Training Centre, London N.W.3
E. G. Tweddle, RGN, SCM, HVCert, Certificate of Child Psychiatry Nursing
Research Interviewer, Human Development Unit, University of Newcastle
Hon. Tutor, Nuffield Child Psychiatry Unit, Newcastle
Christopher J. Wardle, MD, MRCPsych, DPM
Consultant in Child Psychiatry
Clinic Director, Dryden Clinic for Children and Adolescents
Medical Director, Exeter and Devon Child Guidance Clinics
Hon. Lecturer in Child Psychiatry, Exeter University

Contents

Introduction

Inpatient psychiatric hospital facilities for children in Great Britain date back little further than the start of the National Health Service in 1948. Since then some fifty units have come into operation. Little information has been published about the work of these units, and even less about the treatment of particular syndromes and disorders. There is no generally available body of information about the types of children treated, how they are treated or what the outcome is.

This book examines aspects of the work of various child psychiatric hospital units. It is clear that the aims, structure and philosophy of units vary. These variations reflect both local needs and also the interests and skills of those working in the different units. Since there is no set pattern which all, or even most, child psychiatric hospitals follow, it is necessary to look at the work of a number of centres in order to get an idea of the scope of child psychiatric hospitals generally. That is the aim of this book.

It would have been possible to provide a straightforward description of the work of various units, but this might have been dull, it would probably have contained a fair amount of repetition (since units have features in common as well as differing in many respects), and it would not have facilitated the detailed description of the treatment of particular syndromes and types of problems. The latter represents an important gap in the literature. There is therefore only one general description of a unit. Other chapters cover the treatment of various syndromes, each by an author from a different centre. There is naturally included information about how the respective centres operate, so that insights are nevertheless provided into the work and philosophy of the different units.

In any hospital the nurses are important: in child psychiatry units they are of paramount importance. A patient who has had his appendix skilfully removed will probably get better even if indifferently nursed. A child psychiatric patient, on the other hand, will probably not benefit if indifferently nursed; he may well get worse. The milieu and the relationships disturbed children are offered are vital and major parts of the treatment, and in a hospital unit both depend largely on the nursing staff. For this reason a chapter is devoted to nurse training.

No survey of residential psychiatric treatment of children would be complete without a review of the literature. It was at first my intention to provide a comprehensive literature review, but it soon became clear that this was scarcely practicable. There is a large literature on the subject, most of it American, and some of it dating back to the early 1920s. Several books on the subject have been published in the United States and one alone (American Psychiatric Association, 1957) lists 229 references up to 1957. Many of the publications cover common ground, and most are of a general nature. Thus it became apparent that selectivity would be more of a virtue than comprehensiveness. I hope that the main themes of the literature have been covered nevertheless. Only work published in the English language has been included.

This book is a collaborative effort, designed to present a broad view of British practice in the field of the inpatient treatment of emotionally disturbed children. Without the enthusiastic interest of my co-authors when they were approached, and their willing co-operation, it could not have been written. Their contributions speak for themselves, but I must express my personal thanks to them for collaborating with me, and for reacting in so good-natured a way to my queries, comments and suggestions.

I am also deeply grateful to Mrs Edna Collins who has not only typed most of the manuscript – some of it several times – but has also done much other secretarial work in connection with the book. I am grateful to Mrs Ros. Berridge, medical librarian to the Uffculme and Charles Burns Clinics, who has assisted me greatly, and to the librarians at the Royal College of Physicians of Edinburgh who have most efficiently traced and obtained for me some of the more obscure references. Finally I must thank Mr Robert Coates, until recently on the staff of Crosby Lockwood Staples, without whose enthusiastic co-operation the book would never have seen the light of day.

P.B.

CHAPTER ONE

History

Philip Barker

While in Great Britain hospital units specifically for the psychiatric treatment of children have only been established since the Second World War, in the United States some such units have existed since the 1920s. The early literature is therefore mainly American. Nevertheless, emotionally disturbed children have for long received care and treatment in a variety of settings. Before hospital units for them were established in Britain such children were admitted to special schools of various types, industrial schools (later called approved schools), children's homes, mental subnormality hospitals, adult psychiatric units, paediatric wards and foster homes. Children with psychiatric problems still are to be found in such settings, especially subnormality hospitals, special schools (notably, but not exclusively, those for maladjusted children), children's homes and community schools (as the former approved schools are now called). This book, however, concentrates on hospital units designed specially for psychiatrically sick children. In reviewing the literature attention will be given mainly to such units, but work in other types of centre will be referred to from time to time as it is sometimes relevant to the work of hospital units.

In Great Britain it is easy to define a hospital, for it is a centre financed and run by the National Health Service (the 'private' sector of the hospital services is small and, as far as is known, includes no children's psychiatric units). In other countries it can be less clear what is a hospital and what is not, since a variety of agencies, national or local, state-financed or not, may be responsible both for hospitals and for other types of treatment centre. Nevertheless, the distinction is usually apparent, though there seem to be a few hybrid units in the United States.

Early Units in America

The first units to be opened in the United States, in the early 1920s, were provided primarily for children suffering from the after-effects of epidemic encephalitis. In due course many of these units broadened the scope of their work to deal with other psychiatric problems. The early history of residential units in the USA has been reviewed by Beskind (1962). It is clear that by the mid-1930s considerable expertise and a large body of knowledge about inpatient psychiatric units for children and adolescents had been built up. Thus Potter (1934a; 1934b) discusses five years' experience acquired in the children's service of the New York State Psychiatric Institute, New York City. Many of the points in these two important papers are as relevant and appropriate today as when the paper was written.

Potter states that admission for *diagnosis* may be needed in three main situations:

(a) for the investigation of a suspected underlying physical condition;
(b) to assess the ability level, chiefly of children under five or six years of age, in cases where emotional disorder is, or may be, adversely affecting intellectual function and assessment;
(c) where there is an organic element to a child's condition but it is unclear how far the disability is due to resulting over-solicitude or spoiling by the parents.

The Institute admitted children for *treatment* of four main types of problem:

(i) children so disturbed in their conduct that care at home and outpatient treatment was impracticable;
(ii) where severe neurotic or psychotic reactions rendered children incapable of adjusting at home or at school, and where intensive and extensive psychotherapy was necessary;

(iii) where the home situation was so difficult that admission to hospital was required to relieve the tension in the family;
(iv) where children needing residential child care treatment showed behavioural or neurotic symptoms so severe that a period of inpatient treatment was needed before they were placed in a children's home or foster home. This was a numerically small group.

Potter comments with insight on admission procedure, the construction of units for children, their staffing, and treatment methods. The importance of individualising treatment is emphasised. The division of a unit into a section for younger children (below about age nine), and a section for the age range nine to twelve or thirteen, is recommended. The roles of education, occupational therapy, psychotherapy and social work, and the functions of the various categories of professional staff, are outlined. The forward-looking principles described have a relevant application today. There is reference to the use of 'time-out' procedures (not referred to by this name, of course) and to the value of single rooms.

Reports from a number of state hospitals have described the development of children's units in response to demands from community agencies for the admission of children. Thus Klopp (1932) describes how at the Allentown State Hospital there were 266 first admissions of children under sixteen years of age (171 boys and 95 girls) to the hospital between June 1924 and May 1931. Fifty of these had been admitted in the one-year period to 1 May 1931, at which date there were 79 children under sixteen in the hospital. This situation led to the opening, on 1 January 1930, of a special building to accommodate children. Previously children had been treated on adult wards which, Klopp considered, was 'in many respects unfortunate'.

The new building had one floor for boys and another for girls, with a schoolroom, day-rooms, dormitories, offices and various treatment rooms. In the semi-basement there were two occupational therapy rooms, a full-size gymnasium and the children's dining room. Outside there was a playground and a regular programme of play was organised by a trained physical director.

This unit sought to study children as individuals, in the context of their families, and aimed to bring about changes in both the children and the families. Children attended school either in the morning or in the afternoon, the other period being devoted to such activities as music, drama, occupational therapy and so on. While in school the children were given 'straight academic subjects', but initially at a level sufficiently elementary to enable them to gain confidence in their ability to cope with school work. Change in attitude to school tended to be considered more important than the amount learnt.

The importance of a planned, and full, programme is emphasised in this paper which, like Potter's 1934 papers, is an important pioneering contribution to our subject. It was presented at the 1931 annual meeting of the American Psychiatric Association, and it is interesting that in the ensuing discussion (also reported in Klopp, 1932) both Dr Frederick Allen and Dr Earl Bond commented on the need for control by the staff over the intake so that a therapeutic situation could exist in the clinic. The types of children admitted to this unit in those days seem rather different to those found in child psychiatry clinics nowadays, certainly in Britain. Thus the diagnoses in a series of 104 admissions were:

(a) Nonpsychotic:	mental deficiency	34
	environmental problem cases	12
	psychopathic personality	8
	schizoid personality	1
	delinquency	1
	epilepsy	4
	no designation	2
	Total	62
(b) Psychotic:	post-encephalitis (all with conduct disorders)	13
	epilepsy	4
	juvenile general paresis	2
	dementia praecox,	
	catatonic type	6
	hebephrenic type	2
	mental deficiency	3
	manic-depressive, manic type	2
	chorea	1
	undiagnosed	9
	Total	42

This breakdown, even allowing for the use of different diagnostic labels, is very different to recent figures from a British clinic recorded in Chapter 9.

Other early units mentioned by Beskind (1962) are the Franklin School in Philadelphia, the children's psychiatric ward at Bellevue Hospital, New York and the children's institute of King's Park State Hospital.

Many papers have been written by the staff of the children's ward at Bellevue. Bender (1937), describing this unit, emphasised the value of using ward activities for 'group psychotherapy'. She contrasted this approach with that of Potter, who, she considered, looked upon ward life 'as a means of individual observation, treatment and re-education'. Describing the children treated at Bellevue, Bender classified their problems as being in most cases 'neurotic behaviour problems'. These involved:

(a) fear and apprehension growing out of insecurity in family relationships accompanied by inadequate or unsuitable expressions of love;
(b) anxiety and guilt because of their behaviour difficulties which mostly related to aggression, sex problems and the attaining of personal satisfactions.

She saw the need of children in such a unit as being:

free expression of the child's neurotic complexes to the psychiatrist;
relief from feelings of anxiety, guilt, inferiority and insecurity;
demonstrations of affection and approval from the adults who are serving him;
free expression of the child's feelings of affection;
free expression of the child's impulses for aggression;
opportunities for the child to become socially at ease and socially acceptable at his own value;
crystallisation for the child's ideologies which are suitable for himself and the social milieu in which he lives.

Bender considered that these aims could be achieved mainly through group therapy and activities. As well as psychotherapy groups, she described a puppet project, a music project, an art project, group schoolroom activities and group play techniques. More informal and casual groups were also encouraged.

During the 1930s various other children's units were opened. Bradley (1936) claims the Emma Pendleton Bradley Home at East Providence, Rhode Island, opened in 1931, as the first hospital 'planned and especially equipped for the care of children with neurological and behaviour disorders'. As in so many other units, the biggest group of children admitted were those with 'behaviour disorders'. This group was followed by those with 'convulsive disorders' and various other neurological syndromes. The usual preponderance of boys in the 'behaviour disorder' group was noted (the ratio was exactly 2:1). Of 53 children with behaviour disorders who had 'adequate treatment', all but 15 improved; the improvement was considered to be due in most cases to the environment, though individual psychotherapy was used also. The central roles of nurses and teachers are also recognised in this paper. Bradley considered that the most valuable were those who combined 'an attractive, unruffled and ingenious personality with extensive experience among normal active children'.

The boys' adolescent unit at Bellevue Hospital, New York, was claimed by Curran (1939) to be the first unit of its type in America. Curran's paper described its organisation. The maximum stay was thirty days, though a fifth of the patients were readmissions. Between 40 and 50 patients, aged twelve to sixteen, were assessed and given short-term treatment, largely designed to socialise them. Treatment activities included educational sessions, drama, magic activities (the magic being taught to the boys, not practised on them), story-telling, athletics, beadwork and games such as cards, checkers, dominoes, ping-pong and 'parlour' games. Physiotherapy and occupational therapy were used. A main aim of the unit was a comprehensive medical and psychological assessment with a view to recommending subsequent management and placement.

Most of the boys in this unit had shown delinquent behaviour and had been committed by courts. This no doubt partly accounts for the great amount of aggressive and destructive behaviour they displayed in the unit. Curran's paper well illustrates the difficulties which treating such a group of boys in a short-term unit involves.

Non-Hospital Units

As well as strictly hospital units, other treatment centres for disturbed children were emerging during the 1930s, some of them by the evolution or reorganisation of pre-existing institutions. For example, Alt (1960) has described the Hawthorne Cedar Knolls School, New York, a residential treatment centre for disturbed children. Opened in 1906, this centre initially provided rigorous training for delinquent youths, similar perhaps to that which used to be characteristic of many British approved schools. By the mid-1930s the need for more psychiatric involvement, and for treatment rather than training, was appreciated. This led to a turbulent transition period. In 1940 a child guidance clinic was set up at the school, and from 1941 more deliberate attempts to provide a therapeutic milieu were made.

This unit developed into one in which 'specially designed living experience' was combined with psychotherapy, except in the case of some children considered inaccessible to psychotherapy. A large number of the children treated had 'limited internal controls, a reality sense insufficient to inhibit impulsive behaviour, little feeling of guilt, excessive self-love'. Emotional deprivation or rejection was usual in their histories. These aggressive children were treated permissively, restraint only being used to prevent attempts at physical injury. 'Basic in the planning of the living situation for these children is the premise that if they are exposed to considerate and interested adults around them, they will begin to reduce their hostile attitude toward adults and society in general.'

The extent to which the psychiatrist and caseworker prescribed the total milieu for the child varied from time to time. Latterly, however, their function in this area was advisory, the primary responsibility being that of the child care staff under the director, who was not a psychiatrist. The author observes that 'the child care function is the foundation for total treatment'. The experience of this unit is obviously relevant to the treatment of disturbed children in hospital. Nevertheless it is, with its 200 children in cottages, rather different from National Health Service inpatient units.

An example of a hybrid unit is that described, much later, by French (1963). This paper, on the Devereux Foundation, Devon, Pennsylvania, made some general comments on residential treatment programmes for emotionally disturbed 'young people'. The author considered terminology important. He preferred the term *students* to *patients*, and a school atmosphere to a clinical one. A 'rounded, integrated' programme, not one based simply on psychotherapy, was thought to be needed. Attendance at outside schools was considered generally unsatisfactory. This unit was clearly educationally orientated and French, its director, was apparently not medically qualified. In Great Britain it might well have been termed a residential school for maladjusted children, though the paper describing it appeared in the journal *Mental Hospitals*.

Much has also been learnt about the residential treatment of disturbed children from other non-hospital units. Important early work includes that of Aichorn who, in Vienna in the 1920s, brought psychoanalytic principles into the day-to-day treatment of delinquent boys (Aichorn, 1935).

Bettelheim (1950) in his classic book, *Love Is Not Enough*, described the work of the University of Chicago Sonia Shankman Orthogenic School. This school was for severely disturbed children of 'normal or better than normal' intelligence and accommodated 34 children between the ages of six and fourteen. Problems ranged from 'delinquency or a functional inability to read, to childhood schizophrenia'. Treatment lasted two to three years.

Bettelheim aimed for a treatment milieu which would enable very disturbed children to work through their problems in the context of their day-to-day life and relationships with the staff, and in the group. He says: 'In our treatment efforts, which try to embrace the child's total life, we have opportunities for insight into the workings of personality development that fall somewhere between what the artist and the analyst can offer us.' Thus Bettelheim prefers to treat the child by participating in his life, rather than dealing with symbols, as the psychotherapist does. Nevertheless he recognises that some disturbed children are 'so fearful of real personal contact, of real situations, or of realising the meaning or purpose of their behaviour in everyday reality', that they must for a time deal in symbols. Only when these children feel they are dealing in what is 'just talk' can they express themselves freely. For the majority, however, 'dealing with symbols in place of the experience is needlessly time-consuming'.

All concerned with providing a therapeutic milieu for disturbed children should read Bettelheim's book, if only for the care with which children's reactions in all aspects of their daily life are considered. While the efficacy of his methods is not certain, the importance of the all-embracing approach does seem clear.

Developments in Britain

In Britain, too, various non-hospital treatment centres for disturbed children were set up decades before the start of any hospital units. It is likely also that many disturbed children were treated in schools and other units not designed primarily for this type of child. Thus Bridgland (1971), in his comprehensive review of the development of schools for maladjusted children, quotes the following case history. It originally appeared in a pamphlet published for the Home and School for Invalid and Imbecile Children, 10 Gayfield Square, Edinburgh. It describes a case admitted to Dr Howe's school for defectives, founded in Boston in 1845.

> Michael Maher, aged thirteen. This boy was quite unmanageable by any means within the reach of his father or friends. They knew no way to make him obey but that of force or blows. He was formerly a tolerably bright boy, but he had been in this condition for years, and was rapidly growing worse. He seemed to live in continual terror and seldom spoke a word. The first time that I heard him utter a word was one day when his father took hold of him to make him obey some command, upon which, with his knees fairly knocking and his body trembling all over, he screamed convulsively 'Will good boy – Will good boy'. This was enough to show that, whatever may have been the cause of his strange condition, the daily treatment he was receiving was gradually crushing his feeble intellect, and would tend to drive him into hopeless idiocy or insanity . . . The boy, therefore, was taken into our school at once. He is still a little shy, but he has lost all the appearance of terror, he not only comes readily when called, but often goes up to those belonging to the home, and puts his arms affectionately about them, and returns their caresses. He takes his place in class, and strives to imitate all the motions of the scholars, and obey the signs of the teacher. He can select the letters of the alphabet, and understands a few words. He is obedient and docile, and tries hard to learn with the others. He is affectionate and much gratified by any mark of praise or approval. He begins to talk and is rapidly improving in every respect . . . The improvement is mainly attributable to the spirit of gentleness which pervades the household. This has quieted all his terrors and soothed his spirit . . .

It is clear from this and other reports that schools and other residential institutions have for long been admitting and treating emotionally disturbed children. In some of these treatment may well have been along lines similar to those used in present-day child psychiatry units.

In this connection Bridgland (1971) mentions the work of Alexander Devine who 'before his light failed' gave 'some idea of what could be done for disturbed boys by sympathy and imagination', in Glebelands, his school at Mitcham, in the 1890s. The Caldicott community, founded in 1914, also provided a therapeutic environment in which disturbed children were treated. So, too, did the Little Commonwealth, run by Homer Lane in Dorset between 1913 and 1918, and, of course, Summerhill, founded by A. S. Neill in 1924.

It is of interest that the school which Bridgland states was the first true residential school for maladjusted children was founded in 1920 by Dr F. H. Dodd, a psychiatrist on the staff of the Tavistock Clinic. Nowadays, perhaps, he might have set up a children's inpatient unit. Another psychiatrist who started a school for disturbed children was Dr Alfred Fitch, who in 1935 took over Dunnow Hall, a mansion on the Yorkshire–Lancashire border. Fitch ran this school until his retirement in 1952, when a teacher was appointed his successor.

Schools and hospital units for disturbed children have since those days become polarised and have tended to operate in rather different ways. It is unlikely that in the 1970s one would find a psychiatrist being appointed principal of a school for maladjusted children. Similarly, the structure of the National Health Service would make it impossible for a teacher to be the director of a hospital child psychiatry unit. Yet the roles of the two types of unit are similar, especially when the longer-stay hospital units are considered. Undoubtedly each type of unit has much to learn from the other. Referring to staff for schools for maladjusted children, Bridgland (1971) says, 'I know of none who would not consider unconditional love and acceptance of the child (although not always of his actions) as of primary importance. This is not always easy since being loved and being lovable are, to some extent, cause and effect and many children who attend schools for the maladjusted are not naturally either.' This surely applies as much to work in hospital units.

So too must the statement of David Wills (1960): 'In order to live with maladjusted children you have to be the kind of person who can live without them, and indeed without anyone. You have to be a whole, complete person, entirely sufficient unto yourself. Because if you *cannot* do without them, you are dependent on them. If you are dependent on them you and they have reversed roles to the ultimate damnation of both of you.'

The First British Hospital Units

This brief outline of previous work shows that there was a considerable body of knowledge of the residential treatment of psychiatrically disturbed children, both in hospital and elsewhere, when the first units opened in Britain after the Second World War. The first children's unit to open in England was that at the Maudsley Hospital, London. Cameron (1949) gave an early account of it. He described first the physical lay-out of the unit and the criteria for admission. He observed that it 'early became apparent that children actively engaged with an adult constitute an amenable group, however much disturbed, while children left to occupy themselves, or bored, form an explosive mixture, however normal'. The need for a nurse:patient ratio of about 1:1 was recognised, as was the value of school, occupational therapy and voluntary help. The 'paramount' importance of the ward sister was also emphasised.

Nursing staff were given four basic principles to work on:

1. Every child has a biological need for affection.
2. As infants abandon immediate gratification to retain their mother's affection, so reasonable conformity to demands made upon the patients should be obtained in a similar way.
3. Each child has a need for 'emotional outlet, imaginative and creative activity and physical activity'.
4. The assertion of authority by those caring for them is required in appropriate circumstances, and a stable routine is necessary.

The author went on to discuss the importance of staff morale. He described the medical organisation and the approach to investigation and treatment, social workers and psychologists being closely involved in this. The work of the Maudsley Hospital children's department is referred to further in Chapter 4 of this book.

The first two adolescent units opened in England appear to have been at Bethlem Royal Hospital and at St Ebba's Hospital, Epsom. Both opened in 1949. Sands (1953) described the 'juvenile unit', as the St Ebba's Hospital unit was called. It treated adolescents from twelve upwards and seems to have been something of a 'juvenile' version of an adult ward, with considerable emphasis on physical treatment. Thus 48 of 217 patients received insulin coma treatment, 33 had ECT and three were even subject to leucotomy. At the same time the importance of the unit environment was recognised, as also was a role for psychotherapy. The main diagnostic groups were 'schizophrenias, neuroses and psychopathic personalities', about a third of the patients falling into each group. The results on discharge of 217 patients were: recovered, 31; improved, 132; no change, 54. It is hard to know what to make of these results since well over half the 69 psychopathic personalities and four out of the six cases of mental defect are said to have improved.

Warren (1952) described the adolescent unit at the Bethlem Royal Hospital. Sixteen boys' and sixteen girls' beds, in separate wards, were provided. A physician-in-charge led the therapeutic team in each ward and a varied social, occupational and educational programme was provided to suit the wide range of children admitted. The age range was twelve to sixteen. The need for full investigation was found to be as great as in adult wards. Psychotherapy for inpatients, and social work help for families, supplemented the therapeutic milieu. Psychoneurotic disorders, conduct disorders and psychotic illnesses of various types made up the majority of admissions. In about a fifth of the patients the disorder dated back to early childhood. Length of stay was usually from a few months up to a year or so. 'Confirmed delinquents' and children with severe obsessional neurosis had proved the most difficult to handle.

In a subsequent paper dealing with the same unit, Warren (1953) considered a group of thirty-three patients (50 per cent of admissions over the period in question) admitted because of problems of behaviour. Twelve of these were admitted at the request of courts. The author discussed the need to make sure that the group in the unit was a balanced one. Three patients with active antisocial behaviour were considered enough at any one time. Antisocial patients did not corrupt others, but they did tend to be unpopular and shunned. Some children proved unsuitable because of persistent running away or they were removed by their parents. On the whole, however, most of the patients seemed to benefit. The home background was an important factor, and the author considered that careful selection was necessary to ensure admission of antisocial children who would benefit from treatment in a unit of this sort.

The first children's unit in Scotland was the Department of Child Psychiatry at the Crichton Royal Hospital, Dumfries. The work of this large pioneering unit, which opened in 1947, has been described by Rogers (1954, 1965). In the more recent of these papers, Rogers defines the functions of an inpatient unit as diagnostic, short-term treatment and long-term treatment. He considers that *diagnosis* may take up to three months of observation and treatment. He emphasises that a child's assets are as important as the signs and symptoms of disturbance, and should take up at least half of the diagnostic formulation. It is important also to keep the child in the unit long enough to assess his capacity to change. Inpatient assessment helps decide the extent to which behaviour is either reactive or, on the other hand, due to a deep-seated disorder of personality. It can also be useful in cases of epilepsy, psychosomatic disorder and psychosis. *Short-term treatment*, Rogers considers, is mainly to relieve a critical family situation, the child returning home after a few weeks when tensions have subsided. The indications for *long-term treatment* are considered to include certain cases of severe neurotic disorder, severe psychotic disorders, and some children with brain disease or injury.

Rogers (1965) follows with a detailed and valuable account of the treatment used at Ladyfield, as the department was called, and of the ward routine, one of the few such accounts that have been published. Teamwork, an integrated therapeutic plan for each child and free communication among staff are essential. The basis of the treatment is the general nursing care. A complement of eleven nurses for a group of seventeen or eighteen is recommended, though with nine or ten the unit can still be run. Rogers suggests a charge nurse, a deputy charge nurse and two staff nurses, with seven junior nurses. There should be both male and female nurses and attachment to the unit should be long-term.

In handling children, Rogers believes in allowing emotional regression. After finding a level of emotional development at which the child can operate, encouragement is later given to the child to grow up. This progressive policy may result in differential handling of the various children.

School is an important part of the environment at Ladyfield. Rogers described the school work as being done partly in groups of five or six, partly individually or in twos or threes. At the same time group therapy, usually in groups of only two, was carried out by occupational therapists. Rogers believes also that individual therapy has an important part in the total treatment programme. There were no fixed visiting hours, children went home for weekends whenever possible and close contact with the families was maintained. Intensive casework with the families was carried out by social workers.

Further Developments

The opening of the first inpatient children's psychiatric units in America and in Britain was followed by the inception of many more units. This presumably testifies to the usefulness which the first units were considered to have. Thus Roddy (1960) and also Stratas and Schmidt (1960) describe the children's unit of the Eastern State Hospital, Williamsburg, Virginia. This was perhaps fairly typical of many of the state hospital units opened in the post-war years. In this hospital a boys' ward was established in 1954 and a girls' in 1957. The papers outline the development and staffing of this 54-bedded service. The full-time staff are listed as follows:

Physician-in-charge	1
Clinical psychologist	1
Social worker	1
Teachers	3
Nurses	2
Attendants	8

The following part-time staff were also employed:

Occupational therapists	2
Student teachers	3
Clinical psychologists	3
Graduate psychology students	5
Music therapists	2

The unit was considered 'well-staffed', though by current British standards the level of staffing seems low for a unit with a capacity to take 54 children and a patient population which was usually from 30 to 40.

During early weeks an extensive programme of investigation was carried out, followed, if continued hospitalisation was required, by an intensive treatment programme. Seventy per cent of the children received tranquillisers, and all attended group therapy once or twice a week, as well as occupational therapy, school, and recreational and music therapy programmes. More than half the children received individual psychotherapy, and twice-monthly group therapy sessions were held for parents. The age range dealt with was ten to eighteen years.

In 1952 two publications appeared giving details of treatment centres for emotionally disturbed children in the USA. One of these (Federal Security Agency, 1952) lists 36 centres and gives brief details of each. Ten of these units are described in greater detail in *Residential Treatment of Emotionally Disturbed Children* (Reid and Hagan, 1952), which also mentions two additional units (the children's inpatient service of the Langley Porter Clinic and the children's service of the Neuropsychiatric Institute of the University of Michigan). These books give useful data about the organisation and running of the units, but are less informative on details of the clinical material and work, and the results.

The units are clearly very diverse in type, therapeutic orientation, size and aim. Many are far removed from hospital inpatient units of the type that exist in Britain. Only eight of the 38 centres had a psychiatrist as director. In 22 the director was a social worker (two being 'educators' as well); three were directed by psychologists, one by a psychoanalyst and one by an educator. In three cases the profession of the director is not clear. Size varied from 12 to 444 places. The 444-bedded unit (the Children's Village, Dobbs Ferry, NY) had only one psychiatrist on the staff, thought there were also a psychologist, an intern, 10 psychiatric social workers, 18 group workers, 27 teachers and 40 cottage parents; thus the strictly psychiatric treatment must have been very limited. By contrast, some centres were clearly run as psychiatric hospital units for children. Such centres usually have a psychiatrist as director.

In October 1957 the American Psychiatric Association and the American Academy of Child Psychiatry held a conference on inpatient psychiatric treatment for children, in Washington, DC. This was reported in the book *Psychiatric Inpatient Treatment of Children* (American Psychiatric Association, 1957). The foreword outlines the development of inpatient facilities in the United States, starting with the units established to care for children with post-encephalitic behaviour disorders. The first chapter then defines the place of the inpatient unit in its community setting. The conference noted that most such units avoid the use of the word *hospital* in their titles, but it seemed to feel that the use of this term would be helpful. Later chapters discuss 'the plant and its cost', administration and staffing, treatment programmes, research (which the conference considered was an obligation of every unit) and, in a chapter called 'Estimating the need', the epidemiological background of units.

The chapter on treatment emphasises the importance of having parents involved in the treatment process, while recognising that this is not always possible. It goes on to discuss the milieu and its place in the total treatment programme, individual psychotherapy, somatic therapies, the place of education and medical services. The book as a whole is based upon the practice of nineteen centres in different parts of the USA. Its fifth appendix, a list of 'selected references', opens with a preamble which observes that 'the literature on inpatient psychiatric treatment of children . . . is wide in scope and large in volume'. It then lists 229 references to the literature up to that date, spread over 14 pages!

Any administrator or clinician who is planning a new inpatient unit should certainly read this book. The discussion and advice on the structure and siting of units is sound and forward-looking and it is perhaps strange that some subsequently-built British units have ignored many of the recommendations. Only very recently has the Department of Health and Social Security set about producing a plan for child psychiatric inpatient units.

Hylton (1964) examined the working of 21 residential treatment centres and also two therapeutic day schools. Many of these centres had been included in Reid and Hagan's (1952) survey. Of the 21 residential units, 11 were considered to be under psychiatric direction. Administration, fees and costs were examined, as well as aspects of the children's clinical state and social backgrounds. Large variations in costs were found and these were not always easy to explain. But the professional staff: child ratio is an important factor. Medically directed programmes were significantly more expensive than non-medical ones, and public centres than privately run ones. The services provided differed, however.

Progress in Britain

In Britain, a Royal Medico-Psychological Association (1957) memorandum reviewed the inpatient psychiatric needs of children and adolescents. In 1957 there were 11 units, containing a total of 311 beds, and a further 12 units were 'under active consideration'. This memorandum made a number of practical suggestions about the design, organisation and staffing of units and recommended provision of beds as follows:

Children's beds: Not less than 20 beds per 500,000 population
Long-stay children's beds: One unit of not less than 25 beds per region
Adolescent beds: Not less than 20 beds per 500,000 population

Wardle, in 1970, sent questionnaires to all known inpatient and day patient units for children and adolescents in the United Kingdom. He found that by this date there were 52 units. Thirty-three were for inpatients only, 17 were inpatient and day patient units combined and 2 were day patient units. In all, 990 inpatients and 169 day patients were being cared for in these units, in which a total of 821 nursing staff were employed. More recent data are given in Appendix B.

Developing Views on Inpatient Treatment

The expansion of inpatient treatment facilities has led to a corresponding expansion of the literature, and a certain consensus of opinion seems to have emerged on at least some points. Robinson (1947) referred to residential treatment as being of three types. In the first, admission is primarily for *diagnostic study* in a controlled environment. The second provides primarily a suitable *living situation*, and the specifically psychiatric work is designed to help the child make best use of the residential setting. In the third type admission is primarily *to enable the child to participate in psychotherapy*; residence is secondary.

Robinson *et al.* (1947) went on to describe a unit of the third type. This was the Children's Service Centre of Wyoming Valley, Wilkes-Barre, Philadelphia. The children lived in two 'cottages', each with space for up to ten children. Individual psychotherapy was considered 'the core of the process', as distinct from 'the child's adjustment to a resident or placement plan'. The parents' co-operation and participation in casework were considered essential. 'Organic' cases and children presenting withdrawn schizophrenic reactions were not accepted for treatment.

The parent was apparently expected to make the decision whether to have outpatient therapy for his child or to choose 'a plan in which he bodily gives over his child to the treatment centre for a considerable period' (six to eight months). Within the unit, all children had an hour's psychotherapy daily, while the cottage staff were primarily concerned with the children's daily living. Children went out to local public schools. While a close relationship between cottage staff member and child was fostered, this was used to help the child 'take (his) feelings and considerations to the treatment hours', rather than dealing with them directly. As treatment proceeded, 'resident living' became a medium in which he could display his accomplishments. Inner change was thus reflected in group living, and as it proceeded changes in the child's life (for example, the introduction of remedial teaching when it was required) could be made.

The parents arranged termination of treatment, as they initiated it, though the child himself often became aware of his readiness to end treatment in the centre. This paper gives no statistics about the children treated or the results.

The description given by Krug (1952) of the Child Guidance Home Cincinnati, Ohio, similarly emphasises the importance of individual psychoanalytically-oriented psychotherapy. Each child had three such sessions weekly and each parent one. The other major treatment influences, namely child–parent separation and the child's relationship with the unit staff, were also recognised. A permissive environment, within limits, was advocated. The limits extended to behaviour which was 'grossly destructive' to the environment or to the child himself or others in the community. Destructive behaviour was 'firmly blocked in a kindly, protective manner, since otherwise it would give rise to anxiety, guilt or unhappiness'.

Despite the emphasis on individual treatment, Krug acknowledged that children 'sometimes develop their first meaningful relationship in residence rather than in individual therapy'. Sometimes residential workers are able to 'deal more actively at a deeper level in helping the child'. Problems can, however, arise if there are disturbed relationships between staff members, and children can attempt to alienate psychiatrist and residential worker. They may arouse a 'triangular conflict' such as often exists in their family. Residential work can thus awaken unresolved emotional problems in staff.

A further paper by Krug *et al.* (1952) described the inpatient treatment of a nine-year-old girl who had been severely deprived in her life and had petit mal. Individual psychotherapy played a major role in the treatment of this patient at the Cincinnati Child Guidance Home, 250 hours of therapy being provided over a period of 25 months. Treatment was clearly associated with great gains, and it enabled the patient to give up her relationship with a foster mother who had been unable to meet her needs. After two years' treatment, however, the child's dependence on the treatment centre appears to have been marked, though she had 'expressed a wish to find a good permanent home'. This had not been achieved at the time of the report and the authors anticipated 'a somewhat difficult period' as she became 'emancipated' from the Child Guidance Home staff. This paper illustrates the limitations as well as the advantages of this treatment approach.

An important discussion of the theory behind residential treatment of children has been provided by Noshpitz (1962). Like Robinson (1947) he points out that the residential environment can simply be used to support the child while he receives individual psychotherapy. At the other extreme individual therapy is not carried out, and instead the child is placed in a warm, appropriately supportive living environment. The thing most likely to help children in such a setting is the opportunity to form better relationships. This author considers that, unfortunately, we know rather little about the precise conditions in which the most helpful identifications occur, or what is required in addition.

Noshpitz sees the two main approaches in residential treatment as *ego support* and *ego interpretation*. Ego support consists of those aspects of treatment which strengthen and consolidate the ego and help it become better integrated. The aim is to increase the child's sense of contact with the environment, freeing him from fear and the anticipation of danger, and generally helping him learn to interact with the world around him in a more normal way. No interpretation is involved and the child learns through his day to day experiences. This involves skilled care and specific techniques, and requires well trained staff able to deal appropriately with any of the situations which may arise in children with a large variety of problems.

Ego interpretation is also seen by Noshpitz as a function of the staff of the residential unit. The staff may repeatedly call a child's attention to the nature of a defence by 'a steady delicate stream of interpretative remarks'. At the same time there should be systematic control of overt acts, on the theory that, once acting-out is stopped, the 'underlying genetic-dynamic material' can be more easily dealt with.

Noshpitz in the same paper considers also the place of individual psychotherapy. While it is possible for the child under treatment to have his own therapist whom he sees apart from the residential milieu, Noshpitz believes there is much to be said for having a single ward, or group, doctor who both heads the staff and sees the children individually and in groups. Therapy is then not done in regular, scheduled sessions, but as and when necessary, often in crisis situations. The individual sessions thus become a closely integrated part of the total treatment. The doctor's interpretations and tactics are then not just his own; in addition, the other staff are instructed in the line of action needed with each child and the interpretations to be stressed. As the child's ego-functioning improves he has less need for this 'all-embracing' therapy and can be dealt with more appropriately in the individual therapy context. At the same time, presumably, the need for residential treatment lessens or ceases.

Rinsley (1963) pointed out that child psychiatry, unlike adult psychiatry, started out as an outpatient speciality. The development of inpatient units, even if sometimes termed 'schools' or 'treatment centres', meant that workers trained in outpatient work had to adapt to residential settings. Psychoanalytic insights had to be modified also; and the 'obfuscation of professional roles', characteristic of child guidance clinics, courted 'disaster if carried over into an intensive inpatient milieu'. Yet another problem was that of structure. While permissiveness has its place it must be 'dispensed by an otherwise well-structured milieu'. A laissez-faire approach may constitute 'an abysmal error' in children's units, for the child patients' 'normal needs for external controls are exceeded by profound difficulties with readily mobilised erotic and aggressive impulses'. The expression of these impulses is 'the very thing which terrifies them most'. Moreover, Rinsley says, 'lurking behind uncritical, inconsistent or pervasive overpermissiveness is often the misguided notion that controls imposed on *any* child, sick or not, will somehow block his capacity to express himself and his problems; we rather see it, often, as a reaction to more deeply lying retributive, punitive, sadistic impulses directed towards the child.'

Rinsley is thus one of the many authors who stress children's needs for controls. He also believes that inpatient treatment, if it is to induce and maintain 'healthy change' in children, must usually be quite prolonged. At first the child will, towards the hospital staff, 'mount resistances in his compulsion to repeat, within the hospital, those maladaptive ways of dealing with himself and others which he employed outside (hospital)'. These resistances must first be recognised and dealt with, before 'basic, lasting inner change begins to set in'. The patient must face the 'disturbed, painful ideas, feelings and behaviours he brings to and externalises within' the hospital. The capacity of children and adolescents to cover up their needs tends to be less than that of adults. If their needs (for example, for control) are not met they may react by showing increasing anger and bitterness, and by remaining disturbed. They may plunge the ward into turmoil, or they may disappear.

'*Milieu*' *Therapy*

There is a wide agreement about the importance of the milieu. Rioch and Stanton (1953) discuss the nature of milieu therapy, and its value and limitations. Although considering adult psychiatric units as well, they pay a lot of attention to children's units. The importance of group communication is emphasised: staff tensions and disagreements, even though covert, can cause disturbance among the patients in a children's unit (and, no doubt, in units for adults). The importance of groups, including the two-person group of patient and staff member, is also well brought out. The reason for the central importance of milieu therapy in so many child psychiatric disorders is that children with these disorders have, often as their chief problem, difficulties in their group relationships. Thus the task of residential treatment is to help them with group relationships, for which purpose the staff must, through their own relationships with each other, provide a model.

Other work that is important because of the understanding it provides of milieu therapy is that of Bettelheim and Sylvester (1952) and Redl and Wineman (1951, 1952). The latter authors in two books, *Children Who Hate* and *Controls From Within*, describe and discuss many aspects of the residential treatment of children with disordered personalities. These two books, later published in a single volume entitled *The Aggressive Child*, provide a lot of detail about the behaviour and care of these difficult children. Much of the material is derived from the authors' experience at Pioneer House, a long-term treatment unit, very different in many ways from most hospital psychiatric units. Nevertheless much that these books say about the treatment of these children is of general relevance and application.

The authors acknowledged their debt to Bettelheim's (1950) *Love is Not Enough*. They consider the essence of treatment to be slow, gradual personality development, or ego growth, in children who each start with an 'ego that cannot perform' – that is, that cannot provide 'frustration tolerance', the ability to cope with 'insecurity, anxiety and fear', nor 'temptation resistance'. A further nineteen areas of possible ego failure are discussed in *Children Who Hate*, and the need is emphasised to assess these in each child's case, so that treatment can be geared to providing specific help where it is needed.

These books are certainly important milestones in the development of treatment techniques for children with problems of the type concerned. In *Controls From Within* successive chapters deal with the structure of the treatment home, 'Programming for ego support', 'Techniques for the antiseptic manipulation of surface behaviour' (a very interesting chapter despite its unpromising title) and 'Techniques for the clinical exploitation of the events'.

Like a number of other similar treatment centres, Pioneer House closed prematurely, the reason given being lack of funds. It is possible only to speculate on why the community did not provide the funds needed. It seems, however, that getting community acceptance and support for this sort of treatment centre is as difficult, sometimes more so, as running the centre.

Redl (1959b) discussed some of the concepts behind the idea of a therapeutic milieu in a later, interesting paper.

Staff Problems

Schrager (1954), in a paper on residential staff supervision, considered that therapy must be 'incorporated into the fabric of the total culture of the treatment centre'. The latter should not just be 'typical children's institutions', to which a casework or psychotherapy service has been added. Schrager thus stressed the need for skilled and close supervision of the child care staff especially where, as is so often the case, such staff come without previous experience of the work. Aspects of supervision are discussed in this paper in relation to the work at Southard School, the Department of Child Psychiatry of the Menninger Foundation.

Szurek (1951) discussed the relevance of the family situation to the problems of children in psychiatric inpatient units. He also stressed the importance of relationships within the staff group. Work with parents is to be based on the theory that there may be a relation between the child's problems and difficulties the parents are experiencing. Parental attitudes towards staff and hospital may derive from their feelings towards their children. The dynamic significance of these transference feelings needs to be considered by the staff. There is also great opportunity for parents (and children) to act out negative feeling towards their therapists; they may do this by preparing to favour certain staff members, or choosing to confide in some but not in others.

Within the staff group, difficulties can arise from members belonging to different disciplines and also being in different stages of training and seniority. The importance of 'prompt and complete communication' throughout the organisation is stressed by Szurek. Otherwise the disturbance, and the destructive feelings and drives, of the children and their families may affect the environment in a way which makes it less than therapeutic. If staff members are in conflict the patient experiences increased tension. He may succumb to the temptation to divide the authority figures so as to possess each more exclusively, but with the ever-present danger of losing both.

Hendrickson and Holmes (1959) discussed the treatment of patients with severe antisocial behaviour in an adolescent inpatient unit. A social environment was recommended which would ensure 'the failure of pathological character defences'. As their antisocial behaviour lessened, free-floating anxiety, 'psychophysiologic manifestations' and depression were liable to appear instead.

In the unit described, that at the Neuropsychiatric Institute of the University of Michigan, Ann Arbor, a high level of expectation was maintained concerning the patients' behaviour. The patients had to respond to the *verbal* controls of the staff; very definite 'almost Victorian' standards of behaviour were insisted upon; and the whole programme was structured so that the behavioural norms were an unavoidable part of reality. The tendency to group identification of the adolescent patient was exploited to help achieve these ends. In school a standard of performance 'in keeping with community norms' was expected.

A basic philosophy in this unit was that the affection of the staff for the patients is best demonstrated by firmly helping them to abandon their need for direct gratification. A 'too-loving, too-sympathetic' attitude to such behaviour, the authors considered, tends to elicit negative response because 'it indulges those persistent, infantile dependent needs which are most frightening to the patient'. They believed that, in handling negative behaviour, understanding of the dynamics behind it enabled staff to deny the patient the neurotic satisfaction he was seeking. The doctor functioned as both authoritarian-administrator and psychotherapist, since these were both responsibilities of his. The withholding or suspension of privileges might be used but 'seclusion rooms' never were; sedatives and tranquillisers were not considered helpful in controlling delinquent behaviour. Sometimes, if a patient could not respond to the unit's regime, transfer to a closed adult ward was arranged.

Hendrickson and Holmes, like so many other authors, stressed the need for staff supervision to be constantly available, in view of the great anxiety with which adults tend to react to adolescents.

The importance of the control of impulsive behaviour, setting limits and providing 'firm consistency', was also emphasised by Hartmann *et al.* (1968), though these authors were describing the treatment of adolescents on adult wards.

Long-term Treatment

The literature on hospital units for the *long-term treatment* of disturbed children is sparse, presumably because there are few such units. An interesting recent account of one such unit, however, is that of Kahan (1971). The unit concerned, West Stowell House in Wiltshire, England, had previously been run on mental subnormality hospital lines. Reorganisation, and reduction of numbers from 40 to 30, enabled an active treatment programme to be pursued. Kahan's monograph described the treatment of 71 children diagnosed as follows:

Psychotic	21
Psychotic and severely subnormal	15
Disturbed subnormal	17
Conduct disorder	18

It is clear from the case descriptions and other information that these were deeply disturbed children, many of whom would be regarded by most psychiatrists as having a poor prognosis. Many would also probably have been regarded as extremely difficult children to treat or even contain in a therapeutic setting. It is therefore surprising to find that the unit had a staff–patient ratio of only about one to three, and that in 1966–7 the cost per patient week was about £17, much less than that for most child psychiatric inpatient units.

As in so many other units, traditional nurse staffing arrangements were found to be unsatisfactory, so 'it was decided that houseparents should be regarded not as nursing assistants but as unqualified staff nurses with meals provided'. The main treatment approach was 'child-centred intensive care'. This combines 'good parenting' with 'the provision of infant nurture, affection, tolerance, and structure according to the patient's human needs'. To these ends the adults were 'smiling, never frowning, touching, holding and making opportunities for contact'. There was continuous affectionate talk. Impulsive outbursts, incontinence, anger and fearfulness were seen as cries for help of some sort. Close supervision by the psychiatrist of the work of the staff was necessary. Regular seminars and case conferences were held. Communication of this sort took up one-third of the consultant's available time.

The author describes the children's day in detail. Punishment was not used at West Stowell House. Children would sometimes be put to bed, for example if a tantrum was considered to be associated with tiredness. Aggression was dealt with by giving immediate attention to the aggressor as well as to the victim. Children too disturbed to remain in a group were cared for away from the group by a senior nurse, if necessary sleeping apart or even being nursed on their own in bed. This contrasts with 'time-out' procedures which are sometimes recommended as treatment for such behaviour (Brown and Tyler, 1968).

'Regressed nurtural care' was used as a basic treatment for the children who at the same time had child-centred intensive care as their therapeutic background. It was carried out mainly in two therapeutic playgroups. The aim was to provide 'personal emotional contact' at whatever level was demanded. Kahan describes in detail how this is achieved; also how it continues until the patient has passed from withdrawal, through infantile dependence, to a state in which he can achieve an 'on demand' level in social and educational activities.

Regressed nurtural care goes hand-in-hand with child-centred intensive care. Kahan observes that 'many parents have unwittingly aggravated their child's condition by making demands he cannot fulfil or even understand'. This treatment programme aims to overcome the effects of these experiences. Regressed nurtural care leads on to educational activities, at first simple and later more ambitious. Ultimately children can go out to a local school.

The results of treatment, as Kahan points out, are hard to assess.

Especially in long-term treatment, apparent response to treatment has to be weighed against possible maturational changes. Of the four groups studied, the children with conduct disorders did best, those with both psychosis and subnormality worst. Of 47 discharged patients, 24 (11 of them conduct disorder cases) were 'much improved', 15 showed 'some improvement' and 12 showed no improvement. Unfortunately figures for length of stay are not given, except for the 16 children whose case histories are described. Only five of these had been discharged at the date of the survey (May 1966) and the mean duration of stay of this group was 4 years 6 months. The eleven children still under treatment at May 1966 had already been in the unit for a mean duration of 3 years 1 month. The treatment is thus clearly long-term in type.

Summary and Conclusions

This chapter has outlined the development of hospital units for psychiatrically disordered children in the United States and in Great Britain. The units are varied in size, type and the way they operate, but some general agreement has emerged about how units may be run, and examples of different approaches have been given. Most accounts have been of a general nature: despite its size, this literature contains few detailed accounts of the treatment of particular disorders and types of children. Later chapters aim to do this.

CHAPTER TWO

The Aims and Nature of the Inpatient Psychiatric Treatment of Children

Philip Barker

As Chapter 1 has shown, fifty years' experience of the inpatient psychiatric treatment of children in North America, and twenty-five in Britain, have provided an indication of what this treatment can achieve and how units may be run. Before going on to look at the treatment of children with particular types of problem the aims of inpatient treatment will be considered and also how it may fit in with other services and other types of therapy.

Child psychiatry started as an outpatient, rather than an inpatient, specialty. During the 1920s and 1930s it was practised chiefly in child-guidance clinics. Not only were these an outpatient service, but they developed quite apart from the hospital service. The initiative in starting child-guidance clinics seldom comes from psychiatrists; indeed, many pre-war clinics, in Britain at least, had difficulty in obtaining the services of psychiatrists.

Only with the inception of the National Health Service in 1948 did hospital child psychiatry begin to develop in Britain. Before the start of the NHS child psychiatry was practised only in a few specialist hospitals like the Tavistock Clinic and the Maudsley Hospital. Since then it has become generally accepted that the NHS should concern itself with the mental health of children just as it does with the mental health of the adults in the community. Nevertheless, there is still a tendency to omit consideration of child psychiatry services when the health care of communities is being considered. The result is that child psychiatry facilities generally, but inpatient services in particular, are unevenly spread throughout Britain.

What do inpatient units achieve? How many should there be and how should they be run? Warren (1970) in a review of the development of child and adolescent psychiatry in England and Wales, stated that the few units opened in the 1940s proved valuable (though he does not specify in what way), so that subsequently more were opened. In 1970, when he was writing, there were 38 units with 653 beds in the two countries. Warren went on to comment on the haphazard growth of these units. Their distribution throughout the country had been uneven, and they had been set up 'where opportunity offered', developing in different ways and with widely differing functions. This author pointed out that the needs of very disturbed and difficult children, who may also need long-term treatment, had not been met; also that some of these children could not readily be managed with other children, to whom they might be dangerous. This still sometimes led to their placement in adult wards.

Current Policy

The official current policy concerning inpatient units for children and adolescents in England and Wales is contained in a circular from the Ministry of Health (1964). This suggests as an 'initial aim' the provision of 20 to 25 children's beds per million population 'for assessment and relatively short-term treatment', with in addition beds for long-stay treatment, 'at first on the scale of 25 beds per region'. Adolescent beds 'should be increased to 20 to 25 per million', additional to the beds for children. Although it is nearly ten years since this circular was published, most regions are a long way from fully implementing it. In particular, few regions have units for long-stay treatment. Moreover the number of beds recommended for shorter-stay units is only about half that suggested by the Royal Medico-Psychological Association (1957) (see Chapter 1, page 17).

In Scotland a report of a sub-committee (Scottish Home and Health Department, 1962), entitled *Medical Services for Child Guidance*, considered the need for child psychiatric beds. It recognised the need both for units providing observation, investigation and short-term treatment, and for centres treating children and adolescents 'for whom long-term hospital care is required over a period of several years'.

This report emphasised that accommodation for the latter group was 'urgently required', but did not specify the number of beds required. For the first category, however, it referred to the Royal Medico-Psychological Association's (1957) figure of 20 beds for children, and another 20 for adolescents, for each 500,000 population. This Scottish report emphasised the need for non-hospital facilities, notably schools and hostels for maladjusted children. 'Sufficient accommodation of this type is essential to enable hospital units to be used efficiently, and the converse is also true. Ready transfer between hospital and non-hospital facilities should be possible.'

Indications for Admission

The Royal Medico-Psychological Association (1957), as well as recommending the above bed complements, gave some indication of the purpose of inpatient beds. It dealt first with 'observation and investigation' and gave as 'examples of situations calling for inpatient care':

1. children presenting 'as acute problems' and so ill 'that immediate skilled attention in hospital is necessary';
2. instances where distance prevents adequate outpatient investigation, so that inpatient investigation is necessary;
3. psychosomatic conditions when these 'call for inpatient handling by a psychiatrist';
4. some neuropsychiatric conditions of childhood in which inpatient investigation and short-term treatment is needed;
5. psychotic children, who 'frequently present as diagnostic problems and a period of observation and investigation is often essential'.

These categories are somewhat vague, and the report is even less precise in the matter of which children require inpatient *treatment*. A current textbook of child psychiatry (Barker, 1971a) suggests inpatient treatment 'either because of behaviour so severely disturbed as to make treatment or even care elsewhere difficult or impossible, or because of the need to remove the child for a limited period from an adverse social environment, usually the family, occasionally the school'. It sees inpatient treatment as but an episode in the course of treatment, even if it is a prolonged one. Admission is considered to be usually inadvisable for children who have no home or a home so grossly disturbed or unsatisfactory as to be quite unsuitable for the child. This latter point has long been recognised and was emphasised by, for example, Suess and Hoshino (1961), who wrote of the necessity to have 'interested parents or parental figures outside the hospital in regular contact with the patient'. Reidy (1960) similarly stressed the need for contact with families. Some children, he considered, were referred for inpatient care because of the inadequacies of community facilities rather than because residential treatment was the method of choice. This probably still applies today, as does the need, also emphasised by many authors, for the unit to have control over its own admissions. No one unit can deal with all categories of disturbed children and few genuine emergencies occur in this work.

Children without homes often try and make the inpatient unit into a sort of substitute home. Yet a hospital, except perhaps a very long-stay one, cannot play the role of home. Children without homes, or without suitable ones, should be found substitute homes (usually either foster homes or children's homes), and psychiatric treatment should, if necessary, be carried out in the context of the child's life in his substitute home. Such treatment may then involve inpatient or day patient care.

Shaw (1966) considered that the first requirement for admission was 'relationship capacity'. The child should also come from a pathological environment, so that the change to the environment of the residential unit would be a 'positive' experience. Shaw stated that children with neurosis, personality disorder, brain damage, language disabilities and the milder forms of schizophrenia are the ones best helped by residential treatment. He emphasised that a mixed group of children with different types of disorder was desirable. He advised against the admission of 'mental defectives', 'psychopaths' and 'severely schizophrenic' children. By 'psychopaths', Shaw meant children whose capacity to relate has been damaged by adverse experiences in early life.

The indications for admission of children with various classes of disorder are discussed in later chapters.

The Help Given in Inpatient Units

The nature of the help given to the children being treated may include almost any combination of the following:

Assessment and diagnosis
Milieu therapy and the experience of group living
Individual psychotherapy
Group psychotherapy
Behaviour therapy
Educational help, including remedial teaching
Occupational therapy
Speech therapy
Drug treatment
Removal from an intolerable or stressful situation at home or at school
Crisis intervention

In a wider context, inpatient care can be seen as a way of:

(i) altering the family dynamics by the temporary removal of one member;
(ii) demonstrating to the family that a child does have the capacity to change in a way which they may have come to believe is impossible;
(iii) relieving temporarily the family, school or community at large of a child with whom they are unable to cope adequately;
(iv) enabling normal emotional growth and maturation to proceed where formerly adverse environmental factors were preventing this.

Finally, child psychiatry units are places where *research* may be carried out. Indeed, they provide a unique opportunity for the study of disturbed children in a setting which can be controlled, and in which detailed observation is possible.

Most of the specific treatments mentioned above can readily be given to outpatients. This does not apply, however, to milieu therapy, nor to the special sort of group living experience which hospital units can be structured to provide. Behaviour therapy, too, can be incorporated into the milieu of an inpatient or daypatient unit, so that it is used in a way which may not be possible at home or in school. This is discussed further in Chapter 9.

Psychotherapeutic techniques which are suitable in an outpatient setting often cannot be directly transferred to the treatment of grossly disturbed inpatient children. Evans (1970) has pointed out that such children do not have the internalised conflicts of adult neurotic patients. This author suggests a 'reasonably permissive' milieu, which will enable the patients' difficulties to emerge. Some of the tensions which may emerge are unhelpful and are best avoided; others can be examined and used to the advantage of the community. He considers that sources of crisis and tension include:

(a) a contradictory or inconsistent philosophy;
(b) problems arising from staff/patient roles, relationships and conflicts;
(c) staff conflicts (which are inevitable but are better exposed than remaining covert);
(d) conflicts between the aims of patients and those of staff;
(e) conflicts between staff and parents;
(f) conflicts and tension between youngsters and parents;
(g) conflicts and tensions between the unit and its parent hospital;
(h) crises and tensions due to unrealistic expectations (for example in the child who has been severely deprived when younger);
(i) crises and tensions due to poorly developed programmes;
(j) tensions from other sources, for example staff changes, changes of philosophy and imbalance of patients.

The resolution of these conflicts, crises and tensions may be difficult, especially if it is to be done therapeutically. Such problems may be approached by focusing on the patients, on staff relationships, on improving communications, on a distraction or on a scapegoat. Patients are scapegoated more often than staff. This thoughtful paper by Evans discusses these problems, which are matters of central importance in the inpatient treatment process, with insight.

The question of how permissive an inpatient unit should be is often discussed. There is a fairly wide consensus that adolescent units in particular should not be too permissive. Turle (1960) reported on the first nine months' operation of a boys' adolescent unit attached to a mental hospital. Initially permissiveness was the 'governing principle', with minimal controls and an open door policy. The consequence was that the staff were left in the ward while the patients roamed the vicinity committing an increasing number of destructive acts. Eventually a rebellion broke out and the children finally forced the staff to take control. The staff's attitude of 'benevolent neutrality' was changed to one of 'benevolent autocracy'. Probably all children's and adolescent units are faced with the dilemma to which Turle refers in his description of the adolescent position: 'Too restrictive management will drive him to open rebellion, on the other hand, full freedom is not yet acceptable to him and he will either provoke the re-imposition of adult controls or build rigid authoritarian group structures for himself as the study of juvenile gangs shows.' Thus 'adult authority becomes acceptable if tempered with liberal measures'. The authority must be firm but friendly.

An interesting approach to admission and treatment has been described by Bruggan (1971), writing about the unit for young adolescents at Hill End Hospital, England. Here the reason for admission is the focus of work. The indication for the treatment is that the adolescent cannot be coped with in the community.

Initially a staff member discusses the case over the telephone with the referer. This may lead to the second stage, a meeting between unit psychiatrist and social worker and the referring agent(s). A consultation with the family as a group (including the adolescent) may then be held, away from the unit. The family are given information about the unit, and the family situation is explored. A request by the family for admission may follow. If it does, a second meeting with the family is held within a week; this is held at the unit, and the family is shown round. All aspects of admission are discussed. Some families decide at this stage that they can cope; otherwise, a verbal contract concerning admission is established, which includes:

- the reason for admission;
- on whose authority the decision to admit is made;
- the changes necessary before discharge;
- an agreement not to change the contract except at another meeting, which any member present may call.

The adolescent should indicate that he understands the contract, but he need not necessarily agree to it himself, though he may do so.

Help for the Family

Virtually all accounts of inpatient psychiatric treatment of children mention the place of work with the families, but there is much variation in the extent to which families are involved in the treatment. At one extreme the whole family is admitted and treated as a group. This was the practice at the Cassel Hospital, as described in 1961 by Weddell, who writes of the need to cherish the child's tie with his mother, rather than to interfere with it or break it. To this end, the nursing task should be shared with the family 'as members of the nursing team'.

Weddell's paper is one of a number republished in the book *Psycho-social Nursing* (Barnes, 1968), which describes various aspects of the work of the Cassel Hospital. It appears, from a general consideration of the papers in this book, that in many cases children (as distinct from adolescents) were in the hospital secondarily, the primary patient usually being the mother. Nevertheless, the concept of treating the family as a whole, with the acceptance that this may mean admitting the family as a whole, has many attractions. Child psychiatry units have explored extensively the value of separating child and parents for a time, and it seems that this can in certain circumstances be helpful. But treating them in hospital *as a family group* has been little explored, despite the current interest in family group therapy.

An incidental point of interest about the therapeutic community described at the Cassel Hospital is the way the roles of different categories of staff were kept distinct and separate, each group having its own defined responsibilities. Such clearly defined roles are probably as important in child psychiatry units as they are in family units.

At the other extreme are units such as West Stowell House (Kahan, 1970), into which the child is admitted, often for a period of years (see Chapter 1, page 24). This means that the care of the child is virtually taken over from the natural parents, and it is interesting that Kahan refers to staff as 'houseparents', a term not used in most hospital units. This type of treatment may be needed for the more chronically and deeply disturbed children, especially psychotic and subnormal-psychotic ones.

Most units fall between the extremes represented by the Cassel Hospital and West Stowell House. Casework help is offered to parents usually by social workers, while the child is in the hospital; sometimes group therapy or psychiatric treatment is also available to the parents. Shaw (1966) considered that it was not necessary to confine admission to children whose parents could be 'worked with'. Indeed, he believed that to restrict admissions in this way would involve excluding many of the children who could be helped most. The aim of treatment, he said, would not always be to discharge the child to live permanently at home. Some will do better if placed in residential schools, children's homes or other settings away from their own families.

Disadvantages of Inpatient Care

In addition to discussing the value hospital care may have, some of the disadvantages should be mentioned. Hospital treatment, as opposed to care in other institutions, has often been questioned. Thus Benjamin and Weatherly (1947), describing the work of the children's ward of the psychiatric division, Illinois Neuropsychiatric Institute, mention some of the drawbacks. However, many of the difficulties they came across seem to have been a result of the placing of the children's ward on the sixth floor of the Institute building. They considered that there was a need for greater flexibility, more than 'can be introduced within the framework of a hospital'. More space and facilities, including outside play and activity areas, would probably have overcome many of the problems these authors describe. The unit seems to have learnt the hard way many of the practical points which are now well-established, such as the impossibility of admitting an unlimited proportion of aggressive, antisocial children, the need for a relaxed informal atmosphere and the necessity to involve all staff in conferences and discussion of the work.

Subsequently Lourie and Schulman (1952) discussed the role of residential staff. They saw residential treatment as being needed mainly for children 'in whom physical and emotional deprivations have produced changes in personality structure'. They suggested that the personality changes which treatment aims to bring about will be slow to take place. Treatment must be built around the resident staff who make up 'the core of planned living experiences for the child'. These authors saw hospitals, as opposed to 'child-care' institutions, as having limitations imposed by their own traditional staffing arrangements. They 'question the therapeutic effects and possible confusions of so many adult figures who walk in and out of the child's life, with one putting him to bed and another eating with him, and another giving approval or disapproval'. They suggested that the therapeutic usefulness of staff might in such circumstances be diluted or lost.

More recently, a sociological approach to the study of institutions caring for handicapped children has been made by King *et al.* (1971). While none of the units concerned was a child psychiatric one, the study is relevant both because of its methodology and because of the limitations which it reveals in the environment of children in hospitals run on traditional lines.

Four large institutions undertaking the long-term care of children were studied, two children's homes (with 22 units and 36 units respectively) and two hospitals, one for subnormal children (with 16 units) and one for physically handicapped children (5 wards). Wide variations in the patterns of care provided for the children were found. These were quantified using a *child management scale* which the authors developed. This scale was thought to give an indication of how 'child-oriented' the institution was.

The principal finding was that the hospital units were much less child-oriented than the local authority homes. The hospitals tended to fail to provide, for young children, affection, individual treatment, variety of experience and continuity of relationships. They were not harsh or punitive 'but the environment was bleak and the atmosphere institutional'.

The authors 'assume there would be general agreement' that child-oriented practices are desirable, and they are probably right, though the problem of proving their value remains. The main practical point to emerge from this study, however, concerns the apparent causes of the relatively depriving nature of the hospital environments. A number of hypotheses were examined. Management practices did not seem to depend on the level of handicap of the children, the size of the institution, the size of living units or staff–child ratios. There was a tendency for child-oriented units to have greater continuity of staff and to be units where the head had more responsibility for running the unit. More striking, however, was the importance of the training of the head of the unit. There was a lack of child-orientation and low rates of interaction with the children when the head had a nurse training, and the reverse held true when the head had a training in child care.

This finding has important implications for the training, and perhaps also the use, of nurses in child psychiatric units. There would seem to be a need for a similar study of the different sorts of setting in which disturbed children are treated.

Ahnsjo (1969), professor of child psychiatry at Stockholm, considered institutional care generally 'a necessary evil'. He recommended the care of children in small groups of up to eight, with a ratio of up to one staff member to each child. He emphasised the importance of training staff so that they could provide an environment which could change children's 'questions, false concepts and anxiety' into 'affection and a feeling of security'. The importance of providing a stimulating and varied environment without spoiling the children, and the need to resist children's demands and help them learn to accept disappointment, were spelt out. Ahnsjo believed that institutions generally should not accommodate more than 20 children.

Milham (1971), referring to the residential care of adolescents, presents a sort of balance sheet giving advantages and disadvantages. The advantages mentioned are:

(a) In a residential setting social, spiritual and political values can be better developed than in a day setting.
(b) It is a better learning situation for less able children.
(c) It can enlarge the cultural horizons of adolescents.
(d) Closer staff–pupil relations are developed.
(e) Skills in handling authority figures are developed.
(f) Relationships with families can be improved, the institution supporting the child while he is weaned away from his family.
(g) It is possible to manipulate and fragment the informal society of the inmates, to their advantage.

Milham then mentions the following disadvantages of residential institutions for adolescents.

(a) The staff may arrogantly, and wrongly, claim that they provide everything the child needs.
(b) The communities may be too total, and provide insufficient opportunity to escape. Individuality and privacy tend to be discouraged.
(c) There may be a bureaucratic preoccupation with organisation. The institution may become too custodial and insufficiently in touch with the outside world.
(d) The great power the institution has to influence the adolescents' value system may be used to implant undesirable values or, particularly, those which simply reflect the personal prejudices or beliefs of the staff.
(e) There is danger of families being excluded, the community failing to develop a relationship with them. Milham, who is

mainly referring to schools, says he has never found a school at which parents attend staff meetings.

(f) There tend to be too few emotional outlets and a general restriction on emotional life, especially in single-sex communities.

These points are probably all valid when applied to schools, but in hospitals the traditional staffing arrangements, with nurses often working shifts, and perhaps being transferred to and from a unit quite frequently, may have the result that staff–child relationships are not as close as in some residential schools.

The Staff

The staff are the essence of the treatment in a children's unit. In the nature of things children are dependent upon those caring for them, and this applies with even greater force to emotionally disturbed children. Some may make a show of independence and hostility towards adults, but this is usually their attempt to conceal or deny their real needs. The child who can only relate to people in a hostile and aggressive way has almost always had unhappy and unsatisfactory relationship experiences hitherto. But whatever the nature of the child's relationship difficulties (and such difficulties are universal in disturbed children), it is through his relationships in the treatment unit, above all else, that he will be helped. The importance of having staff who can provide this help cannot therefore be over-emphasised.

In most British units it is the nursing staff who have charge of the children for the greater part of the time. They interact with the children quantitatively far more than anyone else, though the child's relationships with his teacher, occupational therapist, doctor, and so on, are important too. In the United States, child-care workers often play a large part in the treatment, but this is not so in Britain, for reasons which are perhaps more related to tradition and administrative considerations than to clinical needs. Unfortunately there has until now been no nationally organised or recognised training in child psychiatric nursing. Thus Wardle (1970), in his survey of British in-patient units, found that only 313 out of a total of 821 nursing staff (38 per cent) were registered nurses and only 73 (9 per cent) had any special qualifications in the care of children.

The importance of nurses in child psychiatry units has long been recognised in the literature. Thus in 1943 Gilbertson and Sutton described how, in a children's psychiatric service, the nurse provides observation and rewards children's behaviour, plays a part in psychotherapy, is largely responsible for the emotional climate and the structure of the unit, provides for the physical needs of the child (a matter of deep emotional significance), learns play techniques, and helps the children with constructive activities. This article also pointed out the importance of the nurse's personality and ability to resolve her own emotional conflicts.

Betz (1945), too, saw the inpatient unit as providing an environment which could significantly influence the course of a child's personality growth and development. She considered the ward personnel, both physicians and nurses, as the main therapeutic agents.

Sutton (1947) noted the necessity for nurses to be clearly involved in the therapy in children's psychiatric units. She observed, 'their contacts with the children and the environment which they provide must be therapeutic or much of the value of hospitalisation is lost . . .'. Moreover, the 'mothering' the children received from the nurses tended to cause children 'to transfer feelings from parents to nurse with great facility'. While Sutton accepted that the nurse could have an individual psychotherapeutic role, she concentrated mainly on the nurse's role in the various ward groups, and on the need for supervision and training. The interesting changes in nursing practice and attitudes in the children's service of the Illinois Neuropsychiatric Institute, over a period of five years, were also outlined in this paper.

Szurek (1947) also discussed the need to involve nurses in detailed discussions of children and their behaviour in an inpatient unit. He described the discussion groups, led by a psychiatrist, in which nurses participated. It is perhaps a measure of the progress and of child psychiatry units, that what he described as a new approach is probably nowadays the routine in most children's units.

The British literature places, if anything, even more emphasis on the role of the nurses, probably because there is not in Britain a separate category of child-care worker to share in the day-to-day care of the children. The sort of nursing required is very different from that needed in other types of hospital, even adult psychiatric ones. This is a possible source of difficulty, for it may not be easy to incorporate the very special type of nursing service required in the children's psychiatric unit into the nursing arrangements for the hospital group as a whole. In the Charles Burns Clinic, Birmingham, for example, it was decided that it would be therapeutically desirable for the nursing staff to take their meals with the children (Barker and Ward, 1972). This was not, however, the practice in any other hospitals in the group, or indeed in the region, and long and complex negotiations were necessary before the desired arrangements were made.

In this connection the report by Bethell (1968) on Merrifield, the children's inpatient unit at Tone Vale Hospital, Taunton, Somerset, is of interest. In 1968 this unit had as its only permanent staff a charge nurse and a deputy nurse, other staff coming, usually for three-month periods, from the parent hospital. This unsatisfactory situation had led to an important development, in that it had been agreed, at the time Bethell's paper was written, that the unit was to have its own matron or chief male nurse, directly responsible to the management committee.* There would seem to be much to be said for administering the nursing services in children's units in this way.

The importance of the nurses in a children's unit is such that Chapter 10 of this book is devoted specifically to it. The more recent literature on the subject is referred to in that chapter, which also deals with the vital question of the training of nurses for work in child psychiatry.

Apart from nursing staff, the personnel employed in inpatient units are largely composed of workers from the same disciplines as staff child guidance clinics. Thus they include psychiatrists, psychologists, social workers, teachers and speech therapists. In Britain only a few clinics have non-medical child psychotherapists, probably because there are at present very few trained therapists available. On the other hand, many units employ occupational therapists, though Barker and Muir (1969) found, when they made enquiries about the inpatient units in Scotland, that this applied to only three of the six then operating.

In America there are in addition not only *child-care workers* but also *group workers*, another category not provided for in the British National Health Service.

The Director

Every treatment centre must have a director, though his title may be that of consultant psychiatrist, consultant-in-charge or something

* In correspondence Dr Bethell has subsequently informed the author that the arrangement eventually worked out was for the nursing officer of the children's unit to be directly responsible to the principal nursing officer ('Salmon' Grade 9).

similar. The central role of the director seems to be generally recognised. Shaw (1966) waxes eloquent on the subject and states that the success or failure of the institution depends almost entirely upon the director. According to Shaw the director controls staff, environment and programme as well as setting the tone of the unit. The treatment centre, Shaw says, 'is a representation of the personality of the director'.

Suitable, and if possible inspired, leadership is without doubt needed in any treatment centre dealing with disturbed children. It seems to be more important that there is consistent dependable leadership and a policy known to all, than that any particular philosophy should be accepted or school of psychiatry followed. The need for good communication is often stressed, and rightly so, but free communication among staff members is secondary to good relationships between them. It is a great help if the staff like each other, and particularly if the director and his staff get on well with each other. Mutual warmth and respect, and tolerance of the failures which all members of staff will from time to time experience, are essential to a well-functioning unit. They should emanate from the director, who must be sensitive to the tensions and stresses in the unit and must ensure that these do not get out of hand. For this purpose regular meetings of the staff are essential. The psychodynamics of a children's unit are complex. This fact, and also the intimate involvement of the staff with the children, were well brought out by Sheimo *et al.* (1949). These authors discussed group formation among children on a psychiatric ward, and traced the activities of a group. The importance of relationships between staff, and of the leadership of the psychiatrist in charge, emerges clearly from this fascinating account of a series of events at the Langley Porter Clinic.

Another illustration of such psychodynamic processes is the following letter received by the author and his nursing colleague:

Dear Dr Barker and Nurse X,

I must express my great concern about the issue of altering staff postings. It is felt among the children that their feelings have not been taken into sufficient consideration. During their stay in the clinic to date the children have become closely attached to several members of staff within the group, and their departure into another group has severely upset several individuals that I know of, and has presumably unfavourably affected many more. I cannot over-stress the point that unless these ridiculous proposals are withdrawn we will continue to pursue a militant course with renewed vigour. Due to well known reasons you would have little power to retaliate, and therefore we are in a position where we can throw the entire clinic into utter confusion. I therefore have set a dead-line of suppertime tonight, after which we will have to seriously consider more militant and aggressive action. I realise your good intentions, but you have overlooked the ties that unavoidably exist between nurses and children. As this is a clinic which contains many depressed or nervous children, I imagined you would realise how important it was that these should not be broken. However, as I was wrong I am pointing it out to you. If, having vigorously examined these proposals, you are disposed to allow the groups to remain as they are. [*sic*] Failing this, more militant action of a more violent nature than before will have to take place.

Yours sincerely
(There follow the names of 10 children)

This letter was a reaction to the proposed transfer of some of the nurses between the different clinical groups (see Chapter 9) at the Charles Burns Clinic.

In fact, some of what Shaw (1966) says about the role of the director of a child psychiatry unit does not strictly apply in British National Health Service Hospitals. Thus, the director does not direct or control the nursing staff, nor select or reject nurses. Much of the administrative work of the clinic, moreover, is the responsibility of the lay administrator. The tripartite administration of Health Service hospitals means that nursing and administrative personnel have been responsible, through their respective hierarchies, to the hospital management committee (now replaced by the 'district management team'), not to the director of the clinic. This could be held to be a disadvantage and it can certainly create difficulties. Nevertheless, if his leadership powers are as good as they ought to be, the director should be able to lead and direct the clinic staff of all disciplines regardless of the theoretical administrative structure. In practice his personality, standing and relationships are what matter most, not the precise powers vested in him.

Why a Hospital?

It is not easy to define which children require help in a hospital rather than in some other type of institution. It does seem that some communities in Great Britain manage to cope with their disturbed children without much use of inpatient treatment. In such areas disturbed children may be provided with help in residential schools or children's homes, particularly if these institutions have psychiatric advice and support available to them.

Yet the demand for hospital care for disturbed children is increasing. In Britain this is clear from the increasing number of inpatient units, and it seems to apply in the USA also: Treffert (1968) has commented on the 'almost alarming' rate of increase in the admission of children and adolescents to psychiatric hospitals. He stated that in 1968 there were 25,000 child or adolescent psychiatric patients in state county psychiatric hospitals, and another 2,000 in private psychiatric hospitals. He went on to say that special units for disturbed children and adolescents had become 'a vital part of the spectrum of services required'.

The need, therefore, seems to exist. Yet it cannot be based simply on the need of these children for 'medical' investigation or treatment of the traditional kind. It is true that there are some disturbed children in whom 'medical' (as distinct from psychiatric) conditions are prominent. This applies to most psychosomatic disorders, some epileptic children and a small proportion of other patients. But the strictly medical aspects of most children's cases do not justify long- or even short-term inpatient care.

It seems that it is the special skills and knowledge of psychiatrists, and the professional colleagues who work with them in hospital, that are the key factors. Rightly or wrongly, hospitals and their staffs are considered to be able to care for and help children so severely disturbed as to be unsuitable for schools or other institutions. Thus, out of the 164 children admitted to the Charles Burns Clinic in a three-year period, and reviewed in Chapter 9, fifty (30 per cent) were children of school age who were out of school at the time of admission. Some had been excluded because of their disturbed behaviour, others were unable to get to school because of neurotic anxiety about going. There were many other children who were causing great difficulty in school and some who were on the point of being excluded; sometimes the threat of exclusion had been temporarily withdrawn in response to a promise of early admission.

The following extracts from referral letters illustrate the expectations that many school staffs have of hospitals:

At a case meeting it was agreed by all present that William needed urgent placement in a medically orientated unit. It was felt that this was necessary not only for the benefit of William but also for the protection of other boys ... The problem is now so acute that we should like William admitted to the Charles Burns Clinic as soon as possible and must regretfully fix ... our mid-term break as the maximum period we can continue to keep him.

(From a letter written by the headmaster of a residential school for maladjusted children)

... We still feel that Nicholas requires extensive curative therapy and we are not able to provide this here ... Nicholas is becoming increasingly disruptive, is by now totally unable to take part in any group activity, or to do any school work of any kind.

(Principal of a residential school for emotionally disturbed children)

I would be very glad if you could take this boy into your children's unit for a period of observation as we feel he is too much of a psychiatric problem to be dealt with here without further investigation. He appears to have what could be described as brain storms, in which he loses complete control and at times dashes mostly out on to the road, or throws violent temper tantrums. He will only co-operate with an adult on a one-to-one basis and in such circumstances will do some school work ...

(Psychiatrist at a residential school for maladjusted children)

Hospitals have other advantages. They normally accept patients however ill they are. Indeed they are seen as places for the more seriously ill. Admission of a child to hospital can also be arranged quickly and informally – provided a place is available and the parents are willing. Admission to a residential school, in Britain at any rate, can be a long and complex matter, because of the administrative procedures necessary. Emergency or crisis admission is difficult or impossible. Hospitals, however, traditionally accept emergency cases, and an inpatient unit can readily be organised to allow for this if the staff wish to provide such a service.

There is often an advantage to the child in being a 'patient'. Many children, by the time they are admitted, have become the centre of much disapproval, criticism or even frank rejection. Being able to look upon themselves as 'ill', and being given the hope that with treatment they can be helped to 'get better', can assist them to overcome the feelings of guilt, worthlessness, helplessness and despondency with which they often enter hospital. In much the same way it can help the attitude of parents, and enable them, and others who have had dealings with the child, to look at the problem differently. Furthermore, admission to hospital is not quite like being 'put away' in a home or 'sent away' to a residential school.

Research

Research should probably be a feature of the work of every hospital child psychiatry unit. The interest of staff in research is apparent from the many papers and research reports referred to in this book. Yet there have been few vigorously scientific studies of the actual treatment processes in hospital units. A paper by Bender (1961), promisingly entitled 'Clinical Research from Inpatient Services for Children, 1920–1957', turns out to be concerned largely with post-encephalitic and brain-damaged children, and also the relative parts played by brain damage and institutionalisation in various clinical syndromes. Thus much of the research reviewed concerns the disorders which children in hospital had, rather than the process of hospital treatment itself. Work done at Bellevue Hospital features prominently in this review, especially the extensive investigation there of 'childhood schizophrenia'.

Goodrich and Boomer (1958) studied therapeutic intervention by staff in a unit treating 'hyperaggressive' children. They used the *critical incident technique* (Flanagan, 1954). This aims to build up generalisations from a large number of concrete events, rather than by starting from a theoretical position regarding the matter in question. In this study staff members were asked to describe an incident involving a child and an adult in which the adult did something he (or she) felt was of therapeutic value. After a year the authors had descriptions of 240 episodes thought to illustrate thirty-one separate principles of therapeutic intervention useful with hyperaggressive children. These were classified under four headings:

(a) Promoting personality change by helping the child to learn to view his own behaviour evaluatively
(b) Promoting ego change
(c) Supporting existing ego controls
(d) Managing one's own conduct as a staff person

This last group, though not strictly interventions, includes principles affecting intervention by staff.

Goodrich and Boomer's work is of interest if only because it emphasises how behaviour and interactions can be studied. Its main limitation is perhaps that in each case interpretation of the value of an intervention is made subjectively by a member of staff or a research worker, who must be strongly influenced by the theoretical orientation of staff and unit. As the authors point out, however, the approach could be helpful in evaluating the performance of staff, in providing material for use in staff training seminars and in providing hypotheses for future studies of intervention techniques. It is clear that there is also needed, for use along with it, a means of measuring change in the children as a result of the intervention. This presents formidable problems; indeed, the number of uncontrolled variables may always prove too numerous for vigorously controlled studies to be possible.

Other examples of research on inpatient populations include the investigation by Pollack and Goldfarb (1957) of orientation for time, place and person in severely disturbed children, as compared with controls, and various drug trials. The latter have led to the construction of *ad hoc* rating scales and questionnaires for particular trials. An example is the behavioural rating scale used by Cunningham *et al.* (1968), in a double blind controlled trial of haloperidol in children in an inpatient unit. Inpatient units clearly provide ideal settings for controlled trials of treatments, both pharmacological and others. Detailed observation of the children is possible, and it is much easier to ensure that treatments are administered regularly and according to the prescribed schedules than it is with outpatients. But for the most part the extensive literature on children's inpatient units consists of general clinical descriptions of patients and of the work done, rather than studies in which a scientific approach has been made to the answering of questions or the testing of hypotheses.

A major reason for the lack of a more scientific approach has certainly been the absence, in most units, of any staff with research as their primary function. There have been, in Britain, no academic units of child psychiatry – apart from the small team which has developed at the Institute of Psychiatry under the leadership of Professor Michael Rutter. The need for such units in at least some of the main child psychiatric centres is urgent if research and teaching are to develop, and the subject is going to progress as a scientific discipline. The need for such units has been pointed out by the Royal College of Psychiatrists (1973) and also elsewhere by the author (Barker, 1973).

Summary and Conclusions

Hospital units for the residential care of children and adolescents with psychiatric disorders are a developing part of the health services of countries of the Western world. They provide a special sort of therapeutic environment and can be places for assessment or for short-, medium- or long-term treatment. They are flexible and can often provide rapid help in a crisis. Most of the help given in hospital could be provided on an outpatient basis, but the special features of inpatient care are the day-to-day living environment they provide for the children, and the temporary separation from their parents.

The hospital unit as a whole must provide a secure and stable situation for its patients. This implies a skilled staff whose relationships and communications are good. The day-to-day care of the children is the essence of the treatment and it is the staff who have the most contact with the children (in Britain the nursing staff) who are the main therapeutic agents. They, and all the staff, are dependent on the psychiatric leadership which is the unique feature of a hospital centre for disturbed children.

CHAPTER THREE

Residential Care of Children with Conduct Disorders

Christopher J. Wardle

> I am afraid that I cannot have Aron at home he is really driving us mad. I just cannot stand any more he is not fit to be at large. He threw a pail of pee over the bunk bed all over the mattress clean sheets in the bed. If he does not go I am afraid I shall be off . . . We have had a scene this morning he put his fist up at me and banged the door. I got hold of his hair and smacked his face after I just sat and cried, something will have to happen as I don't want him at home.
>
> (Letter from Aron's mother)

> Within the environment of an approved school we are able to limit to some extent Bill's violent aggressive outbursts but these are becoming more frequent and more serious . . . He is liable to attack other boys with whatever is to hand. Chairs and bottles have been used on a number of occasions, while fists and feet are commonplace. On Thursday he ran away from an evening activity group on the field; he had attempted violence towards other members of the group, abused the member of staff with the foulest of language and then threatened to throw himself in front of a car. He did lie down in the road but the car stopped in good time . . . On Friday there was a repetition of this incident when the boy was lifted off the road by senior staff who eventually settled him down for the evening although not before he threatened to drown himself in the lake. On Saturday he was given maximum supervision but nevertheless managed to get on to the nearby road to throw bricks at passing cars and neighbouring children. He spent Sunday morning in school with the

> Deputy Headmaster and a couple of other boys and joined a small group for arts and crafts during the afternoon. A complete breakdown followed, when Bill attacked other boys and the members of staff with a chair and other objects, screaming filthy, obscene abuse all the time. Before he was eventually restrained he had torn off all his clothes and had urinated and excreted over them and the floor.
>
> (Part of letter from the headmaster of an approved school)

This chapter will consider the treatment in hospital of children whose behaviour outside has brought them into open conflict with those looking after them and with the guardians of the well-being of society in general.

Like mental illness, conduct disorder is a social concept rather than a medical one (Wardle, 1963), defining children who are not fitting into socially accepted norms of behaviour and who fail to correct their deviation in response to social sanctions. Like many other manifestations of psychiatric disorder and emotional disturbance in childhood, unless the behaviour becomes alarming or annoying to the guardians the child may continue to suffer the sanctions indefinitely without changing the behaviour which evokes them. A characteristic common to all these children on admission is their experience of conflict, misunderstanding and failure in their relationship with adults, so that traditional methods of care and child management which are passable for the majority of happy healthy children have failed repeatedly. It is often because other methods have failed even to contain the child's behaviour, let alone modify it, that we are asked to admit and it is our main task in this chapter to examine methods which have proved relatively successful. But before doing so we will consider in more detail the type of patient to whom they are to be applied.

Definition of Conduct Disorder

The term 'conduct disorder' must be regarded not as a diagnosis but as a descriptive classification of the presenting behaviour problem. In the triaxial classification proposed by a World Health Organisation seminar in 1969 (Rutter *et al.*, 1969), conduct disorder was defined as 'abnormal behaviour which gives rise to social disapproval'. The authors included some types of legally defined delinquency and some non-delinquent disorders of conduct such as fighting, bullying, destructiveness and cruelty. Their exclusion of cases where the behaviour was 'part of any other psychiatric condition or associated with personality disorder' limits their concept very much more narrowly than our own and seems to be at variance with a later part of their definition, in which they emphasise that 'the mere fact that a child has committed a delinquent act is insufficient', and that 'the behaviour must be abnormal in its sociocultural context as judged by the frequency, severity and type of behaviour and by its association with other symptoms' (such as 'abnormal interpersonal relationships'). Barker's definition (1971a) includes persistence and disturbance to others. For the purpose of this discussion we will define conduct disorders as including all those cases in which the child's behavioural abnormality includes the following:

(a) The behaviour is socially disapproved.
(b) The behaviour includes 'acting-out' against people or property.
(c) The behaviour is persistent and fails to respond to normal sanctions.

Acting-out behaviour includes the following:

(i) Stealing, burglary and similar acts
(ii) Destruction of property, vandalism, window-smashing
(iii) Physical assaults on other people
(iv) Intentionally causing discomfort or harm to other people, for example, by swearing, interfering with people's normal progress about their business, threatening behaviour, putting planks on railway lines or obstacles on roads
(v) Wandering, absconding, truancy
(vi) Sexual promiscuity
(vii) Inappropriate public sexual activity, such as self-exposure or sexual assaults

It must be understood that though 'conduct disorder' describes the presenting symptoms, these conditions are likely to be manifestations of a variety of conditions, reactions or situations, some of which may become apparent only after admission. The following is a tentative classification of some of the major varieties (combinations of two or more are common).

1. *Severe Anxiety State – the Cornered Animal Syndrome*

In this syndrome, the underlying state is of severe fear which has not been recognised.

Bob, 13, began truanting because of his fear of other boys. On discovery his father beat him, but when he tried to force him to go to school next day, Bob escaped and barricaded himself in a shed. He threw bricks and bottles at the authorities who approached, and when uniformed authority was brought in, fired a pellet gun at them. When admitted he was clad in leather, studded with spikes and decorated with swastikas. In his suitcase were three pointed kitchen knives, a rubber pipe with nails sticking out and a bicycle chain. He was terrified to leave the doctor to meet the other patients, terrified to go to sleep and clung to the night nurse, and for several weeks refused to leave the safety of his bedroom.

2. *Depression*

(a) *The 'leave me alone' syndrome*. Here the antisocial behaviour seems to be motivated by a desire to be alone. Assaults and obscenities only occur if people approach the patient and try to cajole him to talk or do something.

(b) *'I am no good.'* Often pudgy-faced, overweight, enuretic and failing educationally, these patients seem to welter in their own sense of worthlessness. Their stealing, often of sweets and food, is usually solitary. They seem to seek punishment. Their angry denial of any praise or approval of them or their work is characteristic.

(c) *Suicidal gestures* may often be misinterpreted as antisocial conduct: self-mutilation or broken windows are a commonplace.

Carl, 11, was unusual in that he was arraigned for attempted murder. Desperate about his fear of school and the closing in of authority, in an allotment shed of a neighbour he rigged a string to the trigger of a gun so that it would fire when he sat on a chair, but he lost his nerve and ran off.

3. *Adolescent Psychosis*

An acute psychotic process should always be suspected when the behaviour of a formerly well-ordered individual deteriorates dramatically.

Dot, 12, a conforming, hardworking, though solitary girl, suddenly began swearing at her classmates and attacking them. Eventually she set fire to some school books, rushed out onto the beach and began walking into the waves. On admission she was giggling and weeping alternately, insisted on playing pop records very loud and continuously, and talked earnestly of Krishna to anyone who would listen.

Ed., 15, a neatly dressed, shy, very sober immigrant boy suddenly started truanting and was apprehended, having hit an elderly lady on the head and taken her handbag. Later, when he had attacked another old lady in the hospital grounds, he admitted that voices in his head made him do it.

Hallucinatory experiences must be very frightening and some antisocial conduct seems to be an attempt to shut out or avoid the sensations by hectic activity.

Fay, 13, had to be admitted because of her unpredictable outbursts in her approved school. She would suddenly scream in a fury and attack anyone nearby. She also ran off, enjoyed hectic joyriding and promiscuous sex, flitting from one wild activity to another until caught. On admission she said the only thing wrong with her was that she needed glasses. Eventually she explained her terror at seeing vivid flashing lights and objects coming towards her, and how she could only blot them out by shouting and hectic activity.

4. Organic Cerebral Dysfunctions and Cerebral Dysrhythmia

Although there is no evidence that any cerebral lesions and cerebral dysfunction are a specific cause of conduct disorder, it would seem from our case material that they can contribute in several ways where other circumstances are unfavourable (Wardle, 1967).

(a) Adverse factors are likely to be more frequent in the environment of epileptics (Bagley, 1971). One reason may be that fits evoke unfavourable reactions from the environment.

Gay, 12, a rather plain but friendly girl, was admitted because of repetitive absconding from an approved school. During her wanderings she had stolen considerable sums of money, turned prostitute and when found was performing in a sleazy nude show. She had got to an approved school because she kept running away from children's homes and remand homes.

She got there because she ran away from an epileptic colony. She got there because she was excluded from a day school for the maladjusted because of her wild and difficult behaviour. She behaved in a wild and difficult way there because she felt she was not maladjusted or mad but, 'OK, if "they" thought she was, she would show them'. She had been sent to the school for the maladjusted because she got upset at school when she had started having epileptic fits which frightened her family, the other children and the teachers, and all reacted by wanting to be rid of her. Before the onset of fits her parents were strict but affectionate, and she was a good pupil in an 'A' stream. On admission, the parents wanted nothing to do with her and she was rejecting all adult and socially approved values and codes of behaviour.

(b) Anticonvulsant drugs may cause behaviour difficulties. The effect of phenobarbitone in increasing irritable and aggressive behaviour in susceptible individuals is now so well documented that reference is made to it in the *British National Formulary* (1971). Behaviour disorder can also follow depletion of serum folate secondary to long administration of phenytoin (Reynolds, 1967; Neubauer, 1970).

(c) Modifications in cerebral functions may affect behaviour or emotional control.

Hope, 11, formerly a happy well-adjusted girl, began deteriorating in work and behaviour at school and at home. She clashed violently with her sergeant-major father who became very punitive and angry. This seemed to lead to a crescendo of antisocial behaviour which led to proceedings in court to show she was 'beyond control'. A routine psychiatric examination for the court revealed uncontrollable movements of limbs and tongue, disorientation and confusion. Sydenham's chorea was confirmed on admission.

Jol., 11, had to be excluded from a school for educationally subnormal children because of his over-zealous pursuit of the girls and because when checked by teachers he tended to react by, 'You can't tell me what to do', and by pushing his way past the teacher. Further attempts to check him physically proved abortive because at 5′ 11″ he was as big as the largest teacher in the school. Excluded from school, he spent his days damaging people's motor cars and frightening the police by his menacing attitude when they tried to stop him. On admission, an infantile mind in a huge body proved to be the result of a combination of nurture (neglect and breakdown in family care) plus nature (an extra Y chromosome).

(d) There may be poor frustration tolerance and poor inhibition of aggression.

Kit, 11, was finally referred because of continual truancy and stealing while out of school. His mother had tried to make him go to school, but he would become very angry and threaten to break windows or lash out at his mother. He complained of various rather bizarre physical complaints: pain in left chest and arm, and pain and swelling of his left eye when he was upset. No neurological signs were found except an odd distortion of his left fundus and optic disc. In hospital the unmistakable swelling of his left eye was observed when he was angry, as were the accompanying uncontrollable rages in which he was inaccessible to reason. Three years later a large subarachnoid cyst was removed extending through frontal and temporal lobes to hypothalamus. How much of this behaviour disorder can be attributed to this lesion and how much to environmental influences (an over-protective, over-anxious mother and a violent, aggressive father who often deserted the family, an interfering maternal grandmother who seduced one after the other of the children to live with her and absent themselves from school – two girls refusing school and one girl rebelling in adolescence have also been treated as out-patients) is uncertain.

5. *Conduct Disorder Reactive to Intolerable Stress at Home, such as Severe Chronic Parental Invalidism and/or Constant Nagging*

Len, 14, had been a model only child until his adoptive mother's first cerebral catastrophe. He had been exceptionally tidy and helpful about the house and fitted into his houseproud mother's routine. Her stroke resulted in hemiplegia and speech distortion. Len reacted not by helping more, but by spending more and more time out of the house, partly in a Church Youth Club where he was highly thought of as a leading spirit, but partly with street-corner gangs who became involved in house-breaking and vandalism. His long spells out were punctuated by sessions of angry recrimination and reproach which shortened still further the time he spent at home.

Other children who showed severe antisocial avoidance behaviour had mothers with Parkinson's disease, disseminated sclerosis, incurable carcinoma of colon, progressive muscular dystrophy, hypochondriasis, and loss of both kidneys with survival on dialysis. Constant carping criticism and nagging can have the same effect.

6. Acting-out to Draw Attention to some Serious Wrong

Mick, 13, who had always been Mum's special baby, began truanting from school and staying out late; he stole from home to buy cigarettes to hand round to a much older gang and began feigning injuries and illness to get himself into hospital. On one occasion he came to casualty claiming to have been beaten up by 'skinheads'. While under observation he developed hemiparesis and disturbance of consciousness which disappeared only just in time to avoid the operating theatre. He was admitted after he developed the habit, after seeing a television programme on the subject, of calling out the Samaritans because he was 'desperate' and 'wanted to end it all' and had taken aspirin (first occasion), had taken to drink (second occasion), was going on drugs (third occasion). In hospital he continued to draw attention to himself by all kinds of acting-out – smashing windows, scratching his arms, attacking smaller children in front of staff, and swearing loudly outside the doctors' offices when they were interviewing. This behaviour was particularly noticeable just before and after home visits and eventually he revealed that his mother expected him to sleep with her. Sex instruction and adolescent awareness had made him increasingly embarrassed and worried by this.

7. The 'Fallen Idol' Syndrome

Nan, 14, was apparently a happy, well-adjusted girl until the day she discovered her parents' marriage certificate which indicated they married a month before she was born. She asked her mother about this and felt her mother was ashamed of it ('and so of me'). She began staying out late and dating boys, but her really uncontrolled promiscuity and stealing began when her adored father began an affair with the girl opposite.

8. Conduct Disorder Resulting from a Deficiency and/or Discontinuity of Stable, Secure, Affectionate Care

This runs like a dismal thread through the whole case material as the factor common to almost all the children whose main presenting problem was disapproved and antisocial conduct. The only exceptions were the case of Sydenham's chorea and some cases of acute psychosis and cerebral dysrhythmia where the disruption of internal cerebral organisation appeared to be responsible, or where the unfavourable parental reaction seemed to be evoked by the manifestations of abnormal cerebral functioning, producing a vicious cycle of deterioration in behaviour and family relationships.

Pip, 9, is an extreme example of what can happen to a child. Abandoned at birth, he was collected again at 3 months, only to be removed by a court order at 15 months, neglected and battered. Moved from a nursery to a children's home and thence to a foster home, he was quickly returned to the children's home because at three he was impossible to control, hyperactive and did not seem to learn by experience. Several other foster homes were tried with the same result. At school age he also proved impossible to educate despite average intelligence, and by eight had the distinction of having been excluded from two ordinary schools and two special schools for the maladjusted. From time to time he was claimed by his mother, who drifted about the countryside with his violent, unemployable father. He was admitted on one such visit because his mother complained he was uncontrollable. Unless actually tied up and locked in a room he would be off like a wild animal, stealing anything he laid eyes on, attacking other children for toys and sweets, throwing stones at anything breakable. On admission he was clad in filthy rags, verminous, covered in bruises; his mother shook him fiercely and ordered him to 'Tell the man I never hit you, tell him yer mum loves you'.

Rose, 8, was equally disorganised. Her acting-out took the form of attacking adults in their most tender and embarrassing places with wriggling fingers, she communicated almost entirely with sexual expletives and seemed preoccupied with drawing male and female genitalia and secondary sex characteristics. She pocketed anything she fancied and interfered with everything she saw, apparently uninhibited by anything. Excluded from school, she had to be admitted from her children's home for the sake of the staff and other children. Born illegitimate, although mother was married, the stepfather inflicted grave injuries on Rose during her first year of life, leading to admission to hospital on several occasions; the records of one say she was knocked unconscious and had some form of meningitic or encephalitic process afterwards. After her mother's marriage broke up Rose was placed in a foster home, but when the foster parents moved her mother refused to allow her to go with them and took her with her to a brothel in London. Later, Rose was placed in the care of her grandmother because she was a nuisance to her mother, but from time to time her mother would remove her. Eventually the grandmother was unable to look after Rose and she was placed in a children's home; once again the mother repeatedly interfered. Shortly before admission Rose was found by her grandmother in her mother's flat in London with a number of male clients standing around, blood pouring from her mother's self-inflicted cut wrists, and Rose crouching in a corner swearing at everyone.

We conclude that conduct disorder or acting-out antisocially seems to be the elected method of demonstrating internal tension, stress or other emotional disturbance in children and adolescents who have suffered a deficiency or discontinuity of stable affectionate care through childhood. The internal disturbances can be a response to a real external stress which would evoke anxiety, anger, fear or frustration in anyone, or it may be a response to internal abnormality, for example a change in cerebral rhythm, frightening hallucinations or premenstrual hormonal changes. In many cases the acting-out behaviour is the result of the coincidence of all three types of factor Acting-out behaviour tends to produce a chronic ongoing irritant pathogen of its own by evoking external hostility and internal guilt; this leads to secondary behaviour adopted to avoid the unpleasant feelings these arouse. Since the logical path of stopping the acting-out behaviour appears to be closed, the pathological response to punishment is, as to other stresses, further antisocial behaviour. The frequency of antisocial behaviour in the waiting period before court appearance would appear to support this.

It is hoped that these cases illustrate the variety of problems whose care we are about to consider and the wide range of possibilities which must be taken into consideration in planning their investigation and treatment. Despite the diversity of problems and causes, we believe there can be an overall strategy which can be applied to the treatment and care of all the children in the hospital unit at the same time as a treatment plan specific to each child's individual needs.

Indications for Admission

From the illustrative examples it should be apparent that the children who are admitted present antisocial behaviour well outside the ordinary experience of parents, teachers and even people experienced in the care of specially difficult children – houseparents in remand homes and children's homes and teachers in special schools for the maladjusted and in approved schools. Criteria for admission are difficult to specify because admission is often dictated by influences other than the child's clinical condition. It is probably not a clinical influence which leads to the unusually high proportion of admitted patients who lack the support of two affectionate parents at home waiting eagerly for their return. In considering the admission of these children great care has to be taken that the applying agency is not just trying to get rid of an unwanted problem and that hospital is not regarded as what the social agencies choose to call a 'placement'. This term implies permanency and irrevocability. We feel it is important to insist that all children admitted have a home base to which they can return for holidays, and which will receive them after discharge. For the child to develop the idea that the hospital is his home has grave implications for his future development and behaviour. Home is a place one depends on and returns to.

Those of us specialising in child psychiatry tend to spend more of our time in community and outpatient work than many of our colleagues. It is, therefore, fairly easily for us to remember that most investigations and treatments can be carried out in an outpatient clinic or a day hospital.

The need for removal from the place where the child is at present, because he is a nuisance there, is not a justification for admission to a psychiatric unit, however aggrieved social agencies and parents feel. There must be positive indications, as suggested below, that the child's condition warrants and will benefit by investigation and/or treatment in an inpatient psychiatric unit.

Criteria which are Sufficient in Themselves to Justify Admission

(a) The child's behaviour endangers himself or other people and/or is unacceptable in any non-psychiatric setting because of its bizarre nature or its failure to respond to ordinary social measures.

(b) The behaviour appears irrational or bizarre, or there are clearly recognisable symptoms of a psychiatric illness or syndrome, *and* the investigation or treatment required is not possible as an outpatient or day patient or in the present social setting.

(c) The behaviour is deteriorating or failing to respond to the social measures available in the community, and if the child is not admitted to a psychiatric unit will get worse or damage the child's relationships so badly that rehabilitation will become difficult or impossible.

(d) An essential investigation or treatment can only be undertaken as an inpatient.

Criteria which may Indicate Admission if there are No Contra-indications

(a) Observation day and night away from home would further assessment and appraisal of the child and his problem.
(b) The syndrome the child presents is of a type which has been shown to respond well to the therapeutic environment of the inpatient unit.
(c) It is suspected that the child's present environment is causing the persistence of symptoms.
(d) Outpatient treatment is failing to produce improvement.
(e) Removal to a psychiatric setting will enable the child to recognise his disorganised behaviour as a personal problem to be solved, rather than wickedness.
(f) Repetitive antisocial conduct is being displayed by a child from an apparently stable affectionate background, where the cause is obscure.
(g) Admission will remove the child from a vicious cycle of disturbed behaviour evoking hostility and punishment, which in turn provokes further disturbed behaviour.
(h) Admission will provide a brief truce or breathing space in which relationships which have broken down between parent and child can be repaired.

When a child's antisocial behaviour is controlled in a social setting and no nuisance is being caused, it is sometimes difficult to persuade social agencies that a child is in need of psychiatric inpatient treatment even when it is evident that the child is suffering from a clear-cut psychiatric illness which requires treatment. Social agencies often seem to correlate acting-out behaviour with psychiatric illness and fail to recognise the suffering of a depressed, anxious or psychotic child until acting-out occurs.

Contra-indications to Admission

(a) The child has no home base to look to for visits, letters, pocket-money, and a place for weekends and holidays; and to see as a place to return to when well.
(b) The child has no person (other than an official) outside the hospital who would worry about his well-being and his behaviour while in the hospital.

(c) There is evidence that the child's relationships in the community would suffer as a result of admission, for example he would lose his place in the home or be rejected as damaged.
(d) The child cannot be convinced that he is not being put away or punished.
(e) The antisocial behaviour is confined to stealing of money or goods of value to the child, in a child suffering from deficiency or discontinuity of care and affection.

The Benefits of Hospital Admission

Apart from indications for admission in the child's condition or his environment we should also consider what hospital admission can provide which cannot be provided efficiently in another way.

1. Observation and Investigation

Clearly most psychological and pathological investigations, and most neurological and psychiatric examinations, can be undertaken in an outpatient clinic. Admission enables observation to be made of the child in every aspect of day-to-day life, domestic situations, play and recreation, school, behaviour inside and outside, supervised and apparently unsupervised, and in a diversity of relationships (with caring adults, adults in authority, neutral adults, other girls and boys of all ages and sizes, people giving and demanding, tolerant and controlling, pleased and angry). The inpatient is enabled to demonstrate the nature of his difficulty and how it arises in a situation where the behaviour can be tolerated and prevented from harming either the patient or others, and where it can be dealt with appropriately on the spot by skilled staff.

Admission enables direct and continuous observation of what influences the child's behaviour: of those physical or psychological experiences which evoke it, of those which render the child more vulnerable or less, and of subsequent physical or psychological influences which modify it for better or worse. Apart from the specific behaviour disorder, the child's overall pattern of life adaptation is observed. Over a period of time we are enabled to detect cyclical changes in behaviour and coincidence between behavioural changes and outside events or physiological changes.

A secondary and, to us, unexpected gain is the often quite different picture of the family which unfolds after admission. Defects in the family relationships and caring which were completely concealed in the weekly talking relationship in clinic interviews are quickly revealed by the actual behaviour of parents to the child and each other. Parents who have protested their care and affection for their child fail to make proper arrangements to visit or write – or do write!

> Dear Rona,
> Once again you reveal your characteristic selfishness, do you realise how long and what effort it takes me to earn the money you ask for. Not one little word of love for Mummy, just I want, I want, well 'Mummy' has had enough.

But she hadn't; the letter went on to detail the exact cost of all that Mummy had done for Rona and what Rona had done in return. We now understand, more clearly than any psychotherapeutic interview and/or casework had ever been able to show, just why Rona blew up at home and tried to escape to a drug-taking, but more tolerant, commune.

When Sam's mother told us how slapdash and dirty our laundry and washing facilities were and how dirty, neglectful and untidy her exceptionally fastidious son was, we understood what he was exposed to at home. Five minutes' description by a parent of behaviour or a situation which we have observed ourselves, can be extremely revealing of the parental attitudes to which the child is really exposed. For some reason parents seem able to behave to the staff as if they were members of the family after the child has been admitted, whereas in interviews at home or in the outpatient clinic much is concealed. Most of this is elicited by the actual caring staff, but the parents also seem to identify the doctor-in-charge very much more with their child, and he is likely to be exposed to hostility or other extreme attitudes formerly reserved for the child in the privacy of his own home. The visting social worker gains new insights through the attitudes which the parents reveal about the hospital and the caring staff there. Cracks in the overall family relationships are also revealed; when the scapegoat or imaginary focus of family difficulty is removed, real difficulties in relationships between other members of the family or a new scapegoat emerge, problems in other siblings suddenly appear, or the marital relationship breaks down overtly.

It will be seen that contacts with parents and the rest of the family are an important part of inpatient assessment and that these contacts should not be confined to the consultant or a visiting social worker, as important insights into the family relationships will be missed.

2. *Treatment Procedures which are More Effective in an Inpatient Setting*

Although we have attempted to do so for purposes of discussion, in practice investigation, observation and treatment cannot be separated. Treatment begins, or should begin, from the moment the child leaves his former environment and enters the influence of a new group of people. It may have begun at the moment admission was suggested.

(a) *Relationship building*. We have noted that the primary failure in conduct disorders is a failure in the child's relationships. The child does not care because he feels uncared for or has not experienced care, he does not respect others because he does not respect himself, because he has not been respected. The primary task in these cases is to build relationships in which the child feels cared for and is accorded respect as a person. In individuals whose capacity for formation of relationships has been damaged by repeated disappointments, this can only be achieved by prolonged contact and seems to develop best through very basic activities such as eating, washing, going to bed and such basic emotional experiences as anger, frustration and physical cuddling. Clearly this sort of process can only develop in a residential setting.

(b) *Controlled interaction*. The extent and degree of the child's participation in the various activities of the unit, and the amount of contact with other children, will be determined by the initial observations made of his condition and behaviour. At some stages in treatment it may prove most effective to let the child build up relationships with caring adults in a rather infantile way, away from other children altogether, or in a very small group. Thus unless the child has very good trusting relationships with adults it is never wise to unleash him on a group of children on admission. Gradually the child is allowed to experiment in different settings, moving back a pace if the experience proves too difficult, moving on if successful.

Clearly great flexibility in caring situations is needed, ranging from complete withdrawal, to the security of a single room with a full-time nurse, to complete freedom to be responsible for himself – with the possibility of changing from one to the other quickly.

(c) *Community group therapy*. The major aim of treatment is to remove maladaptive behaviour and to encourage and facilitate adaptive behaviour, not just within the hospital and when the child is observed, but in the community when there is no-one except the child himself to guide and control his behaviour. This requires the development of an understanding of the need to be responsible for one's own behaviour rather than being controlled, and a recognition of the needs of others, and of the necessity to consider these.

The inpatient setting provides an admirable setting for this, provided that the staff understand that they must allow the child to experiment without unnecessary criticism and interference, and that full discussion of the child's behaviour and its effects follows. Group interaction and discussion are the second main plank in our inpatient treatment and will be discussed in more detail.

(d) *Controlled trials of medication and other individual therapy*. Inpatient observation enables an objective assessment of the effect of medication on behaviour in those cases where the clinical condition warrants it. Observation as an outpatient relies on the untutored and sometimes prejudiced reporting of untrained observers, and other influences on the patient's progress may not be known to the clinician. In hospital starting doses can be high without anxiety, and changes in dose or drug can be made quickly as dictated by immediate observations.

The *aims of inpatient care* for severe conduct disorders may be summarised as follows:

1. Temporary removal from an environment which was unsuitable or where the child was damaging or being damaged by his relationships.
2. Provision of an environment where the patient's well-being can be fostered and at the same time his undesirable behaviour can be controlled so that he is prevented from doing too much harm to himself or to others.
3. Provision of a therapeutic environment where the patient can learn more adaptive patterns of behaviour and lose maladaptive ones. This is achieved through formation of good relationships

and controlled interaction in a community arranged to encourage understanding and discussion.
4. Provision of opportunities for the identification and modification by skilled staff of harmful personal and environmental influences.
5. The maintenance of the patient's ongoing development – physical, social, emotional and educational – at the best level possible throughout his stay in hospital.

The Inpatient Regime

A member of a lay committee of a hospital group which included a child psychiatric inpatient unit remarked after a discussion of numerous windows which had just been broken (mainly by one child), 'If I had my way they wouldn't mend them; a month or two of cold draughts would soon teach 'em. Anyway, they wouldn't be here if I had my way – let me get at 'em and I'd teach 'em how to behave!'

It is hoped that the foregoing will explain for him and millions of others with the same attitude why 'they' have to be 'there' and why his rough-and-ready commonsense approach, while possibly applicable to his own healthy, happy children, would not work with the patient who was breaking windows. We hope the foregoing will also have answered the oft repeated questions: (1) Why don't you tell them how to behave? (2) Why do you let them do it? (3) Why don't you punish them? and (4) Why do you provide these awful children with better facilities and professional care than normal children? The answers, if not already apparent, are (1) They know; (2) We don't; (3) It has been proved not to work over and over again; and (4) They need them much more, and society cannot afford not to provide them because the alternatives are much more expensive. The costs which have to be balanced against effective care and treatment in childhood are the costs of maintaining damaged adults in prison and mental hospitals, not to mention the cost to the community of their delinquent and antisocial behaviour, and the cost to the next generation of the products of their failed marriages and efforts at child-rearing (Wardle, 1970; Royal Medico-Psychological Association, 1970). Traditional methods of care and management which have proved passable for the majority of happy, healthy children have failed, and often failed repeatedly, with these children. We will now examine methods of care, treatment facilities and staff deployment which occasionally seem to have been more successful.

The methods described here have been tried out and evolved during the last eight years in an inpatient unit for children and adolescents in Exeter. The unit serves the Devon clinical area and admits all types of psychiatric problem except severe subnormality and isolated subnormality. Despite the absence of restriction on admissions we have run the unit as a therapeutic community with open doors and nurses out of uniform.

At the outset it is important to emphasise that we are not discussing a method of child-rearing and that the techniques are not necessarily appropriate for all children in all settings. The methods we describe have been tried and found effective for very disturbed children in a hospital setting over fairly short periods. While some might be used in other settings with other children, the prospective user would have to consider their effect in relation to the total environment and the overall arrangements into which the methods were introduced. Among other things, we hope to show that introducing these methods is not simple and depends on many factors outside as well as within the unit in which they are used. Difficulties arise in the care of disturbed boys and girls not only from their tendency to act out their emotional tension and distress, but from the reactions of adults to their behaviour on the ward and outside.

The inpatient regime will be discussed under the following headings:

1. Physical facilities and arrangements – play and recreational equipment
2. Daily programme – framework of regular routines and activities
3. Procedure for admission and introduction to the group
4. The treatment plan
5. Setting up a therapeutic community – difficulties – the unit and the outside world – status – the need for the group – evolution of the groups
6. The work of the nurse – introduction to staff on methods of care – staff training – what makes a successful nurse in this setting
7. School
8. Outcome and discharge

The Physical Facilities

Although, in our view, people matter most in treatment of conduct disorders, the physical environment can help or mar the work and morale of the staff and help or hinder the learning processes, emotional development and group interaction of the patients. The buildings and equipment should be designed to foster high morale and efficient working in the staff and, in the children, feelings of security and well-being. They should maximise situations which enable treatment, positive development and learning. It cannot be over-emphasised that treatment depends on good relationships between patient and staff; good relationships can be formed most quickly and effectively in a happy, homely atmosphere where the staff are enthusiastic and enjoying their work and feel they are being given maximum support in their very difficult task.

The building and equipment should be designed to help the staff, minimise frustrations, prevent the staff wasting time on chores not associated with the children and reduce to the minimum time spent restricting or stopping the children. Temptations to activity which will make trouble for the staff or children should be cut out of the design. Equipment, materials or areas which are fragile, dangerous, valuable or otherwise taboo should not be accessible to patients. The relationship between child and staff member can only be damaged if the staff member is repeatedly forced to be policeman or judge because the gardener insists on having his strawberry patch unfenced and next to the play area, or the fire officer insists on having prominent fire equipment and glass-fronted alarms directly linked to the fire station so that beautiful red fire engines and hoards of uniformed men can be summoned by a single blow. Not only does this kind of arrangement force the staff into a negative, restricting role, but it exposes them to demoralising criticism from outside – 'Why can't you control them?' – and wastes their time and emotional energy in numerous profitless directions – watching and restricting before and investigating, explaining and apologising after each crisis which could have been avoided by more sensible planning. The current preoccupation with management and efficiency leads the administration to introduce more and more of these frustrating and dehumanising arrangements, and indicates a failure to appreciate appropriate priorities.

The primary object, then, is to set up a therapeutic environment in which the well-being of the patients and staff, together with effective treatment, takes priority over all other considerations. In achieving this, special consideration must be given to the effect of the design and geographical arrangement of furniture and rooms on the behaviour of patients and staff, as well as to the functions which have to be served. For example, we found that behaviour in the schoolrooms was very much less controlled, and movement in and out of class much more frequent, when the schoolrooms opened directly from the living area of the unit, than when the children had to go out into the open to go to the school area. On the other hand, relationships between teachers and nurses were closer, more harmonious and less marred by rivalry in the first setting. Behaviour at mealtimes was noticeably improved when a dining-room was separated from the rest of the living area and tables laid with cloths and flowers.

We conclude that in planning either physical arrangements or routine organisation, priority should be given to the effect on behaviour, and if possible pilot experiments should be made before irrevocable steps are taken. It is not always possible to predict all the effects of a change beforehand.

Children with conduct disorders do not need a very different environment from other children. They are, however, more likely than other children to find weaknesses and faults in the system and exploit or exaggerate them. They are more readily frustrated and provoked, and they are much more likely to react by destructive behaviour towards the property, the staff or themselves. It is particularly important, therefore, to reduce unnecessary frustrations and temptations, to provide materials which are robust and of good quality, and to avoid breakable materials which might harm the patients or staff. Glass should be as strong as possible but should not appear to be reinforced (by visible wires, etc.) or it creates a punitive appearance and a challenge. If doors have to be locked, the locks and keys should be unobtrusive, of the domestic Yale variety, not great institutional universal locks which create a rift between the keyholders (staff) and the non-keyholders. Keys should be carried and used discreetly, not hanging from a chain or constantly visible. Furniture should be designed to withstand the fiddling, poking and picking of tense children; screws and bolts should not be visible or accessible, but covered in; upholstery should be strong and have no threads to unravel. Modern plastic upholstery is too readily pierced and once pierced the whole is irreparable. Damaged furniture, etc., should never be left, it must be removed and repaired at once as its presence seems to encourage further damage. Furniture and decoration, then, must aim at decreasing the possibility of damage, but *not* at the expense of comfort and homeliness.

Uncontrolled destructive behaviour is almost inevitable at some stage of the treatment of some of these children, but the well-being of the rest of the group must not be irreparably damaged, and it is therefore essential to have a specially designed secure area of the unit where children can be treated away from the rest of the group until they have achieved control and are no longer a danger. This can be achieved by having one or two specially designed rooms with indestructible decoration and furniture and armoured glass observation. A child should never be alone in this observation area unless the presence of a staff member seems to be making things worse, in which case discreet and unprovocative observation through the window will be needed. The child must never be alone and unobserved. We have found effective a suite of two observation rooms on either side of a central office with play and living space and bathing and toilet facilities adjacent, completely separate from the passage of other children during the day.

Two types of activity have proved specially valuable in treating these children and special provision should be made for them in any centre concerned with treating conduct disorders. Cooking and domestic activity contrasts paradoxically with adventurous outdoor activity, yet most of these children are at their best in these two situations. A kitchen should be provided in the living area which the children can call their own and where they can make snacks, toffee, and get themselves a drink of milk or a biscuit as they would be able to in any reasonable home. Cooking is also a valuable activity for building a relationship with the helping adult and as a basis on which schoolwork can be built up. There should, therefore, be generous provision for this activity in the way of equipment and materials. The high level of milk consumption among an older delinquent population (Miller, 1964) is confirmed in our own population; it is vital these children should have access to what they want (but it should be for internal consumption; waste just to demonstrate freedom should not be encouraged).

Various outdoor activities are popular among boys and girls alike provided there is no feeling that success and failure is involved and the adults are enthusiastic and seem to be enjoying them. In the grounds there should be assault course equipment: ropes, tree houses and hide-outs which give a feeling of privacy, but are readily accessible to staff if the need arises. There should also be storage and riding space for wheeled vehicles: trolleys and bicycles, and soap-box carts to be made and raced or crashed, or just tinkered with. Wild moorland and boating waters are not immediately accessible everywhere, but a lodge or hutted camp can make them available to most conurbations for week-end or longer trips. Such trips are well worthwhile as catalysts to building group cohesion and staff/patient relationships.

Daily Programme

A framework of regular happenings and expectations reduces insecurity and uncertainty, both of which may lead to unproductive pathological behaviour, tension, anxiety and testing-out and manipulation of staff. An excess of inflexible rules can be equally counter-therapeutic by preventing the child demonstrating his behavioural difficulties if they are successfully applied, but creating a 'we/them' atmosphere in which hostility to, and evasion of, the staff develop if they are not successfully applied.

The staff should have the security of knowing where everybody should be and what they should be doing at any particular time, and yet have confidence enough to be flexible about enforcing this in any individual instance. A staff member secure in the knowledge that only children with 'reliability' badges are allowed in the grounds unaccompanied cannot be manipulated by the wandering child, who says, 'Dr X said I could', but can listen sympathetically and suggest they work together to get a badge. In contrast, the nurse who shouts, 'Back to bed!' and will not listen to the child who has got out of bed and come down the corridor, may be inhibiting for ever the confidence the therapeutically-minded staff have all been awaiting expectantly.

A sample day's programme is illustrated in Table 3.1. Group meetings at the beginning and end of each day are the community's strength; here regularity is created and maintained and given meaning for the child.

Table 3.1 A sample day's programme

7.30– 8.0 a.m.	Get up, wash, dress
8.00– 8.30 a.m.	Breakfast
8.30– 9.00 a.m.	Bed making, tidy rooms, room judging
9.00– 9.45 a.m.	Group meeting
9.45–11.00 a.m.	School or occupational therapy
11.00–11.15 a.m.	Coffee break
11.15–12.30 a.m.	School or occupational therapy
12.30– 1.00 p.m.	Lunch
1.00– 2.00 p.m.	Free play activity
2.00– 3.30 p.m.	School or occupational therapy or games or swimming
3.30– 3.45 p.m.	Free recreation or refreshments
*3.45– 4.30 p.m.	Group meeting
4.30– 5.00 p.m.	Tea
5.00– 7.00 p.m.	Free play or organised activity, outdoors if possible, with active participation by staff
7.00–	Social activity – visit to fish-and-chip shop or youth club or club activity in unit

Fixed bedtimes according to age

Under 10	8.00 p.m.
10–11	8.30 p.m.
12–13	9.00 p.m.
14	9.30 p.m.
15	10.30 p.m.

* Compulsory for all patients and staff, except for patients too ill to be in the group at all and their nurse.

Procedure for Admission

The main strategies are the following:

(a) Initial interview; child understands need for admission
(b) Support for parent
(c) Selected nurse allocated
(d) Showing round and introductions
(e) Preparation of other patients
(f) Welcome to group
(g) Establishing relations with staff
(h) Initial assessment, first case conference

The initial interview is important because it will establish the attitude the child has about admission. If admission is seen as a punishment, a form of imprisonment, being 'put away', it will become something to fight against and resent. The staff must try to anticipate and understand the child's fears and resentment. It is helpful to have the initial interview in the hospital where the child is to be admitted and to introduce the child to the nurse who will have special responsibility for his care, and to another child who can show him round.

At this first interview it should be established clearly why the doctor thinks the child needs to come in and what the child may expect if he does come in. As far as possible the child should be helped to feel he has a part to play in the decision-making. Even though admission is the only alternative, he can be helped to see that his view has been heard and understood and will continue to be so. At this stage we are establishing the foundations for treatment: the child should recognise that here is a place where children are listened to and their views respected and understood, though not always agreed with.

Fear and hostility about admission may not be confined to the child. Because they blame themselves for their child's difficulties or feel they have failed, the parents may seek to turn their self-blame and anger on those who seem to be setting themselves up as better at caring than they; or, because of their own fear of parting or doing harm to their child, they may panic at the last moment and see all kinds of hidden evils in the hospital. It is vital, therefore, that they should be given as much attention as the child.

Both child and parent should be protected from unpleasant experiences. The visit should be timed and the staff deployed so that the chance of this is removed, and the children who first meet the mother and child should be chosen to suit their needs.

In this introductory stage we have found it important that the child should be mainly with one nurse, perhaps aided by another child. The relationships built up in this first hour or so have proved long-lasting and children have tended to turn to the nurse they first met for support when under stress later. The nurse should introduce the child to other children and to other staff members in an easy, friendly way. Early contacts should not be forceful or too probing. The nurse will have to be careful to protect the child from jealous attacks, particularly by deprived children and children with whom she has close relationships. Particular care should have been taken to prepare vulnerable children for the newcomer, but the whole group should be prepared. At the group meeting before his arrival it is useful to mention it and to anticipate jealous attention-seeking and display behaviour by pointing out that this usually occurs. The way having been prepared, the new child is introduced at the first group meeting after his arrival and if members of the group are demonstrating disturbed behaviour for his benefit, this should be pointed out. We have built up a tradition that new patients are welcomed by the group and the purpose of the group explained to them by some of the patients. One will start and others join in to fill in omissions and make amendments; the group leader can then add a final remark if necessary. We have found that new patients accept the group meeting very readily, and, since each person is named when the chairman goes round the group, he quickly learns who is who.

Deprived and socially maladapted children have remarkable facility for finding other like children and attaching to them. Hardly ever do they relate to anxious, depressed or socially well-adapted children. It is therefore very important that such a child's first contacts are carefully supervised and controlled. Until these children have built up a confident and trusting relationship with the staff members they should not have unsupervised contact with the whole group. Even when the socially maladapted child has been in treatment for some time he can quickly regress to maladaptive patterns of behaviour when in contact with an untreated similar child. Several other unfortunate consequences may follow: sensing the weakness of his own control and jealous that another is going to have the attention he has had, he may derive satisfaction from encouraging the new patient to antisocial behaviour and trouble. Then, seeing the new patient's potential, he may be stimulated to compete; having got into an anti-authority position he will have to join the other boy by rejecting the people who have helped him and by destroying the relationships and fabric which represented his new way of life. The new patient, not having built any relationships, will not know what he is losing and will only see the old stereotype of himself versus authority, and with such a start will find it hard to recognise a different approach. It is best if he makes his first antisocial mistakes on his own, and if the adults are able to deal with them with him alone, uncomplicated by the involvement of other children.

The Treatment Plan

In addition to building up relationships, the early days are a period of active assessment of the child's problems, assets and handicaps. An effective treatment plan depends on this. Special attention will be paid at this stage to the child's habitual ways of reacting to common situations, comparing what has been described elsewhere with what is observed. A variety of situations provides for this part of the assessment: the domestic situations will be observed by the nursing staff, specific work and play situations by the occupational therapists and response to educational situations by the school-teachers. Each will observe and report both maladaptive and adaptive behaviour, making a special note of circumstances which seem to be rewarding and encouraging to the patient and those which are the opposite. From this material will be formulated a programme aimed at modifying maladaptive behaviour and encouraging adaptive behaviour. Paradoxical and neurotic reaction-formation which requires a less direct treatment will begin to become apparent as relationships develop; it is important, therefore, that enthusiastic staff do not make premature attempts at removing maladaptive behaviour before its significance has been fully examined in the context of all the other observations and information available. The social and biological contribution to the child's development and present status must be fully explored.

Within two weeks of admission sufficient data should have accumulated to enable a formulation to be made of the problem and its causes, with a plan for its resolution or modification. The data, behavioural, biological, social and psychodynamic, is best presented at a conference of all the professional staff who have gathered it and will have to put the treatment into effect. Such a conference will include the schoolteacher, occupational therapist, psychologist, psychiatric social worker and nurse who have been specifically concerned with the child and his family.

Although the doctor is finally responsible for the treatment plan, successful application will depend on the staff members most closely involved and these may be quite junior. It is vital that they are present at the conference, and play an active part in it, providing much of the information on which the treatment plan is based and being encouraged to be critical of it. The treatment plan is based on the co-operation of a team, each member contributing separately but linked and co-ordinated by the group meetings of all the patients and staff each day, and by weekly staff meetings. The doctor is responsible for ensuring that the parts form an integrated and co-ordinated whole and that every facet of the child's problem is given attention.

The happy enthusiastic co-operation of the disciplines in this work is an important model for the child and a strength in dealing with children who, through their own family experience, have learned to adapt to adult disharmony and manipulate it. Because of their experience these children are sensitive to adult jealousies and antagonisms and quick to react to them and manipulate them. Since this is the pattern of adult behaviour they are used to, they tend to evoke it. It is particularly important, therefore, that the adults should be aware of this, demonstrate stability, tolerance and friendliness in their relationships with each other, and avoid expressing critical, jealous or angry feelings about other members of the staff in front of the children. Negative feelings and attitudes are inevitable but the most appropriate place for their expression is the conference, not the ward where even a slight hint of criticism or conflict will be perceived by these children. The exploitation of inconsistent and conflicting standards, attitudes, expectations and instructions is another habitual behaviour the child is likely to have learned and may well practise on the new set of adults. To counter this it is essential that all the adults adopt the same standards and attitudes and have agreed their expectations and instructions together. The staff must have that mutual trust which makes it inconceivable for them to believe that another staff member would give a child permission to do something unlikely without communicating with them or that he would express criticism of them to a child.

David, a child who has had three 'stepfathers' and countless housemothers and foster parents, announces to the night nurse, 'Dr X said I could stay up and watch the late night movie.' He will get equal satisfaction from any of the following possible untherapeutic responses: (1) 'Oh, those doctors always letting the children have treats but it is us who have to put up with the results'; (2) 'Oh, did he, dear? Well all right then'; (3) 'I don't believe you, you are a very naughty little boy to tell such lies'; (4) angry criticism of the doctor. All these types of response will encourage continued use of the manipulation he will have become only too familiar with in his previous homes. He will get no satisfaction, but much benefit, from a response which shows that the night nurse trusts her colleagues but does not want to accuse the child of lying because she still likes him: for instance, 'Wouldn't it be lovely to watch the late night movie; next time you must remind him to leave a message for me on the handover book. I'm afraid unless there is something written in it there is nothing I can do'; or, 'That sounds a terrific treat, had you done something special to earn it? I'm afraid he didn't say anything to me; perhaps he meant another night. Shall we have a game of (something the child likes) instead?' If the child insists that what he said is true, it is important for the night nurse to offer to contact the doctor and if the child still insists, to do so. Again this requires that the night nurse feels this child's problem is worth taking trouble over and that she trusts that the doctor will too. If the doctor snaps back, 'What the h . . . did you interrupt my leisure for to ask me that', the child's manipulation will have been rewarded.

Trust and communication good enough to counter such practised manipulation can only be achieved through very frequent contact in open and unfettered group discussion. A night nurse was chosen as an example because the night nurse is most likely to be, and feel, isolated and get least opportunity for identification with the staff team. Permanent night staff should be allocated paid time to attend staff conferences regularly, and at least some night staff should be rotated from the regular day staff.

Social Factors. The social worker plays a vital role in the initial assessment by uncovering the child's experiences of care and family life, the impact of society on him and his impact on society. In treatment, again, she takes a vital role:

(i) Through frequent contacts with the parents (or substitutes) she will attempt to help them to modify pathogenic attitudes and child-rearing techniques and to become more sympathetic and positive in their attitudes.

(ii) As the child progresses he will be allowed trials at home. Preparing the family for this and early follow-up visits are essential for subsequent planning.

(iii) The social worker provides the link with other social agencies, such as probation officers and social services departments. Plans can go wrong unless careful attention is given to communications with all concerned in the community. The social worker is responsible for inviting the appropriate community workers to conferences.

(iv) Rehabilitation and discharge. Inpatient treatment can seem completely successful until the child is exposed to his old environment. The social worker assesses the capacity of the family to receive the child back and, in the many instances where this will be lacking, makes alternative arrangements such as placement in a hostel or foster home. An important contribution to successful rehabilitation is her knowledge of the facilities which are available and her good relations with the staff concerned with placing children. With school-leavers a job is an important preliminary to discharge, and here again the social worker's knowledge of local facilities (employers and youth employment officers) and skill in dealing with them is needed. Before discharge, school-children may be given a trial in a local school; communications between the hospital school-teachers and the outside school will be important, but we have found that the social worker may be able to maintain a precarious situation by regular visiting and, in some cases, by accompanying the child to and from school. This link will be useful when the child returns to the community.

(v) Trial in the community. The social worker will prepare the way for this and make frequent visits and contacts with all those in the community who may make or mar the success of the trial. In the first week or so daily contacts may be needed. She will also ensure that the child and his family attend for follow-up, bringing them if necessary. Children are often very reluctant to return, fearing readmission, angry at rejection, not wishing to be reminded. Parents, too, often seem reluctant, perhaps for similar reasons and because of an illogical idea that the hospital was the cause of the breakdown and so contact with it could cause a relapse. The social worker can help the child and family over these resistances. Contact with employers is tricky; sometimes visits or enquiry help, but sometimes they arouse anxiety and focus undesirable attention on the employee patient. They may be resented by the patient and lead to a harmful paranoid attitude.

Biological factors may sometimes contribute to the development of conduct disorders, and their presence may undoubtedly interfere with successful treatment. Full consideration should be given, therefore, to the child's physical status and particularly to factors which could influence behaviour either by their direct influence on the organs of behaviour, or indirectly by adverse effects on adaptation or social acceptance. The Oseretsky tests (Rutter, 1969), the Wechsler Intelligence Scales and the EEG have proved particularly useful additions to a full clinical examination.

Although conduct disorders have appeared to be associated with various disorders and defects, for example cerebral dysrhythmia, the extra Y chromosome (Borgaonkar *et al.*, 1972) and premenstrual hormonal disturbance (Dalton, 1960; MacKinnon, 1959), it is difficult to see how these conditions alone could actually cause an individual to perform an antisocial act. Examination of our case histories confirms the observation (Pond, 1961) that in antisocial children with neurological dysfunction the same kinds of family and social disadvantage are found as in children with antisocial disorder in the absence of physical abnormalities. The physical abnormality may act by making the child more vulnerable to specific situations. Thus, the hyperactive child seems particularly vulnerable in a restricting, perfectionistic family; the slow-learner, in a family with high expectations. The unusually large child or the child with poor inhibition of aggression is particularly vulnerable in a family where quarrelling and physical punishments or aggression are frequently seen. The undersized or immature child is vulnerable in a situation (such as school or street-corner society) where physical strength or sexual development are over-valued, leading to a feeling of inferiority and to compensatory behaviour. Advanced physical or sexual development render children vulnerable if their circumstances (for example, neglect) bring them among older companions with whom they have to compete.

Physical factors, genetic or acquired, may also render the child vulnerable by the behaviour they evoke. A damaged child may evoke excessive protection and mothering, in which case he is unlikely to present conduct disorder but, on the other hand, the same damage may evoke hostility. A baby damaged at birth may be separated from his mother during the first two or three crucial days when primary attachment behaviour should be evoked from the mother (Russell-Davis, 1972), or neurological damage may lead him to be floppy or less responsive, making him less easy to love.

Finally, physical factors may be influencing the child's ability to adapt and learn here and now; examples include cerebral dysrhythmias, the drugs used to treat them and their side-effects, and hormonal imbalances associated with menstruation and diabetes. These conditions have first to be treated in order that the other methods can begin to succeed.

It will be clear from the foregoing, however, that many of the physical conditions are chronic or unchangeable, so that the main treatment has to be directed at helping parents and child to accept the condition and learn to adapt to it more effectively, avoiding situations where the vulnerability becomes a handicap.

Medication. There is no evidence that any medication has a specific effect on conduct disorder and, as with physical disorders, it is difficult to see how it could have. Drugs which decrease inhibition are clearly to be avoided as they increase the likelihood of acting-out in a vulnerable individual. Barbiturates tend to increase irritability and lower frustration tolerance, and there is some evidence that they interfere with learning processes (phenobarbitone is particularly harmful in all these respects). Drugs which are potentially addictive or habit-forming should also be avoided, and in giving drugs in tablet form to older patients one must be aware of the danger of hoarding for antisocial purposes (for example to sell, to take as a suicide gesture or to give to other patients out of malice or misdirected kindness).

Anticonvulsants can have a dramatic effect on improving uninhibited and explosive behaviour in a few cases; we have found it impossible to predict which cases will be helped by which anticonvulsant. Phenytoin, primidone, carbamazepine, beclamide and sulthiame have all proved useful.

Chlorpromazine and the other phenothiazines we have found of little value; in small doses they lower inhibition, very large doses may tame aggression but the resulting doping interferes with the learning process and development of relationships. Very rarely it may be necessary to sedate a child heavily because he has become completely beyond reason. In this case it seems kindest to use large doses of chlorpromazine combined with sodium amylobarbitone for a day or two of prolonged sleep.

Stimulants of the central nervous system have no obvious place in treating conduct disorders. Antidepressant drugs will be indicated if depression is the underlying condition. Replacement therapy may be needed where vitamin B12 and serum folate are abnormally low (Neubauer, 1970); yeast has been suggested as a safe alternative (Eastman and Jarcar, 1971) but some doubt has been expressed about the efficacy of replacement (Moir *et al.*, 1971).

Extremes of size can be particularly difficult for girls at puberty and both precocious puberty and very late onset of puberty have been associated with promiscuous acting-out among our cases. Physical treatment has little place in the treatment of reactions of this kind. Sometimes simple discussion of sexual information relieves the whole situation. More often, prolonged discussion is needed to give the child confidence to reveal underlying guilt and anxiety. The physical problem is seldom the whole answer.

Psychotherapy. Traditional psychotherapy based on psychoanalytic theory is usually thwarted by children with conduct disorder because of their tendency to avoid strong emotions and to act-out under stress. Acting-out which seems to be designed to draw attention to something may be helped by individual psychotherapeutic interviews which eventually give the child confidence to reveal the stresses.

> Mick, 13, advanced in puberty, repeatedly drew attention to himself by open antisocial and delinquent acts like window breaking, getting drunk, openly bullying little children. Eventually, like a homing device, the acting-out got closer and closer to the therapist, her windows were broken, her car tyres let down, and finally he revealed his guilt and disgust that he was sleeping with his mother whilst his father slept in his bed. The delinquent acts continued until the social worker tactfully managed to get these sleeping arrangements first revealed and then altered without divulging Mick's confidence.

Children who seem unable to use individual psychotherapy are those who have been totally deprived of the opportunity to relate to one individual in the past. A prolonged period of intensive nurture of a much more basic kind, coupled with progressive behaviour expectations and training, seems more appropriate.

Group therapy is said to be contra-indicated for children who steal outside the home, are aggressive or sociopathic (Ginott, 1961; Slavson, 1943, 1947, 1955). We have found that these children cannot tolerate small formal groups and indulge in a variety of avoidance behaviour and acting-out which nullifies any therapeutic endeavour and rapidly forces the therapist into an authoritarian position. Informal activity, particularly in the open air, tramping over the moors, climbing or messing about in boats, provides a setting in which group work can be done. The community group also appears tolerable, perhaps because it is more structured (Slavson, 1947).

Formal conditioning techniques have not proved appropriate. The formalisation of behaviour-modifying techniques which form the basis of operant conditioning has proved useful in helping the nursing staff formulate effective plans for treatment and in evaluating what they are doing.

The use of 'time out' has proved useful in all group situations where children were becoming disruptive or their undesirable behaviour was becoming contagious. The period out must be brief (3 minutes) and unrewarding. It is important that no warning is given beforehand and that removal is swift and quiet, otherwise other children will vie for this special attention and the child will be rewarded by other children's attention to their screams and antics before removal is effected. A 'time out' room near the main centres of activity – school and living space – is needed; too long a journey reduces the efficacy of removal, but the journey and the 'time out' place should not be in a centre of population.

Longer periods of removal are needed if the child's antisocial behaviour in the group is damaging the relationships of other children with the staff by causing repeated demonstrations of negative attitudes and relationships between adult and child. The removal should be to an area where the child can be given secure care and enjoy relationship with nursing staff, but motivation to return to the group must be maintained. Morale and hope for return must also be maintained by offering rewards and the prospect of further rewards for improvement. A child who feels more secure and comfortable away from the group may learn to seek removal and avoid the stress of trying to return. A child who keeps failing will give up trying, and a child who sees no hope is likely to deteriorate to increasing depredations on the staff and fabric. The extremes a negative policy can lead to are described in the log-books (*c.* 1810–15) of the Bethlem Hospital where a young patient of 14 had been placed 'below' in irons and was described as 'even tearing up the straw with his nails and teeth and clawing at the stones'. Equivalent behaviour is still to be seen in resident establishments where one punishment follows another, ending with some form of locked, isolated detention room.

> When unintentionally the effect of our removal policy led him to feel totally friendless, Sam secreted a match in his dressing-gown and set fire to his mattress. Fortunately, his past good relationships served him in good stead and this 'flare distress signal' alerted us to the need for positive encouragement and reinforcement procedures, and the avoidance of the use of negative ones, so that from 'rock bottom' as it were, he made rapid improvement.

Rehabilitation to the community. As the child progresses, contact with the outside community plays an increasing part in social rehabilitation. In the initial stages volunteers come in to organise social and recreational activities; later they take children back to their youth clubs or to other outside activities. Volunteers have to be selected carefully.

Some are only coming because they themselves have problems in relationships or in order to indulge their voyeurism. Clearly the models they themselves provide are important, though it is surprising how selectively purist and critical the children themselves can be, complaining in the group of volunteers who swore or smoked on the ward and totally rejecting a couple who 'just came to snog'. Enthusiasts with special skills like model-making, canoeing or music-making are particularly welcome, but the single-minded perfectionist is not.

When the children first go out into community activities vigilance is needed because regression to maladaptive behaviour and relationships is likely. The boy who on admission could only relate to other boys by boastful talk of his drug-taking seemed to have completely forgotten this pattern of behaviour in our community group, but relapsed into it on his second visit to an outside youth club. He nearly got the whole unit barred by his extravagant tales of the drug-taking there, and attracted police enquiries by trying to sell his trimipramine tablets! Girls from a family background deficient in affection and a social background deficient in ethical standards are particularly vulnerable when making their essays into the community. Their first contacts are likely to be unattached young men also deficient in inhibiting background experience who appear only too ready to take advantage of an opportunity. Sexual activity has evolved to be gratifying and, once a sexual liaison has been established, little any residential unit can offer can compete as an attraction. Perhaps worse still, the relationship outside seems more powerful than those inside which are now marred by the child's feeling of guilt, so that relationships within the unit may not be helpful to the child and old friends become enemies who are thwarting gratification and evoking unpleasant guilt feelings. Fortunately these outside liaisons tend to break down because of the personalities involved, but it is still best not to let them develop.

On return from the shops, a discreet check of acquisition against expenditure is wise. If the child has stolen, very early detection and skilled management seem the most hopeful for preventing a relapse. After detection the child must be helped to return the goods personally with the support of his nurse. A telephone call to the manager before setting out is helpful. After the goods are returned a general air of relief or celebration is in order and no further action. Stealing is occasionally helped by group discussion where it affects relationships with the group, but the initiative must come from a child. A staff member who has lost something may announce it but to force the group to action about it has proved disastrous. Staff must learn to look after their things and must understand that it is very harmful to their relationship if their carelessness leads to a child being tempted and exposed to the group's anger and his own guilt.

Setting up a Therapeutic Community

The therapeutic community has been defined as the exploitation to the fullest advantage of the therapeutic potential which resides in all members of a multidisciplinary treatment team and the patients gathered together under one roof at a particular time (Jones, 1962).

The discussion so far will have indicated that our aim is to provide an environment which children will enjoy, in which they can feel at ease and in which their problems are likely to be revealed and dealt with, not concealed or suppressed. We advance the hypothesis that characteristics which increase the therapeutic efficacy of a unit include:

(a) A warm, family-like atmosphere.
(b) Minimum inessential formality. (By inessential formality we mean expressions of rank and status, titles, uniform, separate staff toilet and eating facilities, keys, etc. We do not mean adults pretending to be children or abrogating their responsibility.)
(c) Maximum staff and patient participation and cohesion in control of their environment and in everything which is done. This is achieved:
(i) by group discussion of changes which affect the group (for instance, rearrangements of beds or school groupings, damage to fabric or loss of property, who shall go swimming or be free to go out unaccompanied, a staff member leaving, a new patient coming);
(ii) by active involvement in physical arrangements: meal-preparing, cleaning, decorating, mending. Neither staff nor children should be able to feel passive recipients of attention in an environment which is outside their control.

To attain these aims the unit should be autonomous, only occasionally needing to call on services from outside in the same way as a family living in their own home would have to. Permanent domestic staff, handyman and gardener would be included in the establishment and they would be important members of the therapeutic team. The children would be encouraged to participate with them in cooking and cleaning, making and mending. Unhappily, the climate of opinion is likely to thwart achievement of autonomy. Administrators believe that centralisation and pooling of resources leads to greater efficiency and economy, trade-unionists jealously guard the boundaries of job demarcation, and the professionally trained, their status.

As we were establishing our own unit the organisation of three hospitals in our group was being centralised: gardeners, supplies, engineers, and so on, were all removed from the peripheral hospitals to a base from where their activities were controlled and synchronised. All requests for equipment have to go to base via appropriate channels, and repairs are undertaken by a team which invades the ward from time to time. Similarly, the cleaning is undertaken by a cleaning team which tours round with mass cleaning equipment.

The child who has been told by a visiting workman that he 'ought to be in Borstal not hospital', may feel resentful and remove the workman's ladders or push the newly puttied window out. The child whose attention-seeking behaviour has been painstakingly coped with and ignored, may at last find herself with a gawping appreciative audience, unwittingly cheering on each new excess. The nurse trying to deal with this in the approved way may be hampered by embarrassment and unhelpful suggestions and remarks and may regress into an authoritarian pattern and so make matters worse. In any case, carefully built-up relationships can be strained by this unfortunate conflict in front of an audience of strangers. Worse still, the unruly behaviour, rudeness and destructiveness of 'all' children in the unit is reported back to base, not by one person but by several. Even when the incidents are not exaggerated this can have a number of undesirable side-effects:

(a) The unit develops a reputation in the rest of the hospital group as a place where there is no control and the children are allowed to be rude and destructive – that is, a bad place to work. Possible consequence – difficulty in recruitment of staff.
(b) The children get a reputation as all antisocial and not deserving to be helped. Possible consequence – reluctance to do things for the unit, delays in repairs and so on; management committee unwilling to spend money on toys and things for the children's enjoyment.

(c) The staff of the unit get a reputation of not controlling the children properly. Possible consequence – demands by the management committee and senior nursing staff for more discipline and authoritarian type of control, which if introduced lead to more disturbance and interfere with therapy. Even if these are resisted, the criticism of the nursing staff and doctors may result in lowering of morale and irritation, with a less therapeutic atmosphere and handling, which in turn results in more disturbance.

We feel there are strong arguments for reducing to the minimum visits to the ward by strangers not in the control of those running the ward. The doctor or nurse must be able to direct or guide those who do come.

There is little place for the outward display of status in a therapeutic environment. It is important that the child be able to take the role he needs at the moment, with the adults around, and not be rebuffed; yet at the same time the adults must remain adults and maintain control of the situation as a therapeutic one for everybody in the group. This requires very special qualities of personality as well as training. The worker must be sure of his own status as an adult person, and not need props or outward display and assertion. It is very difficult for nursing staff to accept that rudeness and swearing and other attention-seeking behaviours are more likely to persist if too much attention is paid to them. It is difficult to accept that the nurses' status will not be permanently damaged if they desist from asserting it by such remarks as, 'You can't speak to me like that', or, 'Do what you are told'. Equally it is hard for some nurses to realise that relationships cannot be built by buying friendship with laxity, nor will they be damaged by sensible firmness and control, for instance by preventing a child from some undesirable act.

One of the most difficult achievements in the therapeutic community seems to be this balance between relaxation and tolerance, and the possibility of self-expression on the one hand, with the provision of reasonably efficient organisation of the ward with a framework of control and sensible limits on the other.

Many have pointed out that a major factor in emotional illness and antisocial behaviour is faulty function in relating to other people. This is particularly so in the problems of childhood. Working with groups enables one first to see where the faults in relationships lie in actual practice, and then to enable the patient to see these faults through the eyes of fellow patients so that he can gradually remedy the faults, practising new skills in a sheltered environment where the slings and arrows are tempered by the guidance of the group leader and by the knowledge that everyone else is going through it too.

Authority is a strongly entrenched tradition in most hospitals and is clearly invaluable where patients are critically ill and need specific skilled treatment along clearly defined lines. Didactic authority is incompatible with the therapeutic community, and indeed with group therapy, yet leadership is essential. Resolution of this kind of conflict is a strength of the group approach. Particular areas of conflict which have to be resolved include:

(a) Balance between providing a homely flexible environment on the one hand and efficient organisation on the other. This is particularly difficult if the organisation is institutional and part of a larger central organisation not represented in the group.
(b) Balance between relaxation, tolerance and allowing self-expression on the one hand and a framework of control and sensible limits on the other.
(c) Preservation of the decorations, furnishings and equipment and control of destructiveness without tyranny, punishment or driving disturbance underground.
(d) The conflict between preservation of hierarchical structure and need of staff for status and the provision of a relaxed atmosphere in which relationships can be explored, social difficulties acted-out and social adaptation learned.
(e) The conflict between the individual's freedom and therapeutic needs, between his needs and those of each other individual and between the needs of the individual and of the group.

We discovered the value of groups for resolving such conflicts when crises began to develop within a few weeks of opening eight pilot beds in 1965. Children were complaining about nurses nagging and bullying and restricting them, and nurses were complaining about the rudeness, swearing and antisocial behaviour of the children. A 'them' versus 'us' situation was developing rapidly and the consultant was being called out of his bed to arbitrate too often for his comfort. The increasing use of tranquillisers and bed rest was clearly not an answer and their effectiveness was being reduced still further by injudicious staff who used them as a threat. When 'seeing the doctor', 'treatment' and 'injection' are viewed as punishments it is time to inspect the lines of communication. A weekly group meeting conducted by the consultant reduced these tensions, and in the ensuing seven years, group work has evolved as a major therapeutic strength of the unit.

The use of groups has been allowed to vary according to the needs of the population from time to time. Group decision-making permits great flexibility. At present there are eight types of group in operation:

(i) A daily community group of all the children and staff in the unit
(ii) Smaller community groups held in the evenings by the children and nurses in the different living areas
(iii) A weekly review group attended by the consultant, teaching and occupational therapy staff, nurses and all the children, at which progress is reviewed and new plans made for the next week
(iv) Emergency groups which can be called by a child or staff member at any time by ringing a bell in case of a grievance or injustice or injury or a special plan
(v) Weekly staff conference (all staff invited concerned with the particular child under review)
(vi) Meeting of nurses on arrival each morning to plan the day
(vii) Weekly meeting of doctors with nurses
(viii) Weekly lunch of all the staff that can get away, usually doctors, teachers, occupational therapists and some nurses

The most important of these is the daily meeting of the whole community. Everyone working in the unit that day, the consultant and unit officers and all patients are expected to be there punctually at 9 a.m. The chairman (usually a child) will have been elected at the end of the preceding meeting. The minutes are read by the consultant who is responsible for recording what has been said. The chairman then names each person in turn round the circle asking them if they have any suggestions, complaints or problems. Anything may be said but all remarks are supposed to be addressed to the chair; this is an attempt to minimise cross-floor battles and asides unheard by all the group, since the aim is to expose interpersonal conflicts, not foster them. It is also a simple way of avoiding the setting-up of other authority figures by the group, and it enables people in leadership positions, for example, senior nurses, teachers and doctors, to fade into the background.

From time to time the group has applied sanctions to avoidance of the meeting or late arrival (for instance, loss of privileges for the day) or for repeated interruption. Threats, acting-out and name-calling are barred. At one time we used a token system; tokens could be voted for approved or improved behaviour and taken away for disapproved behaviour. Taking away tokens turned out to be disrupting, time-consuming and counter-productive, and has been dropped. The consultant, as secretary, can intervene by asking questions about the minutes or raising points of order, and in this way can maintain a therapeutic control over the group interaction if necessary.

Occasionally the group has called for the removal of a disruptive member and children have been barred from attendance, but it has been recognised that if they are barred they are in the position of outlaws, a very anti-therapeutic and anti-community position. 'Little groups' in which really disruptive people could learn how to use the big group were created with good effect in some instances, quiet removal by a nurse with no attention paid by the group in others. On the whole, the group has learned that attention paid to the disruption increases the disruption.

This group deals with the day-to-day progress of each individual, interpersonal conflicts, damage to fabric, lapses of behaviour, improvements and good deeds. The group tries to explore and understand the reason for lapses and to help the individual see how he impinges on the whole group. Reparation, sanctions or a plan for overcoming the lapse in the future may be discussed. It is important that scapegoating and outcasting are avoided: this is safeguarded by the child's special nurse always supporting him unless she brings up the problem, in which case the child's doctor does.

The group can become quite sophisticated in both dynamic and operant conditioning techniques for dealing with behaviour problems, and this meeting has proved a suitable situation for their application because everyone knows how and why and what has happened and is to happen, leaving little room for manipulation.

Development of the present situation was slow and arduous, with resistance from staff and patients at all stages; it is therefore interesting that new patients and staff accept it readily, though both can find frank discussion of their mistakes a threat. Initially, the staff found the frankness and equality of expression threatening to their status and interpreted the consultant's readiness to accept criticism of the unit and staff as acquiescing and agreeing with the children. Remarks intended to support a very disturbed child were interpreted as a policy decision or a criticism of the nurse who (correctly) raised a problem. It proved necessary to emphasise that policy decisions and such matters as changes in ward organisation and treatment must be ratified at separate staff meetings. (Separate staff meetings to support the staff are essential, especially at the development stage, but they can present problems. Before the introduction of successful integrated community meetings, staff meetings and case notes were regarded with hostility and suspicion by the children. The level of tension and disturbed behaviour was noticeably raised during staff meetings and children would hang round peeping in or attention-seeking. Now, at a community meeting children will suggest that a problem should be discussed at a staff meeting.)

We conclude that group meetings are essential to the successful running of a residential unit for children and adolescents. Once a week is probably not frequent enough and we have found daily meetings plus extras were needed for really adequate communication and treatment. To be effective, attendance at community meetings has to be compulsory for every member regardless of status (in the case of staff) or mental state (in the case of patients).

The main functions of the group are:

(a) Avoidance of build-up in interpersonal conflict and group tensions
(b) The exposure and avoidance of 'them' versus 'us' situations
(c) The exposure and avoidance of bullying and secretive, undesirable or exclusive clique-formation and of scapegoating
(d) The fostering of social learning and adaptation
(e) Leading each individual to face reality
(f) Keeping everyone informed
(g) Carrying out effective multidisciplinary planning which involves all members of the community

The Work of the Nurse

Since the role of the other professional staff is well defined, we will concentrate on the work of the junior nurses. These are the staff who are in closest and most continuous contact with the children and therefore can have the greatest influence on the therapeutic endeavour.

The nurse has, first, the task of relationship-building and then, in the setting of this relationship, that of helping the child to increase profitable and adaptive behaviour and to decrease maladaptive behaviour which harms him and those around him. Both tasks require more skill than would be likely to be available to any one individual nurse, so she will require the full support of the therapeutic team throughout each stage. The following basic rules about relating to children are offered to all nurses during their introductory training and reinforced at subsequent discussions on practical issues. Failure to follow one or other has proved to be the most frequent cause of crises:

(a) Your aim should be the creation of a happy, warm atmosphere and good relationships together with the establishment and maintenance of reasonable standards of behaviour. Your natural kindness and commonsense are the basis for success, but there are pitfalls anyone can fall into who is not in the know. Many of your patients would not be in your care if they responded to everyday handling, sanctions and punishments.
(b) Good relationships are based on understanding and sympathy for the other person's point of view even if you don't agree with it.
(c) The way you speak and the words you use matter. Think before you speak, try to make your expression and tone of voice convey friendliness and understanding. Try to work out the most positive and friendly way of saying things and avoid cutting, unkind or critical remarks.
(d) What the child is saying, whether statement or question, may not mean what it seems at first hearing. Try to understand what underlies it by keeping the question open, seeking amplification.
(e) When a child seems to be behaving badly or being rude to you, do not react at once by overt criticism and anger; there is always a reason which you need to find out. Stop the undesirable behaviour, but then find out what caused it – not, 'What do you think you are doing, you naughty boy?' but, 'Goodness, this is my nice Lenny isn't it? What has gone wrong to make a good boy like you do this?'
(f) When you check someone, remember never to let him lose face

in front of his peers. If you do he will have to regain it either by continuing or by doing something worse to show he doesn't care and you can't control him. He may get no gratification from you, but he will from his peers.

(g) Never subject a child to face-to-face confrontation, particularly in front of other children. Where there has to be a clash allow the child an escape, a little time or a face-saver of some kind, and if possible remove him quietly and have the clash in private. You cannot win in public.

(h) Name-calling and derogatory remarks are obviously taboo, but be careful that what you are saying isn't one in disguise.

(i) Try to remember that ordering children about separates you from them and may create a situation where you move further and further apart, you becoming increasingly punitive, and the children increasingly rebellious. Your authority depends on your good relationships and a background of goodwill on both sides. In the absence of the goodwill of the inmates, even prisons cannot contain the prisoners without extreme cruelty. Getting angry or increasing the loudness of what you are saying only serves to create an unpleasant atmosphere and is likely to arouse the unfavourable responses which it did at home. Try whispering.

(j) Be aware of the effect the child is having on you. Young people tend to bring out fear and resentment in adults when they do not obey and respect us at once. It hits our self-esteem so we react badly. We may get irritated, shout, start throwing our weight about, and stop people from doing things for no reason.

(k) Be aware that fear and feelings of inferiority are often hidden behind surliness, aggressiveness and bravado, and do not be tempted to 'take him down a peg'.

(l) Be aware that older children resent being treated like children yet they also need to regress; they hate being talked down to, yet often misunderstand if you use too difficult words or phrases.

(m) The following almost always upset children and make matters worse: threats, shouting, taking offence, showing anger or distress, protests about ingratitude, selfishness or inconsiderateness and other negative criticisms.

(n) The following almost always help children and improve matters even in the worst situation: a warm, friendly, encouraging manner; quiet speech, genuine reasonableness and understanding; being positive, emphasising the child's good points.

Sustained enthusiasm for this difficult, often apparently unrewarding task can only be maintained by very strong support from the multidisciplinary team. Frequent staff meetings are vital, not only for planning and communication, but to foster and sustain group morale and sense of purpose. Nurses' notes are valuable beyond their value in communicating information about the patient's progress. They also focus the nurse's attention on what she is doing and form a basis for subsequent discussion in a multidisciplinary setting, so preventing isolation and a feeling that all that the nurses are doing is babyminding for the other professional staff.

The nurse's responses to the child's behaviour require frequent review and discussion, particularly when a specific type of undesirable behaviour is spreading, or when it occurs more frequently with specific nurses, as this indicates that something about the staff response or way of handling it may be contributing. It must be borne in mind that the response which reduces the behaviour in child A may be a factor in triggering off the same behaviour in children B and C.

Lyn, having been let down by her mother, came back in acute distress, smashed a window and cut her hand. Kindly, sympathetic attention was given and it did not seem inappropriate to mention Lyn's misfortune to the rest of the group, until we observed the spate of window-smashing and arm-cutting which followed among other deprived girls.

As well as a caring attitude about people, it is essential that the nurses show very positively a caring attitude about standards of behaviour and care of the environment. A relationship built on a laissez-faire attitude will show its weakness when improvements in behaviour control are expected. The nurse may be tolerant of disturbed behaviour and continue to accept the wrongdoer, but will always demonstrate in some way that there is a better way. The toys are always put away when the game is finished, at first by the nurse but gradually with more and more help from the child. On the same lines, messes are always cleared up and broken things mended. The caring attitude of the nurse about the physical environment is gradually taken in by the child in the same way as the caring attitude for people. The amount of work involved in this caring for the physical environment should be reduced to the minimum by efficient, easy-to-manage equipment and arrangements, so that caring for people can always come first.

Acting-out presents particular difficulty to nursing staff, and if it worries the staff it can become contagious. The following acting-out behaviours occasionally swell into epidemics; the solution to all of them lies in calm discussion, emphasis on seeking the cause, continuing to apply the positive treatment principles and avoidance of panic reactions and special measures. A big increase in any of them always indicates that someone is being dictatorial and unreasonable, or that the children have a guilty secret of some kind (sex or smoking or stealing) and are seeking to place the staff in an authoritarian position so that they can justify themselves as hard-done-by and repressed.

Attention-seeking	– climbing on roof, locking self in
Depredations	– window-smashing, plaster-picking, furniture cutting, curtain-pulling
Self-mutilation	– scratching, tattooing
Suicide gestures	– pin-swallowing, drug-taking
Running off	
Aggressiveness, swearing	
Stealing from staff or other patients	

The nurse must be trained to recognise the underlying implications of behaviour, asking herself what is the child trying to communicate and why ordinary channels of communication have broken down. Good observation and communication, anticipation and understanding will reduce acting-out to a minimum. Clashes are then most likely when expectations are being raised and support being reduced. Some clashes are inevitable and should not be avoided if the child is to learn to accept frustration. Where the clash is inevitable the group has to be prepared or protected and the strategy discussed with the whole team beforehand.

Planning and discussion should not be confined to crises: regular attention should be given to the ward routines and arrangements. The nurses should be encouraged to advance new ideas and experiments and to re-examine the present way of doing things with a critical eye. Staff conferences enable the nurse to reappraise her work through other eyes. The detached observer can often see significance and meaning in behaviour and incidents not immediately apparent to those personally involved. Similarly, listening to other people's experiences may have significance for one's own work. The conference considers the dynamics of behaviour and interpersonal interactions, but it is also a useful forum for planning active intervention to modify behaviour either of the group or of a single individual.

Much of the success of the nurse in modifying antisocial behaviour can be attributed to caring relationships she builds up: the child feels cared for and begins to learn to care for other people, he feels respected and so learns to respect first the nurse, and then others. But without expectations of desirable behaviour this would probably be insufficient. The nurse provides models and standards of behaviour and through her relationships begins to reward approved, and not to reward disapproved, behaviour. The child likes her and therefore wishes to imitate her (Stayton *et al.*, 1971). Sometimes it is necessary to make this process explicit, to define goals and, equally important, to define rewards, because these are not always as clear as seems at first sight. This definition of goals and rewards and discussion of techniques is a frequent function of nursing conferences. In other contexts (ordinary schools and schools for the autistic) it has been noted that the details of how rewards like praise and punishment are distributed affect which behaviours are encouraged and discouraged (Bartak *et al.*, 1971). It is with these details that we have been concerned in our case conferences. We wished to bring some order into what tends to be a haphazard hit-or-miss procedure. If not planned, staff responses in institutions have tended to be indiscriminate (Beuhler *et al.*, 1966).

From the child's point of view, the ideal would be for the same nursing staff who got them up to be there still at bedtime. This is quite impossible unless the conditions of employment are to be altered radically. We have been unable to envisage a system which would meet the needs of the children and allow acceptable time off for the nursing staff. Meal-times, evening recreation and bedtimes have proved the most difficult to cater for, while during school hours the nursing staff are under-employed. When the staff are able to eat *en famille* with the children, they have all observed a great improvement in behaviour and group cohesion. The staff have to sacrifice a break in privacy and comfort in doing this and should be compensated by being allowed the meal free and given time off at some other time. An immense gulf between 'them' and 'us' is created by having staff standing round watching the patients feeding, even if they are administering needs. In these circumstances, unpleasant remarks about the food and unpleasant behaviour like food-throwing, knife-twanging, fork-bending and wandering about become common, as if to emphasise the gulf.

Bedtime has long been recognised as a difficult time (Bettelheim, 1950). We have observed the very high proportion of incidents of destructive and antisocial behaviour between 8 and 10 p.m. (Wardle, 1969). It is therefore unfortunate that the hospital nursing hours should traditionally be arranged so that the nursing staff is decimated at 7 p.m. We have tried to overcome this to some degree by employing evening staff from 6 until 10 p.m. This works well if some of the regular staff are willing to work a late shift periodically, so that there is some continuity of care.

Once again, we find a conflict between the needs of the child and effective treatment and the undeniable needs of staff for reasonable working hours and personal privacy. We must accept that, because of this, child care in a hospital or any other residential setting staffed by paid staff must lack the essential ingredient of good family care, namely whole-time commitment to the child's needs. These inadequacies and others have been discussed very fully elsewhere (King *et al.*, 1971).

School

Even if not actually excluded, these children have usually had unhappy experiences of school and education by the time they are admitted. Some will be entrenched in an attitude of hostility to teachers and all their works, others will have learned to avoid education as a situation where they meet failure and criticism. Most will have some degree of retardation in verbal and academic skills. The task of overcoming educational handicaps in the face of active resistance or passive avoidance is formidable. Clearly it is useless to repeat the orthodox approach to teaching which has not only palpably failed, but in some cases actively contributed to the problem.

Clearly the first task must be to get rid of the resistance and build up positive motivation. The child comes with the expectation that he is going to have unpleasant experiences and, in particular, that he is going to experience failure. It is essential, therefore, that his experiences of this new school are pleasant and that he experiences success and no failure.

Elsewhere it has been suggested that the method of teaching is not as significant as the motivation. If a child wants to learn something he will do so no matter how it is taught (Neill, 1962). Our experience seems to confirm that helping the child to want to learn is the primary task. The warm and enthusiastic relationship of the teacher with the child and an atmosphere of well-being and co-operation in the school are the tools.

The school aims to be a happy, informal place in which opportunities for learning are offered but not forced on the child. The teacher's skill is directed first at getting to know the child, his assets and debits, his areas of success as well as his areas of difficulty. The child must see him as someone who genuinely wants to help and accept him, and who will not jolt him with unkind criticism and reminders of his inadequacy. False praise has no place, but genuine pleasure in the modest achievements of someone who has achieved nothing before certainly has. The teacher must know how the child can succeed and help him to do this, being most careful to avoid failure. Failure in front of other children is particularly galling, so that initial assessment and remedial measures should be in private. In the group the teacher must help the child avoid exposing his inadequacy to other children, for the inevitable consequence will be the adoption of a bravado, 'couldn't care less' attitude which will block any further progress. Rewards and public praise for specific achievements are to be avoided as they are nearly as bad as criticism for those who do not get the reward. Praise and reward, if used, must be for progress relative to previous personal achievement, not relative to other people's achievement.

Subjects are not taught unless a child specifically asks for this, for instance to take an examination. Interests are aroused through a diversity of books, pictures, displays and activities scattered apparently haphazard about the rooms; topics arise through discussion of the child's interests. The teacher seizes opportunities as they arise in discussion of the child's interests. The teacher seizes opportunities as they arise in discussion through his knowledge of the child's needs.

As the child progresses some pressure can be exerted towards remedying basic deficiencies; for example, 'Yes, I would be glad to help you with your model, but first I think we ought to try a few of the sums which were holding you up in your measuring'. Pressure is needed to overcome the inertia which besets most people when faced with a task requiring some pain or effort, even when they want to achieve, but it must be at the right time: if too early, it entrenches resistance; if too late, the habit of avoidance is established. Pressure will only succeed if the child really wants to try despite apparent resistance. Recognition of this covert wish to try is an important skill. When it is too late, adolescents often complain, 'If only they had made me do it'.

To summarise, the basic skills of a teacher in this setting are:

(a) Accurate assessment of assets and debits
(b) Creating positive motivation
(c) Creating an environment which stimulates appropriate interest
(d) Recognising and seizing opportunities
(e) Knowing when to apply pressure

Outcome and Discharge

The severity and type of disturbance of conduct before admission does not always predict the behaviour manifest after admission. In part this may be because the child is removed from the stresses which evoked the behaviour and from opportunities to indulge certain types of behaviour. In addition it seems likely that opportunities for alternative expression of difficulty, through verbalisation and through group and individual interaction in a sympathetic and protective environment, remove the need for more serious acting-out. Certain characteristics have been identified in those children who tend to act-out after admission and are slower to respond (Wardle, 1969).

Ten nurses were asked to rate on a four-point scale what 50 children cared for in 1968 were like to look after. 'Very difficult' scored 4, 'difficult' 3, 'so-so' scored 2 and 'easy' scored 1. The ratings were combined and an average score calculated for each child.

In this analysis a child was defined as having a broken home if his natural parents were not living together before admission. EEGs are done routinely on admission; the EEG was defined as abnormal if it was reported as showing excess of slow waves for age or focal or epileptic features. The consultant reporting has no clinical contact with the children, and ward behaviour is not mentioned on the request card.

In making comparison we have given the average score for the group and also the number of children in each group scoring 2 and over. This latter is perhaps the most meaningful figure as the scores were strikingly bimodal, with only six scores between 1·7 and 2·3 inclusive.

Younger children tended to be regarded as easier to manage (Table 3.2), those aged 13–14 presenting the greatest difficulty. Girls tended more often to be regarded as difficult (Table 3.3).

Table 3.2 Age on admission related to difficulty

	Age on admission			
	14	*13*	*12*	*11 and less*
Average difficulty score	2·1	2·0	1·9	1·5
No. of patients	17	10	12	11
Difficulty score > 2	9	6	5	3
Difficulty score < 2	8	4	7	8

Table 3.3 Sex of patient related to difficulty

	Male	*Female*
Average difficulty score	1·8	2·0
No. of patients	31	19
No. with difficulty score > 2	12	11
No. with difficulty score < 2	19	8

Patients admitted from other residential establishments were usually admitted because they could not be managed, so it is not surprising that they were all regarded as very difficult by our own staff (Table 3.4). Those from approved schools proved particularly difficult because they introduced an alien 'them' versus 'us' attitude. In 1968 only three children were from approved schools – the only three to have average scores of 3 and above.

An investigation of children and their management in approved schools might throw some light on why children admitted from them are so particularly difficult.

Of the 104 serious ward incidents in 1968, 56 took place between 3 September and 25 November. These are the dates of admission of Amanda from an approved school and her transfer to an adult ward. Amanda was

Table 3.4 Source of admission related to difficulty experienced by staff during stay

	Whence admitted		
	Residential school or institution	*Own home but excluded from school*	*Own home*
Average difficulty score	2·7	2·3	1·5
No. of patients	10	10	30
Difficulty score > 2	10	7	6
Difficulty score < 2	0	3	24

not responsible for all the incidents, they just seemed to happen when she was awake. She seldom broke glass, but more panes of glass were broken during this period than the whole of the rest of the unit's history. Her speciality was in finding the weak spots of staff and children and exploiting them. Breakers became smashers, petty pilferers became active, weak nurses collapsed, strong nurses became authoritarian. When she was involved personally in an incident it was a really serious one: for example, she succeeded in getting a senior male nurse to imply she was a prostitute, fought him violently and when apparently calmed in her room set fire to it. It was her combination with two other girls from severely broken homes which made it quite impossible to keep her or them, although she seemed to be improving. One very disturbed patient against the group can be managed by the group, but if she succeeds in forming an anti-group clique or manipulates the group, it ceases to be effective. An audible sigh of relief went up in the group when it was learned she had been transferred. With trepidation all asked, 'Will she be coming back?' Incidents continued for a week, then petered out. In December there were 14, compared with 73 in November.

The main problem leading to admission is clearly related to behaviour after admission. A very high proportion of children were regarded as difficult who had exhibited antisocial conduct before admission. In contrast, almost all children admitted with predominantly neurotic symptoms, school phobia and behaviour or habit disorders confined to home, were regarded as easy and were very rarely involved in incidents, even when the ward was very disturbed (Table 3.5).

Table 3.5 Main problem before admission related to difficulty experienced by staff during stay

	Main problem			
	Neurosis, school phobia	*Antisocial conduct*	*Psychosis*	*Other*
Average difficulty score	1·3	2·5	2·3	1·5
No. of patients	17	16	8	9
Difficulty score > 2	1	14	6	2

The difficulty of managing children from broken homes fits our observation that the children who find most difficulty in accepting the therapeutic environment, and the possibility for relationships offered there, are those whose past experience of relationships has been most adverse, and particularly those who have learned faulty patterns of adaptation in other institutions.

Table 3.6 Relationship of home background and EEG to behaviour while in hospital

	Intact home		*Broken home*	
	Normal EEG	*Abnormal EEG*	*Normal EEG*	*Abnormal EEG*
Average difficulty score	1·3	2·1	2·2	2·4
No. of patients	18	14	7	8
Scores above 2	0	9	5	7

The other group of children who find adaptation difficult are those who are prevented from adapting by cerebral dysfunction. Children from intact homes, who had shown severe tantrums and conduct disorder in their homes, usually settled well. The exceptions were a few with abnormal EEGs who were aggressive, impulsive and unpredictable or psychotic. With the exception of these patients who respond to anticonvulsants or tranquillisers, drugs are of little value except as a temporary expedient. Amanda was no problem while she was asleep, but large doses of phenothiazines did not stop her machinations if she was ambulant.

Difficulty in the ward does not necessarily predict outcome. Stormy initial relationships may develop therapeutically more rapidly than initial passive acceptance. Two types of patient seem to progress more slowly and to be more difficult to discharge to the community area:

(a) those children with the combination of cerebral dysrhythmia plus an incomplete family to return to;
(b) children with no roots in the community and no family to return to. These children tend to develop a discontented dependency on the hospital and retrospectively admission can be seen as mistaken, since it has substituted a pattern of invalid dependency for conduct disorder.

A date for discharge should be set when planning admission. Community social agencies must appreciate that admission is not a 'placement' and that roots must be maintained in the community. There must be a bed in the community to which the child can go for weekends and holidays and the child's guardians must accept that they must take the child if he is discharged. Some reluctance to do this may be encountered if the child has been very difficult, but we have found it is unwise to admit children unless this is agreed. Schools seem particularly loth to believe that a child they have excluded is fit to return after treatment; in conferences the teachers will reiterate the behaviour of months or even years before as evidence for their refusal to give the child a trial. In such circumstances persuasion is not in the child's interest as the reluctance and expectations of trouble are likely to be justified.

Close early supervision of the child is essential, even when discharged to favourable situations. Too often a honeymoon period, in which the child is described as no trouble or perfect, is followed by breakdown. Then it is revealed that there has been trouble from the start. People in the community, whether foster parents, schoolteachers or employers, tend to fall into several stereotyped traps in accepting children from hospital. Perhaps, expecting difficulty, they are pleasantly surprised by the apparent ease of the first days and make the mistake of ignoring or overlooking misdemeanors until they get out of hand; they then make the second mistake of clamping down, with disastrous results; and finally, and only when it is too late, they seek advice from the psychiatric team. But by this time, they have made up their mind to reject the child anyway and relationships on both sides are irreparably damaged. As we have emphasised earlier, contact must be insisted on against all resistance. The children most likely to break down are those where the community agent sees himself as 'saving the child from that terrible psychiatric hospital' and believes that the hospital is responsible for the child's problem.

Once the duration of a patient's stay in the unit exceeds the average length of stay for all patients it may have passed the therapeutic optimum. The child begins to lose optimism about leaving and to become over-dependent, his motivation may become increasingly directed at remaining in hospital and avoiding the stress of new uncertain experiences outside. With the longer-stay patient, active steps must be directed to maintaining enthusiasm for return to the community.

From protective, specialised care and schooling in hospital to an unspecialised care in the community can be too large a change to make in one move. Several strategies are possible to avoid breakdown because of this. If the main breakdown is likely to be at home, attendance as a daypatient can continue for a while after discharge home or into a children's home or hostel near by. If, on the other hand, school is the main difficulty, the first step may be to establish successful attendance at a local school before discharge home.

For older patients who are ready to start work we have felt the particular need for a half-way house or hostel where group support can continue in the evenings and at weekends. Working adolescents find it very difficult to take time off for outpatient appointments, and one hour a week is inadequate to support them through inevitable crises, even if appointments are kept. We have found that the final step of leaving hospital is particularly difficult for adolescents who have got jobs, and fear of leaving often leads them to give up a job in which they were succeeding.

The return to the community of children admitted from approved schools presents some problems. The approved school is seen as a punishment, so to return there when improved is seen as a grave injustice. The approved schools are reluctant to have the children back, partly because of their previous difficult behaviour and partly because they feel the child will have difficulty in accepting their methods, having experienced the therapeutic community method. Reclassification was a successful solution in one case, return home in all the others. Only two girls have actually returned to their original approved school and both did very badly thereafter.

Duller, antisocial children, particularly those of subnormal intelligence (intelligent quotient below 70) find it difficult to adapt to group discussions and the therapeutic community and transfer to special schools or inpatient services for the subnormal should be arranged as soon as the nature of the problem is discovered; they will meet increasing frustration and experience of failure if they remain, and are likely to try to solve this by disruption of the therapeutic activity of the group. This is a disruption which we have found cannot be resolved by the techniques we have described. Intelligence may be an important predictor of outcome since, in contrast, children of higher intelligence have seemed more able to make use of the group discussion method and derived satisfaction and encouragement from relations with staff.

The criteria for an unfavourable outcome in delinquents (Gibbens, 1961; West, 1967) seem to be the criteria for admission to our inpatient units, notably truancy, wandering, poor school, educational and behavioural record, absence of stable and affectionate family background. Children referred to child-guidance (outpatient) clinics for antisocial behaviour have been found to be more deviant in their adult adjustment than other referrals and control subjects not referred to child-guidance clinics (Robins, 1966). Progress and outcome in conduct disorder are difficult to evaluate; as behaviour like arson, assault, stealing or housebreaking may only occur rarely there is no indication of the continuing presence in an individual of the potential for them unless he is placed in a situation where they are likely to occur. The consequences of a positive response to such a test are serious for the community and the patient. To some extent this problem can be overcome in microcosm in the therapeutic community with less dire consequences, followed by cautious progressive trials in the community with acceptance of reversals.

Our present clinical follow-up indicates that a relapse is particularly likely in those patients whose antisocial conduct was to be expected because of very adverse family experience (Wardle, 1961). Patients who have made least progress and are in most danger of becoming chronically in need of continuing residential care are those with evidence of persisting cerebral dysfunction in the absence of any satisfactory roots or attachments in the community. If we accept the ethological concept of limited critical periods for establishing attachment behaviour (Russell-Davis, 1972), then even intensive attempts to establish it may fail if too late. Good prognostic signs are the ability of the child to form relationships with the staff of the unit, to demonstrate his difficulties and above all to talk about them in a group setting.

Follow-up studies are lacking and needed. They should attempt to relate definite behavioural phenomena to specific social factors and child-rearing experiences. Pseudo-disease concepts cloud the central issue, which we consider to be the identification of the determining and modifying influences on specific patterns of behaviour.

Summary and Conclusions

Conduct disorder is not a disease or even a group of diseases, but defines a cluster of repetitive behaviour patterns which are antisocial and disapproved. The causes are multiple, though a factor which seems common to all is impairment of the ability of the sufferer to care enough about other people because he himself has not been cared about enough in childhood. Our description of an inpatient regime for children with conduct disorders indicates that no single approach is applicable, and treatment must be based on a complete appraisal of the social, biological and psychodynamic contributions to the child's development, and his presenting assets and deficits. Deficiency of stable, secure, affectionate care is a common factor, but some children are rendered more vulnerable by cerebral dysfunction or by a coincidence of multiple, adverse factors. Treatment is based on a therapeutic environment in which the child can experiment behaviourally in an accepting environment where relationship formation and discussion of social interactions are encouraged.

Setting up a genuinely therapeutic unit in which this can occur is not a simple matter of costing, providing a suitable physical environment, adequate equipment and staff establishment; these take very much second place to overcoming the many interpersonal difficulties raised by setting up such a unit, not only within the unit, but in the hospital itself. Such a unit is a challenge to the personal resources of all those involved. Within the unit much can be done by selection and training of staff and by the use of group techniques. We must seek solutions to the problems raised by the therapeutic community in the larger community around. Perhaps this too is a matter of maximising accurate communication and informed discussion. The alternative is isolation or very drastic alteration in the selection of patients. It is suggested that we could predict those patients who are likely to cause disturbance and destruction, but we have also shown that they can be improved in this mixed setting. If we exclude them we have an easier, perhaps cheaper time, but at whose expense? The cost of damage to the hospital structure and equanimity by such patients must be balanced against the long-term cost to the community of avoiding it. Nevertheless, we must balance the cost to other patients of admitting the most extreme cases, and special facilities are needed in a unit taking such cases so that temporary isolation from other patients is possible if such children are interfering with the treatment of the other patients. The more deficient or discontinuous the child's experience of stable, secure care, the poorer is the prognosis. Cerebral dysfunction and poor intellectual function also worsen the prognosis.

CHAPTER FOUR

Neurotic Disorders with Special Reference to School Refusal

L. A. Hersov

The diagnostic category of neurosis or neurotic disorder appears in most classifications of childhood psychiatric disorders. Classification of deviant behaviour and emotions facilitates communication between professional workers and allows comparison between observations made in different clinical settings, nationally and internationally. Diagnosis should be based on careful enquiry, observation and assessment, which should lead to a thorough understanding of the individual patient. With this information a diagnostic formulation can include the biological, psychological, social and cultural antecedents and determinants of the particular psychiatric disorder and its relationship to the processes of normal development. While most child psychiatrists would agree about the usefulness of the diagnostic category of neurotic disorder, and its main characteristics, there would be less agreement about origins and aetiology and least agreement, perhaps, about the most appropriate treatments.

Neurotic Disorder in Childhood

The distinction between those disorders which result mainly in suffering for the child, the so-called 'personality problems', and those which create disturbance for other people, the so-called 'conduct problems', was made many years ago (Ackerson, 1931; Hewitt and

Jenkins, 1946) and supported by later studies using more sophisticated means of data collection and statistical methods (Achenbach, 1966; Patterson, 1964; Quay, 1964). Peterson (1961) identified two types of disorder: in the first there was a tendency to express impulses against society which he called *conduct problems*. The second included a variety of elements suggesting low self-esteem, social withdrawal and dysphoric mood, which he called *personality problems*; these elements were in marked contrast to those found in conduct problems. All these studies were operational and empirical without commitment to any theory of origin of the behaviour, but psychoanalysts with a very definite but different theoretical viewpoint have also made a similar distinction (Freud, 1966).

In the triaxial classification of mental disorders in childhood (Rutter *et al.*, 1969) the category of neurotic disorder is used for conditions in which there is an abnormality of the emotions not accompanied by marked personality disorder or loss of reality sense (as in psychosis). Disorders in this category include states of disproportionate anxiety and depression, obsessions, compulsions and phobias (which are abnormal in their developmental context). 'Hypochondriasis' and 'conversion hysteria' are also included. In the framework of this classification the diagnosis is made on the overt condition of the child and has no implications as to aetiology, or mechanisms of production of symptoms, but merely describes the form of symptoms. Epidemiological studies in the Isle of Wight using this method of classification have shown the prevalence of neurotic disorder to be 2·5 per cent; girls were more often affected than boys (Rutter *et al.*, 1970). The reverse applies in conduct disorders, that is, abnormal behaviour giving rise to social disapproval (Rutter *et al.*, 1970), which are more frequent generally and occur more often in boys. At the descriptive level there are also instances of 'mixed' neurotic and conduct disorders, but this group as classified has much in common with the 'pure' antisocial (conduct) disorders and very little in common with 'pure' neurotic disorders (Rutter *et al.*, 1970).

Clinical Diagnosis of Neurotic Disorder

Among the common features of neurotic disorder are complaints of feeling generally distressed, specific and general fears, overt anxiety, variable moods of sadness and unhappiness, physical complaints, lack of self-esteem, poor social relationships, difficulties with schoolwork, and those more clear-cut manifestations such as phobias, obsessions and compulsions. In arriving at a judgement of the significance of these complaints the clinical-diagnostic approach (Rutter *et al.*, 1970) emphasises persistence, duration and severity of abnormality in behaviour, emotion and relationships and their effect on the patient, his or her family and the community. The child's behavioural and emotional response is evaluated in relation to what would be expected in a child of this age and stage of psychological development, as well as its appropriateness to the time and place of occurrence and life-setting. There is no attempt to determine the extent of internal conflict.

Anna Freud (1970) has commented on the misleading and deceiving nature of manifest symptomatology from the psychoanalyst's viewpoint. Symptoms are very significant for diagnostic classification – indeed the diagnosis is wholly decided on manifest symptomatology – but they are relatively unimportant for the purposes of the technique of therapy. Symptoms are mere symbols of inner mental turmoil, responding fairly easily to many types of therapy but equally easily replaced by other abnormalities, apparently different, but expressing the same latent content and just as disabling for the patient. The question of the validity of this theory that removing or suppressing symptoms without modifying underlying causes or internal conflicts results in 'symptom substitution' has been much discussed (Yates, 1958, 1962; Bookbinder, 1962; Speigel, 1967). In childhood the issue is further complicated by the fact that some developmental disorders, such as nocturnal enuresis, respond to symptomatic treatment at that point in their natural history when remission can be expected, without any apparent appearance of other symptoms. Indeed, the evidence to date for symptom substitution is very slight.

In phenomenological terms, widely different symptoms and behaviour may be given the same weighting but this is not the case in psychoanalytic psychopathology. Symptoms may be a transitory response to some developmental stress, or a fixed defensive pattern hindering further development of stable features of personality structure (Freud, 1970). The following is a definition of psychoneurotic reactions in terms acceptable to those working within the psychoanalytic frame of reference: 'This category is reserved for those disorders based on unconscious conflicts over the handling of sexual and aggressive impulses which, though removed from awareness by the mechanisms of repression, remain active and unresolved. Such neurotic conflicts are ordinarily derived from earlier conscious conflicts between the child and significant persons in his environment such as parents and siblings.' (Group for the Advancement of Psychiatry, 1966, p. 229).

Anthony (1967) has commented that such conflicts belong almost exclusively to the pre-school years of childhood; in later childhood they become internalised, encapsulated and relatively chronic, although many of the milder reactions resolve spontaneously. Kessler (1972) observes that when psychoneurosis is categorised in these terms it implies a level of social and intellectual maturity rarely reached before the age of six or seven years. When the conscience becomes an internalised part of the personality, so that the child suffers guilt and anxiety which are no longer based on fear of external detection or punishment, the child is rendered vulnerable to internalised conflicts from which escape is not easy.

Chess (1969) views psychiatric disorders in children on a continuum from normality to sociopathic character disorder. The interaction between the child's personality attributes and important aspects of family and community environment gives rise to stresses and strains which are dealt with by the child in different ways. The concepts of reversibility and fixity of behaviour and symptoms are crucial to this scheme of classification. A reactive behaviour disorder is readily reversible under environmental manipulation or very brief direct treatment. When the difficulties have become fixed patterns which the child brings even to favourable circumstances, the term 'neurotic' is appropriate. Rigidity of pattern is the distinctive feature, and the beginnings of adult neurosis lie here in early compulsions, phobias or hysterical reactions. The patterns cannot be altered by modifying the environment alone. Notions of repeated traumatic exposure leading to distorted perceptions of people with reinforcement of these perceptions by the reactions of significant persons are used to explain the progression towards fixity and rigidity.

Chess also questions both the view which regards neurotic symptoms as a technique for reducing anxiety and the elaborate schemata of motivation in neurotic disorders derived from psychoanalytic studies of adults. She believes that in young children a simpler explanation in terms of child–environment interaction can account for all the facts, though motivational factors may have to be invoked in older children. In her longitudinal studies (Thomas *et al.*, 1968) she and her co-workers did not find overt anxiety prior to symptom formation; instead it developed as a secondary phenomenon, as a consequence rather than a cause. She regards some of the neurotic reactions of childhood as representing immature versions of adult neuroses. This is in keeping with general clinical experience that the older the child the more the pattern of disorder approximates to the adult pattern. Age is an extremely important variable, for symptoms should only be called neurotic if they are inappropriate in terms of developmental stage and if they interfere with the child's happiness, overall functioning and relationships in everyday life.

Behaviour therapy (Eysenck, 1959) is defined as the correction of psychological disorders through the systematic and explicit application of the principles of learning (Ross, 1972). Problems of classification and diagnosis have not worried the exponents of this method, for most agree with Eysenck (1959) that the presenting symptom is itself 'the neurosis' so there is no point in searching for causes. Similarly, a detailed knowledge of the child's history is unnecessary in planning treatment. Skinner (1953) also considers the disagnosis or label of 'neurosis' as an explanatory fiction and rejects the notion of a neurotic state within the individual. In his view, people behave as they do because of environmental contingencies which can be observed, controlled and manipulated so that the behaviour can be significantly and permanently modified. For the purposes of behaviour therapy the symptom is regarded as a form of maladaptive behaviour in which the behavioural responses in the individual's repertoire are emitted under inappropriate circumstances. Responses which are developmentally adaptive at one stage may not be so at another, or they may be adaptive in one setting and not another (Ross, 1972). The environment determines what is adaptive in almost all circumstances and the *current* conditions under which behaviour occurs are important. Corrective action, i.e. 'treatment', involves learning, unlearning and relearning so that responses will come to be emitted only in appropriate circumstances. Behaviour is the focus of therapy and, according to the theory, learning of behaviour takes place either through respondent or operant conditioning and sometimes in complex interaction between the two (Lazarus *et al.*, 1965). Avoidance behaviour maintained by fear reductions may lead to what is labelled 'school phobia', a refusal to attend school that may entail either fear of school (true school phobia) or fear of leaving home. These maladaptive responses have been modified or eliminated by behaviour therapy (Lazarus and Abramowitz, 1965; Garvey and Hegrenes, 1966; Chapel 1967).

The contrast between the latter approach and that of psychoanalysis has been the source of comment, for 'analysts have always been proud of the distinction that theirs is a causal therapy aimed directly at the conflicts and stresses which are hidden in their patients' personalities and underlie their symptomatology' (Freud, 1970). The same authority makes mention of parents who are only concerned with removing the disturbing manifestations in the child, and so are at cross-purposes with the psychoanalyst who would like time to reach deeper conflicts. This is a general and not uncommon experience in clinical work with the parents of children with neurotic disorders such as school refusal. Suggestions that the origin of some of the child's difficulties may lie, not in school, but in the child and at home are seldom kindly received and attempts to work along these lines may be resisted. Taking the child into hospital often strengthens the parents' wish or need to believe that the problem is entirely of the child's making and that they are exonerated. The parents' behaviour often shows that they do have mixed feelings of hostility and guilt about their own part in their child's disorder but these are often so distorted that they may prove very difficult to understand and clarify. It is not surprising that for some parents the limited aim of behaviour therapy may be much preferable to the uncovering and probing methods of psychodynamic therapy.

In a discussion of symptom classification according to psychoanalytic psychology, Anna Freud (1970) emphasises how accurate diagnostic assessment should lead to a choice of treatment method. She remarks that the specific type of disorder is too often inadequately matched with a specific type of treatment and that it is futile to expect any single therapeutic method, deep or superficial, to prove effective for a range of different disorders. This plea for more precision in diagnosis, leading to better matching of treatment and disorder, may be applied to clinical practice generally.

Over the years the traditional methods of individual psychotherapy and casework, which were strongly influenced by psychoanalytic principles, have been extended by the addition of group therapy and family therapy, group and conjoint (Skynner, 1969; Brown, 1972). Various psychotropic drugs are now used either alone or in combination with psychotherapy and casework. Behaviour modification techniques can also be used in treating individual children, and the same principles applied to helping their parents manage disturbed behaviour.

Residential treatment of children with neurotic disorders in a hospital setting should include all these methods, sometimes singly, more often in combination, as appropriate. In theory it should also be possible to incorporate them into a living setting for treatment in which various professional disciplines play their part in providing an individual programme for each child and his or her family. In practice, problems do arise in providing a therapeutic environment for a varied group of children of different sex, chronological age, and stage of biological and emotional development. Psychiatric inpatient units usually contain a mixed collection of patients with conduct, developmental, psychotic and neurotic disorders. Units which specialise in the treatment of single conditions, e.g. neurotic disorder, are few and far between. The treatment needs vary greatly, and maintaining an individual programme for each child, while adhering to a general routine plan for a whole ward, puts great strains upon the professional staff.

Structure and Setting of Inpatient Units

What are the characteristics of hospital inpatient units and how do they differ from other residential treatment units? Robinson (1957) has defined the inpatient unit as a psychiatric treatment service in a medical institution, or unit of a medical institution. Its function is the diagnosis and treatment *in residence* of children with psychiatric disorders. It provies a twenty-four-hour, and most often a seven-day-week, service for children whose family situation, severity of emotional disturbance and behaviour make such a service the *treatment of choice* in contrast to outpatient or other treatment.

A brief description of the children's inpatient unit at the Maudsley Hospital will give a picture of one unit, established in 1947 and the first in Great Britain. The unit admits a maximum of twenty-five children of both sexes with an upper age limit of around twelve to thirteen years. This limit is not fixed by chronological age, for degree and extent of social, emotional and biological maturity will influence the decision whether a child is young enough to be suitably placed with other younger children or would be better in an adolescent unit. Children are admitted with conditions ranging from developmental disorders through neurotic and conduct disorders to psychoses. Children with idiopathic epilepsy or epilepsy associated with cerebral damage are also admitted. The balance of different disorders is crucial to the smooth and effective working of individual treatment plans and needs constant watching. Most of the patient care is carried out by the nursing staff in a ratio, ideally, of one nurse to one patient.

In addition there is a special school, recognised by the Department of Education and Science as efficient to deal with maladjusted pupils, within the unit. It is staffed by specially trained teachers and has its own head teacher responsible for all the education services within the different units of the joint hospital (the Bethlem Royal Hospital and the Maudsley Hospital). All children, unless they are utterly unable to profit from the school setting, attend school daily for up to six hours, five days a week, throughout the year. There is also an occupational therapist providing this specialised form of treatment for the children. The usual clinical team of psychiatrist, social worker and clinical psychologist are engaged with each child and his family throughout the child's stay in hospital, but are integrated into the ward organisation in a different fashion from that on the outpatient service.

Details of how a treatment plan is arrived at and implemented in the individual case will be discussed later in the section on 'school refusal'. However, in order for any treatment plan to be effective by mobilising the therapeutic resources of the unit, an involved system of communication between all professional disciplines has come into being. This includes, in addition to ward rounds, the traditional diagnostic and decision-making meeting taken by a consultant in the ward, other meetings three times a week lasting one hour for all staff engaged on working with the children, led by a senior registrar, and daily handover meetings of the different nursing shifts presided over by the charge nurse. There are also weekly meetings between social worker and nursing staff to discuss problems that arise with families of the children in hospital, and weekly meetings taken by the senior registrar with junior nurses to teach principles of child development and behaviour in relation to management problems on the ward. The aim of these meetings is to ensure that all concerned know as fully as possible what is happening with each patient, and the direction, aim and extent of the particular treatment plan, so that there is uniformity of purpose and consistency of practice. The children and nursing staff thus feel more secure, there is less room for manipulation by children and their families, and any crises, such as suicidal acts or threats, running away, paranoid accusations by parents, and so forth, are dealt with effectively and rapidly.

General Indications for Inpatient Treatment of Neurotic Disorders in Children

An inpatient unit can only solve some of the problems of psychiatrically disordered children who have not responded to other efforts at treatment. Too often parents and child are given an unrealistic picture of what to expect in an effort to 'sell' admission. It is much better to spell out the objectives and limits of any treatment plan, to let the parents and child look over the unit before admission, and to handle the difficult first phase of settling in with tact and sensitivity. In neurotic disorders this phase is often concerned with difficulties in separating, with homesickness and manipulative attempts by children to control parents and staff.

It is not appropriate to use an inpatient unit with therapeutic aims and resources purely as a place of custody and containment. In the majority of cases of neurotic disorder, admission of a child to hospital should be one phase of treatment with the eventual aim of reuniting child and family. It should not be used merely as a prelude to, or in waiting for, boarding-school placement as a maladjusted pupil. If this is done hospital admission may be felt by the child to be a 'sending away' or punishment for past misbehaviour, and may become associated with feelings of anger and projection which get in the way of the positive identification necessary for the success of residential school placement. There are bound to be instances where a decision about boarding-school placement is taken while the child is in hospital. This is because the assessment of the child's needs in hospital, and an appraisal of family strengths and weaknesses, has led to a considered decision that an experience at boarding-school would continue and expand the gains from inpatient treatment and provide a setting for further development which cannot be provided at home. Once the decision is made the plan must be worked through with the child and family.

Admission to an inpatient unit is usually recommended when the child's symptoms are evidence of severe pathology which has not responded to other methods of treatment. The assumption is that, while the child continues to live in his everyday environment, the family environment is itself such a pathogenic factor in supporting and maintaining the disorder that it blocks effective treatment. Exposing the child to a healthier environment should then make treatment easier. This often happens, but admission sometimes has the effect of taking the emphasis away from the child's personal conflicts and the need to deal with them, thus leaving the new environment to do all the work. It may also lead parents to feel that they have no part to play in further treatment so that they withdraw into becoming mere visitors or bringers of gifts. Their former hostility to the patient becomes displaced onto the nursing staff over day-to-day care, state of clothes and other comparatively trivial matters. Nursing staff can react quite sharply to the implicit criticism of their caring skills, unless they are helped to understand that this criticism is the family's way of coping with their feelings of failure and guilt concerning their child. Such difficulties can be forestalled if the parents are involved in the treatment plan from the outset, given an active part to play and helped to understand that their responsibility continues while their child is in hospital.

Admission to hospital has been used by some (Rose and Sonis, 1959; Gair and Salomon, 1962) to test the child's and the family's capacities to mobilise resources in response to the experience of separation which admission involves. It is argued that the way the patient and his family cope with the situation shows how far they are open to modification and treatment. There may be an emotional deadlock which keeps the child's symptoms going: for instance, some children involve a parent in obsessional rituals in which the parent masochistically submits to the child's controlling demands. These dramatically disappear when the child comes into hospital. In other instances the child's disturbance plays an important part in family interaction and the presence of the disturbed child maintains the balance of family forces, at the same time gratifying the child and reinforcing the disorder. While the child is still within the family no progress can be made in outpatient treatment; hospital admission upsets the balance, sometimes allowing positive moves towards healthier functioning. In other circumstances it may prove very stressful to the parents, particularly if there is an apparent dramatic improvement in the child, and when this happens the parents may remove the child from hospital, arguing that with improvement no further treatment is necessary. Many of these families never return for help even if this is offered. It is possible that the tolerance for deviant behaviour is increased while the more obvious disturbance in the child diminishes, so that a new balance of forces is achieved at a level of function which is not so handicapping as again to bring the child to the notice of the school services.

Specific Indications for Inpatient Treatment

It is probably true to say that the majority of children with neurotic disorders are treated as outpatients, usually by a combination of methods including environmental modification, individual psychotherapy, casework with one or both parents and, in appropriate cases, medication with psychotropic drugs. In some clinics the techniques of family group therapy are used. The majority of children are never referred for inpatient treatment either because there are no facilities available or because outpatient treatment is considered effective enough.

When children with neurotic disorders are admitted it is most often because outpatient treatment has not achieved the desired effect. The reasons include irregular attendance which interferes with the therapeutic alliance or prevents it ever becoming established. In these instances it is hoped that admission will ensure regular treatment in addition to the benefits of a therapeutic environment. It also tacitly reduces the parental influence on treatment which may have taken the form of interference with regular attendance or negative attitudes to treatment which affect the child's co-operation. When in hospital the child is protected to some extent from these attitudes and his own positive feelings about being helped are supported by the nurses, teachers and others who value their own efforts and those of others in helping him get better.

Anxiety Reactions

A characteristic feature of neurotic disorders is that the child is aware of feeling anxious. The anxiety may be diffuse and free-floating as in anxiety reactions, and when chronic it is often associated with apprehensiveness in the mother, sometimes verging on frank and crippling anxiety. There is a good deal of communication of anxiety within such families and uprushes of more intense anxiety are poorly tolerated. If these are manifest as night terrors and as panic attacks during the day, the family as a whole may become so disturbed that the normal control of anxiety breaks down; a reverberating cycle of communicated anxiety may then be established which cannot be contained by outpatient therapeutic procedures or by drugs. In such instances it is often helpful to admit the child to hospital, thus breaking the cycle of 'contagious anxiety' (Anthony, 1967), and allowing both child and family to regain their nerve. The child who has been suffering a good deal and showing it by clinging, demanding behaviour, leading to sleepless family nights and limitation of activity during the day, is often greatly relieved to be in a calm supportive atmosphere. Here adults who are not overwhelmed by his distress can effectively relieve it by bringing out the worries and half-expressed fears, and by providing a programme which will strengthen the healthy aspects of the child's personality and activities at the expense of the neurotic ones.

Hypochondrial Reactions

Hypochondrial reactions are another type of neurotic disorder in which hospital admission is often the appropriate method of treatment. There is the opportunity for a detailed physical examination of the patient and additional investigations where necessary, bearing in mind the dangers of causing iatrogenic symptoms by too zealous and basically unnecessary investigation. The whole procedure reassures all concerned that there is no organic disease, yet at the same time may reveal minor physical defects which handicap the child and which can be taken into account in the treatment programme. Children can often be reassured to some extent by their doctor who, having done the examination, can then deal with the child's repeated complaints of vague aches and pains and the anxious anticipation of future illness. This attention-gaining behaviour, so effective at home, does not have the usual effect and is slowly given up. Identifications are built up with healthy adults, unlike the often ill parents and siblings. The child can then abandon the role of the sick one which ensured escape from routine and from any demands at school (where social and educational failure may have led to a loss of self-esteem). Similarly, he will no longer need to avoid situations where he would experience social disgrace.

The hospital school is important in restoring self-esteem. Life in hospital protects the child from the intrusiveness of anxious parents who often magnify and maintain the conflicts and complaints of hypochondriacal children. It also allows the cutting-down of excessive medication, often ineffective or inappropriate, and replacement by tranquillising drugs when anxiety is acute and sleep is disturbed (Anthony, 1967).

Obsessional Disorders

Obsessional disorders usually occur in pre-adolescent children and take such forms as counting and touching ceremonials or recurrent thoughts, washing compulsions, doubts, timidity and depressed mood. The child with an obsessional disorder, unlike an adult, does not or cannot keep his ruminations to himself or conceal his rituals. Instead he may force his parents, usually his mother, to take part in the rituals, answer repetitive questions or meet his compulsive needs with some attention to detail. Mothers who are themselves compulsive may fit in with these demands but others become impatient and hostile, trying to resist their child's demands usually by reasoning, later by punishment. Hospital admission can be a means of intervening in the struggle. The child's obsessional behaviour in hospital is often markedly diminished, especially as other activities are set up to break into rituals such as handwashing, often lessening the underlying anxiety and tension.

Depressive Phenomena

Depressive phenomena in children have been the subject of much discussion by child psychiatrists. There are many who do not believe that a clinical entity of depressive illness or disorder, comparable to that seen in adults, occurs in children before puberty. Many will accept that depressive reactions are more likely to occur in adolescence (Chess, 1969). On the other hand, children do often show mood disturbances, including short-lived states of sadness which are experienced as painful, and more enduring states which can be reasonably described as depressed mood. The notion of 'depressive equivalents' or accompaniments where the depressive affect is held to be replaced by hypochondriasis, hyperactivity, acting-out behaviour, or even obesity or anorexia, is less convincing. In cases of persistent depressed mood arising from inappropriate or adverse environmental circumstances, treatment focusses on this aspect; but where depressive affect is associated with social withdrawal, self-depreciation and self-accusation, anti-depressant medication on an outpatient basis may be effective in older children. When it is not, and if the family is unable to cope with and support the child, admission to an inpatient unit is indicated. If the clinical picture also includes instances of attempted suicide the patient should certainly be admitted.

Hysterical and Conversion Reactions

The literature on hysteria in childhood does not compare in quantity with that on adult hysteria and there are marked differences of opinion as to the frequency of the condition. Some insist that it is an everyday phenomenon, so including a host of somatic symptoms such as headache, abdominal pain, vomiting, hiccups and histrionic behaviour, while others limit the diagnosis to more clear-cut instances of contracture, aphonia, amblyopia, the so-called 'conversion hysteria', and to those cases where there is an hysterical prolongation of a symptom or sign occurring originally as part of an organically determined illness.

Caplan (1970) used the following operational definition of hysteria in a study of cases seen at the children's department of the Maudsley Hospital: 'Those patients with a disorder involving somatic symptoms (not referable to the autonomic nervous system) which were thought to be emotional in origin. Thus abdominal pain, nausea, vomiting and the like would *not* be included, whereas paralyses, abnormalities of gait, disorders of sensation, blindness, deafness, aphonia, fits and fugues would, if considered to be due to an emotional disorder' (p. 34). The author eschewed the type of psychological mechanism concerned in his definition.

Caplan matched each index case with a control for age, sex and year of referral but with a diagnosis of either anxiety state or unspecified psychoneurosis in order to compare cases and controls on a number of clinical and demographic variables. His aim was to determine which features, if any, predispose towards a diagnosis of 'hysteria' and 'hysterical conversion symptoms'. He found that children so diagnosed were less likely to have symptoms of general emotional disturbance than controls but more likely to have a family history of 'hysteria'.

Caplan's findings were that the rate of referral of pre-pubertal children with diagnosed 'hysteria' was 0·3 per cent, considerably lower than the rate for equivalent children referred to the psychiatric department of a paediatric general hospital (0·99 per cent) and for pubertal and pubescent children referred to the Maudsley Hospital (1·8 per cent). A most significant finding was that 46·4 per cent of all the cases, who were referred mainly by specialist physicians rather than general practitioners, were found to have an organic illness related to the presenting symptom either at the time of discharge from hospital or at follow-up four to eleven years later. Of the somatic disturbances diagnosed as 'hysterical conversion symptoms', amblyopia was most likely to be due to an organic cause.

It is of interest that a higher number of index cases than controls was treated as inpatients, reflecting the opinion that they were more severely ill or presenting diagnostic problems requiring assessment and treatment in hospital, often after a period in a general hospital. This is in accord with clinical experience that it is grosser forms of hysterical and conversion reactions which are referred for admission, rather than the milder disorders which are usually part of a mixed neurotic disorder with depressive, obsessional or phobic features. Treatment was mainly individual psychotherapy with the patient and casework or psychotherapy with a parent. Anthony (1967) has commented on the number of different treatment procedures which have been successful in hysteria, most of them incorporating some method of suggestion. He believes that the use of hypnosis with children, especially girls at puberty, has iatrogenic dangers. He points out that insight therapy aims at uncovering the neurotic conflict leading to the conversion, so helping the child to 'reconvert'.

Kanner (1957) asserts that environmental manipulation is sometimes more successful with hysterical children than with adults. Hospital admission certainly represents a great change of environment from home. In hospital a situation can be constructed where 'escape with honour' from the disabling symptom is often possible (Gold, 1965), and strong reinforcement of normal activity and behaviour can be provided. Caplan (1970) found that most of the children with substantiated hysteria in his series recovered completely from the presenting disability either rapidly (less than 9 months) or moderately slowly (more than 24 months).

Phobic Disorders

Phobic disorders in children, that is, morbid fears, need to be differentiated from healthy fears or normal developmental fears which diminish or disappear as the child grows. It is the persistence of this infantile fearful tendency that characterises the neurotic in the making (Anthony, 1967). The phobic states in children which are commonly referred for psychiatric help are animal phobias, death phobias, insect phobias, noise phobias, and school phobias.

In psychodynamic terms the child displaces the content of his original conflict onto an object or situation in the external environment which has some symbolic significance for him, and among the objects or situations are animals, school, dirt, disease, high places, elevators and dying (Anthony, 1967). The same author states that phobic children are often a pleasure to treat in that they are generally alert, inquisitive and resourceful in the therapeutic situation and make full use of all the symbolic equations in play both consciously and unconsciously. Here psychotherapy is the treatment of choice but psychotropic drugs which reduce anxiety may be helpful in cases of death phobia and of dark phobia when getting off to sleep is a problem. In phobias with acute onset and clear-cut precipitation, abreaction followed by, or in conjunction with, psychotherapy may be effective. Monosymptomatic phobias are nowadays treated, very often successfully, with methods such as systematic desensitisation and other methods of behaviour therapy (Ross, 1972). Both psychotherapeutic and behaviour therapy approaches are used when the child is sufficiently disturbed to warrant hospital admission, but the majority will still be treated as outpatients. School phobias are one pattern of response in the general category of refusal to attend school and as such are considered in a separate section of this chapter.

Plan of Treatment in Inpatient Care of Neurotic Disorders

Any treatment plan must be based on a comprehensive diagnostic formulation. This will include a description of the particular neurotic disorder for which admission has been thought necessary. Symptoms and behaviour are considered in terms of the distress they cause the patient as well as their effect on family, school and community. A detailed physical examination will reveal any physical handicaps, major or minor, which interfere with adaptation to demands of school and peer group and may be a source of feelings of deep shame and sensitivity on the child's part. Clumsiness, poor co-ordination and poorly developed perceptual skills can prove quite severe handicaps to competence in games and school work. Muscular development, body size and factors such as obesity are relevant to self-concepts of attractiveness and ability to compete with others. They also affect grouping in the ward. Level of intelligence and academic attainments have usually been assessed, but further investigations may be necessary to elucidate the reasons for educational retardation. Psychologist and teacher will together plan the educational part of the treatment scheme with this information in mind.

The family's part in treatment must be clarified at an early stage, otherwise they may withdraw from participation at the beginning and prove difficult to engage later on. The social worker is the main link with the family, but her role overlaps that of nursing staff who will also have important contacts with the patient's family. Who does what and when needs to be carefully discussed; parents may otherwise exploit this undefined area of contact and play one member of staff against another, often with the patient joining in. Inter-staff recrimination is a potent cause of failure to reach treatment goals and may recapitulate aspects of the home situation for the patient. In certain instances a particular nurse may be in the best position to work with parents and there are definite advantages when a nurse has the authority and skill to do so.

The relationship of professional staff to the parents of the child in hospital needs constant discussion, including the question of 'visiting' by parents (Christ and Wagoner, 1966). Each family situation needs to be considered on its own, and the reason for each particular decision discussed repeatedly with the parents and child. Limitation of 'visiting' which is thought to be in the child's interests may have a totally unexpected meaning and consequence for the parents, confirming them in their half-expressed view that they are the cause of the illness. This may arouse feelings of anger and criticism towards professional staff, leading either to complaints about food, clothes, cleanliness or lack of care, or tense rivalry between parents and nursing staff. On the other hand, the parents may withdraw and remain in only superficial contact with the ward staff. The latter situation is the less taxing and it is all too easy to accept it, only to discover that unrecognised family factors are holding up progress so that unnecessary time and energy has to be spent bringing the family back into therapeutic contact.

In one sense treatment begins before the child's admission to hospital, for care in discussing the reasons for this with parents and child, and arranging for them all to visit the ward and school prior to admission, can avoid many of the anxieties and uncertainties which arise when preparation cannot be lengthy and detailed. The actual experience of being shown around, having questions answered, meeting the staff and seeing the children in school and at play does much to restrain fears and fantasies about 'mental' hospitals and 'mad' or 'bad' children.

One innovation which has proved particularly useful is the pre-admission home visit. Once admission is agreed to, the parents are asked whether a team from the hospital ward may visit them in the four to five days prior to admission. The team consists of the psychiatrist who will be responsible, under consultant supervision, for the day-to-day care and treatment of the patient, the social worker and the particular nurse who will be the focal figure for the child during his stay in hospital.

This home visit allows the family to meet the clinical team on home ground and not at a disadvantage. It reduces the psychological distance between home and ward and enables the clinical team to form an appreciation of the family, including siblings and relatives, in their home setting. The nurse establishes contact with the child on familiar ground and particularly asks to see the child's bedroom and special toys and possessions. The child is invited to bring a special toy into hospital with him and the choice and questions about this are talked through with the nurse. On admission the parents and child are met by the same staff and the mutual trust and confidence earlier established eases this situation considerably. In our experience it is particularly helpful in mitigating the tensions arising from the difficult period of separation in cases of school refusal who are treated in hospital.

Once in hospital, the treatment plan for each patient is formulated in terms of ward life generally, school experience, occupational therapy, psychotherapy, psychological procedures such as desensitisation or operant training, family casework, medication, special investigations and long-term plans for future schooling. Certain general points apply to the treatment of all types of neurotic disorder, but specific approaches are required for particular disorders. Allocation to a particular children's group on the ward is made on the basis of age, size and general level of maturity in social relationships and behaviour, and each group is the responsibility of a staff nurse with several junior nurses or nursing assistants. Each patient has a particular nurse whom he may have met at the pre-admission home visit or when first admitted, and who was responsible for supporting him through the admission procedure, introducing him to other children, explaining the limits and routine on the ward and generally acting as a figure for attachment and reassurance until he became settled.

Neurotic children make use of this relationship in a dependent fashion at first, but later mixed feelings may emerge and it is the nurse's task to help the child by tolerating the expression of negative feelings. Nurses who are unused to this may need much help from senior nursing staff and others and the daily ward discussions are important here.

Whenever possible, an attempt is made to help a child develop some competence or even skill in an activity which he had formerly avoided or had not previously experienced. In the case of school refusal the child is often competent and even academically advanced in school, but behind contemporaries in games, model-making or visiting parks, galleries or zoos, because of over-protection and restriction at home. The nursing staff will then elicit what the child would most like to do but believes that he is unable to do and a definite attempt is made to provide a chance of mastering this desired new skill. Confidence and new-found competence are generalised to other activities, and parents encouraged, if not pointedly advised, to provide the same opportunities on weekends at home.

The same principles apply in the school situation. Although the situation is freer than in a conventional school, the emphasis is always on a steady progression of work so that the level on admission is maintained. For children who are backward, intensive remedial help is also provided. A teacher rather than a nurse may be chosen as the focus of the patient's developing relationships, perhaps because teachers are more familiar to children than nurses. In many instances teacher and nurse can work together by defining the areas of interaction with the patient; however, rivalry can develop and this may need clarification by some senior person, either head teacher, charge nurse or psychiatrist in ward discussion.

Occupational therapy activities may be provided individually or in a group, depending on what is appropriate at the time. This is another area where new experiences and activities can be provided and new skills learnt in motor or perceptual spheres, and there is also the chance of helping patients adapt to a social group through the medium of shared activity.

Behaviour modification procedures include systematic desensitisation of specific phobias and the use of implosion which can reduce obsessional rituals by reinforcement of normal behaviour, so that abnormal behaviour gradually decreases. Neurotic eating patterns in the form of faddiness, excessive slowness, or fixation to infantile eating patterns, for example bottle feeding, can be helped with reinforcement and extinction techniques.

The social worker has an important role in an inpatient unit. She provides an individual on-going therapeutic relationship with the family, a link between nursing and other staff and the family, a contact between child and family, and a link between social and educational community agencies and the ward staff. For this reason she should ideally attend all meetings, discussions and ward rounds about patients, so as to be aware of changes in the treatment programme and to inform staff what changes are taking place in the family and what alignment of family forces now exists. There is often considerable change in parental relationships following admission of a child and these can easily become pathological and anti-therapeutic unless work is done from the outset. Sometimes this must be done on the basis of home visits, particularly where other members of the nuclear family who never visit the patient are exerting an influence at home. Work with both parents, with whole families and with one parent, all have their place. The clinical psychologist may join the social worker when there is a need for parents to continue behaviour-modification techniques being used in the ward.

Place of Psychotherapy in Residential Psychiatric Treatment

The place of individual psychotherapy in the treatment of children in hospital has undergone changes as concepts of residential treatment have altered. Noshpitz (1962) has described how residential work was earlier considered effective to the extent that it made a child available for psychotherapy, so that a style of therapy evolved that attempted to reproduce the traditional analytic situation where the child in a healthy home is taken to see the analyst. He describes how this evolved in time into two approaches to treatment, namely ego support and ego interpretation. The tactics of treatment involve the whole residential staff and not merely the therapist, and Noshpitz remarks that providing ego support is a complex task requiring highly trained staff capable of understanding the theory of ego functions and able to work specifically on strengthening the patients' ego functions.

Weiss and Cain (1964) have described the difficulties of psychotherapy with a group of school phobics treated in hospital. They mention strong unyielding defences, denial of problems, reluctance to talk and resistance to play in interview and grim oppositional silence rendering their internal fantasy life inaccessible to exploration or interpretation. Barker (1968) comments that individual psychotherapy played a relatively small part in the inpatient treatment of six severe cases of school refusal and was supportive in nature. He mentions that in spite of their above average intelligence the patients stand out by their reluctance to communicate either verbally or in play, so that interpretation was little used, but discussion of family relationships was possible in some cases. Coolidge *et al.* (1957) have also found that older school phobics presenting in adolescence are resistant to psychotherapy and show a striking lack of fantasy material in therapeutic sessions.

It may be that these difficulties apply particularly in certain types of school refusal. Weiss and Cain and Coolidge *et al.* observed that patients in one of their two described groups were more accessible to psychotherapy in that they were younger, with more acute onset symptoms, apparently less profoundly disturbed and with a better outcome in terms of return to school. In the second group of cases with what amounted to a personality disorder the difficulties in treatment seemed to arise as much from an inability to relate, and a lack of fantasy life, as from reluctance to participate in psychotherapy.

These factors have a bearing on the place of individual psychotherapy in the inpatient treatment of neurotic disorders generally. The opinions of experienced workers (Greenwood, 1955; Shaw and Lucas, 1970; Redl, 1959a) show that effective therapeutic interaction is possible using different methods and professional staff other than psychiatrist or psychotherapist alone. Bettelheim (1966) has remarked that, although the residential treatment situation is an application of the psychoanalytic search into the workings of the unconscious mind, 'it is much harder to do when the patient is not lying in relative quiet on the couch but is engaging in the wide range of activities of the abnormal child'.

It seems that the goals of psychotherapy in inpatient treatment may not need to include the modification of basic character structure and the resolution of major unconscious conflicts. If this is so, psychotherapy is one of several therapeutic approaches available for use at any time during the patient's period of treatment. When the use of this method is indicated by the patient's symptomatology and capacity, the aims of psychotherapy can be realistically modified. The child can be helped to tolerate emotional stress and develop stronger and more effective defences against anxiety, without solving the underlying unconscious causes of the neurotic conflict. Within the psychotherapeutic relationship the patient can be helped to accept his hostile and negative feelings towards family members, and his peer group, and to feel that his positive feelings are valued so that he feels less bad in himself about his hostility. The psychotherapeutic experience can focus on 'here-and-now conflicts' in the ward in relation to other children and the staff and in relation to home and school. In both settings the patient is offered a chance of new kinds of human relationships rather than the constricted, anxiety-ridden experience with his parents, and in this sense psychotherapy is re-educative rather than uncovering.

Inpatient Treatment of School Refusal

The literature on 'school refusal' or, as some authors prefer to call it, 'school phobia', continues to proliferate. There are many reasons for this which Eisenberg (1958) has summarised most elegantly when he writes: 'Beyond its own intrinsic importance, school phobia serves as a paradigm of neurotic disorders in children, for it illustrates with special clarity the relation between symptoms in the child and the psychologic structure of the family. The principles of its treatment highlight general considerations in the psychotherapy of emotional disorders. Only if the physician, the school authorities and participating social agencies co-ordinate therapeutic efforts is rehabilitation of the family unit likely to be successful'. Good co-ordination and appropriate treatment very often lead to a successful outcome, but some cases do not respond to these social measures and outpatient psychiatric treatment. For such cases admission to an inpatient or residential hospital service has been advocated (Warren, 1948; Weiss and Cain, 1964; Barker, 1968).

At present both 'school refusal' and 'school phobia' are commonly used to describe persistent non-attendance at school other than truancy (Hersov, 1960a). This author regards 'school phobia' as only one type of symptom pattern within the general category of 'school refusal' (Hersov, 1972). The latter includes a wide range of clinical disorders and individual and family psychopathology which are far from being a homogeneous group (Hersov, 1960b). The cases of early onset in primary school-children are very different clinical conditions from those occurring at puberty or in early adolescence. The range of conditions is from neurotic disorders through personality disorders to, in some cases, borderline or frank psychotic disorders. Precipitating factors may be mainly external in the form of threatening or shaming school experiences or a change of school. They may be more closely connected to an illness, accident or operation befalling the child, or a family event such as physical illness, death of a parent or relative or the occurrence of psychiatric illness in a parent. Actual or threatening marital breakdown can also be a precipitating factor.

Many writers (Johnson *et al.*, 1941; Davidson, 1961; Coolidge *et al.*, 1962) stress the causal role of the parents, especially the mother, commenting on their ambivalence, inconsistency, immaturity and dependency on their own parents. Kessler (1972) queries this on the grounds that the same kinds of parental psychopathology, attitudes and handling have been found in very different psychiatric disorders, that school refusal does not run in families, and that parental over-protectiveness may follow rather than antedate school refusal. She therefore considers that the affected child must have some special susceptibility. She is also critical of the notion that separation anxiety always occurs in school refusal connected with the fear of loss or death of a parent, pointing out, as have others (Frick, 1964), that many such children can leave their home for places other than school, or tolerate parents leaving them alone at home. Experience in treating children with school refusal leads Kessler (1972) to suspect that the individual psychopathology of girls with the condition may be quite different from that of boys, in that boys are more generally immature and dependent with less sexual involvement. In discussing the principal means of dynamic psychotherapy she mentions (1) child–therapist relationship, (2) work with mother, (3) spontaneous play with conversation, (4) release and acceptance of feelings, (5) interpretation – all aimed at treating the underlying cause rather than the overt symptom. Within the same psychodynamic framework, Sperling (1961, 1967) distinguishes more precisely between 'induced school phobia' arising from pathological parent–child relationships where the parent is treated, and the 'traumatic or common type of acute school phobia' in which the child is treated.

In recent years behaviour modification approaches to treatment have been used where the child's behaviour and other clinical phenomena meet descriptive criteria for a phobia, that is, a special form of fear out of proportion to the demands of the situation which cannot be explained or reasoned away, is beyond voluntary control and leads to avoidance of the feared situation (Marks, 1969). Only those cases in which refusal to attend school is due to fear of school can strictly speaking be called 'school phobia', although fear of leaving home may also manifest itself as school refusal (Ross, 1972). Here the maladaptive avoidance responses would be eliminated or modified by desensitisation techniques (Garvey and Hegrenes, 1966; Chapel, 1967) or by a combination of operant and respondent conditioning approaches (Lazarus *et al.*, 1965). Proponents of this approach point out that school refusal is a complex of behaviour in which the avoidance response to school may originally have served to reduce fear but has then become reinforced, maintained and complicated by events at home when the child is not in school (Ross, 1972). When this occurs over a long period of time the total situation becomes chronic and extremely difficult to treat. Even clinicians with a totally different theoretical viewpoint, who have struggled to treat children with long-standing school refusal, will agree with the accuracy of this observation.

This brief survey of views on classification and treatment shows that there is no one treatment of choice and that an accurate diagnosis and formulation must pinpoint what the relevant psychopathology is, taking into account the age and sex of the child. With the advent of newer methods of treatment aimed at 'target' behaviour there is even more need for clear identification and differentiation of the many factors that enter into 'school-refusal'.

Indications for Inpatient Treatment of School Refusal

In general, the criteria for taking any child with psychiatric disorder into treatment will depend on the following:

(a) Frequency of symptoms or occurrence of disturbed behaviour
(b) Number of symptoms and areas of life in which symptoms show themselves
(c) Degree of handicap or social disadvantage imposed by the symptoms
(d) Degree of impairment of functions such as learning, playing and developing independence appropriate to age
(e) Suffering or discomfort imposed upon the child by the symptoms

(f) Persistence of symptoms or behaviour over time and intractibility to the usual measures of comfort, reassurance and support.

Scrutiny of the scanty literature on inpatient treatment (Warren, 1948; Weiss and Cain, 1964; Barker, 1968) shows that the following are the main reasons for deciding to admit a child with school refusal into residential treatment:

1. Early onset of school refusal and persistence on and off over time, leading eventually to a complete breakdown of school attendance.
2. Resistance on the child's part to entreaty, persuasion, recrimination and punishment by parents and pressure from teachers and educational welfare officers.
3. Parents' inability to maintain effective control over the child in getting him to attend school, so that physical struggles and violent resistance on the child's part are followed by guilt, mutual recrimination or compensatory over-protection on the part of the parent or parents.
4. Increasing social withdrawal and isolation on the child's part.
5. Outpatient treatment becoming increasingly hampered by the child's and parents' inability to separate from each other, or the parents' inaccessibility to casework.
6. In the last-named circumstances, where treatment as an outpatient lasts so long that the child suffers secondarily in terms of academic retardation because of the time he spends off school.
7. Where a lengthy period of thoughtful, well-planned outpatient treatment has proved ineffective (Kennedy, 1965).

The indications for admission discussed so far are mainly negative or anti-therapeutic aspects of symptomatology and family structure. It can be argued that there are also positive reasons for hospital admission over and above the failure of outpatient treatment, so that in certain circumstances hospital admission is the treatment of choice.

Significance of the School for the Child

One viewpoint is that school and learning are libidinally determined from the first for everyone, thus compelling the child to sublimate his instinctual energies. Faced with new objects and activities which test the mobility of his libido, he has to abandon earlier more or less passive feminine energies in order to be active and successful (Klein, 1924). If the demands of school life are looked at in terms of ego-functions the school can be seen as the first testing-ground set up by society which lies outside the secure atmosphere of home. Going to school involves the first separation from home and the submission to outside rules and standards. These are applied in a situation from which there is no escape and over which the child has no control. For the first time the standards by which the child must abide are set up by a non-parental authority, and loving and protective parents are unable to help and support their child as hitherto.

Attendance at school symbolises the acceptance of the responsibilities of growing up and of increasing independence of the family. It enhances the young child's feeling of importance, but it also means giving up the privileges of early childhood. Also, the unrelenting reality of school is a new and demanding situation which puts pressure upon children in many ways. It brings the opportunity of learning new skills, but it may also mean facing more competition and perhaps relative failure compared with previous experience of ready recognition and success. It introduces new experiences and situations for which the child may have been totally unprepared. He is now judged, not by intention or previous record, but by his actual performance within a peer group and in the classroom. He is in intellectual competition with others and is judged by qualities over which he has no control, such as intellectual level, social status and racial group. Competitive physical games and contact with different rougher children are the rule. The teachers he meets have varying personalities and attitudes, some patient and tolerant, others short-tempered, critical and verbally punitive.

The majority of children will weather these storms of adjustment so that school in time becomes a place of industry, achievement, pleasure and success. Other children will have problems of school adjustment. These may stem from the child's own dread of inferiority and sense of shame over failure, combined with an intense need to become competent and achieve in learning and social skills. Disappointment over this, coupled with painful school experiences with teachers, may be main causal factors in school refusal. Other children can meet the educational requirements of school, yet are unable to cope with the demand for separation from home and entry into a peer group.

Leventhal and Sills (1964) have put forward a relatively simple, parsimonious interpretation of school phobia which states that these children over-value themselves and their achievements and try to maintain their unrealistic self-image. When their 'power' is threatened in the school situation they suffer anxiety, avoid the threat and try to maintain their narcissistic self-fictions. A permissive mother frequently serves as a refuge. (In behaviour modification terms the mother reinforces the avoidance behaviour by her handling of the child at home (Ross, 1972)). Leventhal *et al.* (1967) conceptualise treatment in terms of strategy and tactics which require assessment of the ability of family members to take part in and achieve success in a 'show-down' when pressure is brought upon the child to return to school.

Fleck (1972), writing on basic and essential family functions, lists as one of them the emancipation of offspring from the family. This must occur physically and geographically as well as psychologically and socially. To be successful the final separation must not be abrupt but follow increasing steps towards separations between parents and child. 'Through separation experiences the child learns and grows: he becomes more able to avoid the same impasse and less vulnerable to, and threatened by, subsequent separations or emotional distance from others. This mastery must be facilitated by the opportunity to observe, imitate, and eventually internalise how other family members cope with frustration and "separation anxiety"' (p. 192). Among the steps towards independence are the first school entrance, camps or other experiences of being away from home. The emotionally unhealthy family is unable to accept and further these normal experiences of separation by the child, indeed the child is often made to feel guilty if attempts to separate are made as part of normal development.

It has been shown that children with school refusal have significantly less experience of separation from parents than truants and children with psychiatric disorders other than school refusal (Hersov, 1960a). It is also true that many mothers of children with school refusal are still dependent on their own parents and have not resolved the problems of emancipation and forming a separate family unit of their own (Davidson, 1961). In these instances admission to an in-patient unit with a setting for special education may help the child achieve separate development and the sense of achievement in school. A further advantage is that hospital admission reduces the amount of reinforcement of avoidance and maladaptive behaviour provided at home and gives an opportunity of learning different and more effective patterns, which are then reinforced.

R, a boy aged 12 years 5 months, was referred by GP as an emergency in October 1971, for reluctance to attend school of long duration which had gradually increased in the last year till he was missing some days a week, often because he said he was too ill to attend. In addition he was complaining of nausea and stomach-ache in the mornings before school, waking early at 6.30 a.m., going to the toilet four times every morning and having to sit on the toilet seat four times. He was unable to eat a normal breakfast, cried every morning in bed before getting up and would spend an hour during the evening before each school day checking that his school bag was complete and that he had not left anything out. He had urinary frequency on every school morning and required constant reassurance from his mother. He would go to school with three friends if driven there by his father but would have to be pushed out of the car weeping and protesting. He seemed most worried by mathematics and general science and with his mother's intervention had obtained a protective letter from his housemaster. This said he was under strain and needed to be treated with kindness and understanding. This he showed to different masters whenever he felt worried, but in spite of this support he gradually became worse and began to return home after getting half-way to school.

He first attended school at the age of 5 years but disliked it from the beginning. His mother thought it was because he disliked being away from her. He reacted badly to the change from infant to junior school; he seemed very afraid, and his mother had to go into the classroom with him each morning. He appeared convinced he would be unable to cope with school without her help. When he moved to his present comprehensive school he seemed overcome by the size and impersonality of the school, often complaining of illness in order to stay at home. The parental description of his personality was a mixed one, contrasting his sensitivity to suffering of others with boyish interests such as cycling and games with friends. His closest relationship was with his mother. They often reassured each other that all would be well in times of difficulty and thought about each other a lot, he about his mother when at school and his mother about him when he was away from home. His parents denied that he was in any way fearful or over-dependent.

The family were in a state of crisis when first seen, not only over the problem of R's school attendance but because the father (aged 55) was suspected of having heart trouble and had recently been declared redundant after 37 years with one firm. He was depressed, wept easily and was very preoccupied with his difficulties. His wife (aged 52) was a chronic worrier who had required hypnotics to sleep for the past 13 years. Her father had died of Alzheimer's disease in a psychiatric hospital at the age of 61. There was an 18-year-old daughter born after 14 years of marriage. She was described as happy, stable and successful. The patient's infancy and early childhood were apparently normal, although the picture emerged of a rather clinging toddler who later lacked confidence at school. Family relationships were close, with the mother as the dominant personality. She had coped well in the past but now appeared anxious and tense, possibly with depressive feelings which she denied.

At the initial interview the boy was reluctant to separate from his mother and attempted to control the situation by getting her to stay with him and the doctor. He talked with reluctance about his school problems, focussing on the difficulties in his work and the teasing he experienced. He was guilty about causing his mother worry, but not upset by the effect on his father. His drawing of his bicycle was accurate and detailed but he left it incomplete after he made a mistake over drawing the wheels and went on to something else. Physical examination showed that he was in good health, prepubertal and with no neurological abnormality.

The initial diagnostic formulation was of neurotic disorder with incipient school refusal and minor compulsive rituals in an only boy and youngest child of elderly parents. He appeared of average intelligence with some possible learning difficulties at school. There was a long-standing history of dependence upon mother and difficulties in adapting to school which had increased since the move to a large comprehensive school so that non-attendance was becoming an increasing problem. Family tension was high, centering on the boy's behaviour but also affected by the father's ill-health and redundancy at work.

The treatment plan at that stage was to mobilise resources at home and at school to ensure firm handling of immediate return to school, while offering psychotherapy to the boy and casework for his parents. It was hoped to explore the boy's anxieties about school and home and to unravel the strengths and weaknesses of the reciprocal relationship between him and his mother. A full psychological assessment was arranged and further information sought from the school. The family doctor was advised of the father's depression and concern about his health and asked to arrange an appointment for him with a cardiologist.

The treatment was unsuccessful in that the parents and a school counsellor were unable to get the boy to attend school in spite of the use of minor tranquillisers to allay his anxiety. The mother had become depressed and, although she responded well to anti-depressants, her attempts to manage the situation at home remained ineffective. The boy and his parents attended weekly for five weeks during which time school refusal became outright and unresponsive to all efforts. At this stage inpatient treatment was offered with the aim of breaking the deadlock at home in which both parents were becoming increasingly despondent and hopeless about the boy, who was himself beginning to withdraw from social relationships and his usual activities outside home. Much preparation was needed to help the family accept hospital admission. Stress was laid on the experience of attending hospital school and the experience of being away from home among a peer group yet supported by his doctor and other in-patient staff.

Admission was an upsetting experience at first with much weeping and calling by R for his parents to take him home. The parents were equally tense. R's entreaties continued, but the nurse quietly but persistently pursued the line of describing exactly what would be asked of him in the ward and at school. After a while R understood that his behaviour was not evoking the hoped-for response so he began to show interest in the other children. The latter were positive and supportive and he was re-assured that no-one was older or bigger than he. His questions were now about how long he would be staying in hospital, and his dependence upon this particular nurse was shown by anxious enquiries as to whether she would be on duty the next day and would come to his aid if he needed her. He now enquired what the teachers were like in the school, adding that he preferred women teachers to men.

After the admission routine was completed he was taken straight into the school. At first he was tremulous and afraid but settled into work with encouragement and began talking to the boy at the next desk. He was given much praise for his efforts to overcome his fears and began to look quite proud of himself. He joined in a football game.

However, during the next week, while he went into school without difficulty, he remained anxious, tense and at times tearful, enquiring about going home and offering to go to his former school from hospital. This was agreed to and for two days he attended escorted to and from school by a nurse. On the third day he left school and telephoned his parents from a friend's house asking them to take him home. They did so and were unwilling to bring him back to hospital. He continued to attend school regularly after this without any major difficulties for the following six months, during which time he attended as an outpatient for psychotherapy while his parents were seen in joint interviews by doctor and social worker. There were two occasions, both on a Monday morning, when R did not go to school because of apparent illness and his mother could not decide whether to make him go or not.

Attempts were made in the joint family interviews to help the parents look at how their over-protection of and over-identification with R made it difficult for them to handle him firmly and consistently. They were given direct advice on how to deal with actual problems of behaviour and R's attempts to manipulate them over school issues. This they could accept but remained throughout most resistant to any attempt to discuss family relationships and their relevance to R's behaviour. They continually returned to their theme that the reasons for his difficulties lay in the school not at home. By now the father was re-employed, had been reassured about his health and the crisis in his life had passed. The mother's depression improved a good deal, but she remained unable to look at her relationship with R in spite of earlier bringing out her ambivalent feelings, including hostility to R for making her feel so angry and helpless. She was, however, able to express warm positive feelings to social worker and doctor and take up the decision to end treatment on the basis of contacting the hospital if the need arose again.

Comment. The treatment of this case of school refusal was carried out on the basis of active intervention using resources at school to try and ensure attendance. Pressure to get back to school was set up and maintained from the outset, while joint parent interviews and individual psychotherapy continued. The progress of treatment was reviewed every week and, when attempts failed to get R to school, hospital admission was advised and the feelings about this worked through prior to admission. The aim was a short-term period in hospital with return to attendance at the former school while R was still in hospital. R of his own accord telescoped the procedure considerably so that the goal was achieved much earlier than expected and without the general improvement in anxiety about separation from home which had also been a hoped-for result of inpatient treatment. Admission helped to resolve the crisis at home, which had made any plan of management ineffective, so that the parents were in a better state to take up the responsibility for R after he left hospital, admittedly against advice. Fortunately this event did not affect the on-going therapeutic relationship with parents and patient, which remained concerned with practical problems of management when all other approaches towards deeper understanding were blocked or denied by parents.

L, a boy aged 10 years, was referred to the children's department of the Maudsley Hospital in May 1969 with a view to admission. The referral letter described a childish, fatuous manner, giggling fits, and inability to give a good account of his difficulties apart from a dislike of school. L's mother was most concerned about her inability to get L to go to school and by his odd behaviour when 'he pulls faces at me and runs away'. The referring psychiatrist was of the opinion that the boy was verging on a psychotic breakdown which was no longer held back by phobic defences, so that he was displaying inappropriate affect, becoming unmanageable and showing possible delusional misperceptions.

When first seen as an outpatient for assessment the problem, as verbalised by the boy's mother, was of outright school refusal of three months' duration, following on a long history of frequent absences from school since the age of four years. The patient apparently came home one day from school saying he had fought with his boy friend; the next day he came home saying he was not going back to school and he had stayed at home since. His behaviour at home was odd, different from that formerly shown. He acted aggressively to his mother and the family pet, and would be on the floor grimacing and belching if frustrated. A knock on the front door made him hide in a cupboard. Each morning he would get ready for school, answer the door to his friends, yet be unable to go with them. Forcible attempts to get him to school had led to struggles and his running away.

L had always been a timid child and since the age of four years had suffered recurrent attacks of illness, lasting two to three days, about once a month. These episodes were marked by the sudden onset of headache, anorexia, stomach cramps and vomiting and sometimes pallor and pyrexia, and resulted in two to three days in bed off school. These attacks never occurred at weekends or during holidays and were more severe at the beginning of each week.

The family consisted of his mother, aged 51, in good health, working as a part-time canteen assistant. There was a maternal family history of haemophilia and a 26-year-old brother to the patient suffered from haemophilia and paranoid schizophrenia and lived at home. L's father died, aged 45, from lung cancer when L was four years old. He had been very close to L, who was ten years younger than his next sibling. A sister, aged 28, was married and living away from home. Another sister, aged 20, had suddenly left home because of the intolerable behaviour of her schizophrenic brother. Up till then she had been a source of great support to the patient.

When first seen it was noted that L had slept in his own bed in his mother's bedroom since his father's death. He suffered from frequency of micturition and had wet his bed from three-and-a-half till six years of age. His concentration was poor and he would sometimes sit rocking in a chair and suck his thumb. He had difficulty in pronouncing his Rs. He had school friends, but since the school refusal began would not go outside the house in the daytime.

Physical examination showed a plump boy in good health with no physical abnormality. He was of average intelligence but retarded by over 18 months in reading comprehension and accuracy. He also had difficulty with the basic elements of arithmetic. A school report obtained when he was first seen gave details of babyish behaviour when he first began school, persistent low attainments all round and a tendency to sensitivity and tearfulness in the junior school when questioned by a teacher. His school also remarked on the persistent pattern of absence over the years, but had done nothing about it. The diagnostic formulation was of a neurotic disorder with school refusal, ostensibly precipitated by an argument at school but more probably related to anxiety and loss of support at home following a much-loved sister's departure. The behaviour of his paranoid schizophrenic brother towards his mother was another source of concern. The patient was academically retarded, mainly due to many absences from school. His personality development was influenced by his ordinal position as the youngest in the family, with a gap of ten years between him and the next sibling who acted in a maternal role toward him. She reinforced the maternal over-protectiveness following the father's death when L was four years old.

Initially, treatment was begun on an outpatient basis with the aim of dealing with L's anxieties and helping his mother to be consistent about school attendance, even if he complained of illness. In spite of support from school authorities and her oldest daughter, the mother was unable to ensure L's attendance and so accepted the offer of inpatient treatment. The aim was to try to reduce the over-close relationship between patient and mother which allowed him to control and manipulate her by his behaviour and complaints of illness. Although over-dependent in many ways, he was still able to make and maintain peer relationships outside the home. It was hoped that these could be encouraged and developed in the inpatient ward group. Throughout the stay in hospital emphasis would be laid on group activities, although he would also be having individual psychotherapy while casework contact was maintained with his mother.

On admission to hospital L was anxious and wept and clung to his mother. With firmness and sympathetic handling he eventually parted from his mother and went into the main play area. He showed no interest at first in the other children or nurses and stayed very close to the nurse who had been assigned to him and was to induce him into the ward routine. He remained in this state of hostile passivity until his mother began to say goodbye to him. He again wept and entreated her not to leave him, but soon after her departure became involved in games with the other children and became much less tense and anxious. He was noted to be meticulous about washing and keeping his clothes in order. His first night he slept well.

He remained in hospital for nine months and went to the hospital school without difficulty from the first day of entry. At school he tried at first to avoid conventional school work, particularly when there was a chance of failure. He was particularly anxious when doing arithmetic, more at ease when reading. When in a group of children at school he would say defensively that he could not do his work but was then easily able to attempt the same work when alone with one teacher. He became very dependent upon and attached to the occupational therapist, wanting to be near to her and seeking her approval at first. For much of his stay he seemed happier in the company of adults, although he was reticent about his feelings. These showed up as tears when his mother visited him, and the first weekend at home proved stressful for both him and his mother.

L's mother was seen fortnightly by the social worker who helped her with her distress over his hospital admission. She emerged as a warm, trusting person who talked about the loss of her own father when she was four years old (the age at which L lost his father) and told of how she had to look after her mother as she was the eldest girl in the family. Since her husband's death, looking after her children has been a great burden, especially the schizophrenic son. She felt his behaviour had driven her 20-year-old daughter out of the house and was now making life intolerable for L. She had found herself turning to L more and more for companionship. She received some of this in a relationship with a man friend who lived in the house but would not marry her, nor even enter a sexual relationship with her. She felt frustrated and thrown back onto her closeness with L. She was later able to see how this closeness must have been alarming yet gratifying to the boy, coloured as it was by her sexual longings.

It also became clear that there was a great concern about illness in the family, both mental and physical. Besides the patient's brother, a paternal aunt had died in a psychiatric hospital. There was also the issue of haemophilia as a familial disease. The mother was able to bring out her concern about L's earlier illness, but could not readily accept that this had led to over-protection on her part. She was, however, able to eject L from her bedroom. She tended to focus on the schizophrenic member of the family as being the 'cause' of all the difficulties, saying that he should move out of the home into a hostel. Attempts to do this had been made in the past by the mental welfare officer responsible for his care, but had not been successful because of his resistance to leaving home.

While L was in hospital he continued to be careful and meticulous with his possessions, anxious about not missing his evening bath and generally co-operative and easy to manage. Gradually his attachment to adult staff diminished and he entered more into the group life of the children. He had been put on a diet and medication to reduce weight which he gained after admission to hospital, and as he slimmed down he became more acceptable to the other active athletic boys; this clearly enhanced his self-esteem.

At this stage of his treatment attempts were made to strengthen the identification he had made with a particular male nurse. He became quite possessive of this man and through his support was able to learn to swim, and to stand up for himself in arguments with other boys. In occupational therapy he played out his feelings about the advent of his sister's new baby.

These were clearly ambivalent and after the hostile aspect emerged he was noted to be more clinging to his mother at weekends.

Psychotherapy did not prove easy with L. He was unable to express feelings with the authority ward figures, including his doctor, nor was he able to produce any fantasy material. For this reason his doctor saw him mainly on a supportive basis for short periods; the ward environment, particularly through the various staff members to whom he had become attached, was the basic therapeutic agent.

His mother wished him to return home and attend his former day school, and after a difficult start he was able to maintain regular attendance throughout the summer term, after discharge from hospital. This was despite a substantially unchanged home situation, as the schizophrenic brother remained in the house.

Comment. This case history illustrates another benefit of long-term inpatient treatment. Here the emphasis was on the therapeutic milieu and the deliberate use of certain individuals to whom the patient related. This was done as a matter of choice in preference to psycho therapy. The outcome was successful not only in terms of return to school but also in increased independence and academic achievement, though the patient remained vulnerable to stresses at home and was liable to regress to a dependent state.

The two cases described illustrate the following principles of inpatient treatment of school refusal:

1. Parents and other family members should be involved if possible; this helps prevent manipulation by the child.
2. Many difficulties are either avoided, or revealed so that they can be worked through, by careful preparation for admission. This may involve a pre-admission home visit.
3. The mutually hostile dependency of parent and child is a central problem to be dealt with. Threats and bargains may have formerly been the rule but must now be resisted.
4. The child should enter the unit school on the day of admission, preferably supported by his nurse. He often does well once settled in the school, to the benefit of his self-esteem.
5. Psychotherapy can be difficult, and milieu therapy is often the main treatment.
6. Liaison with the school the child is to attend after discharge is a prerequisite, whether the child goes out to it from the hospital for a period, or is discharged to start at the school, with support, subsequently.

Outcome of Inpatient Treatment of Neurotic Disorder

The problems involved in the study of the effects of treatment have been well discussed by Robins and O'Neal (1969). These include the need for a control group, so that a treated experimental group can be compared with an untreated control group having the same complaints, symptoms and diagnosis. Presence or absence of treatment, or the recommendation of a particular treatment, is never random so that selection variables enter into any study. These may depend on the beliefs of the physician recommending treatment as to the effectiveness of one or other treatment, the receptiveness of the child and family to the offer of treatment and their own belief in its effectiveness. Attitudes are known to vary with socio-economic status, indeed the treatment offered may be very much influenced by the social class of the family.

The paucity of studies of the outcome of outpatient treatment reflects the difficulties mentioned above and it is not surprising that no reliable study of the effectiveness of inpatient treatment has been carried out. It would be difficult to match different outpatient units and so compare the outcome of treatment with different therapeutic regimes. As indicated earlier, it is usually the more severely ill patients who are offered inpatient treatment, so that comparison groups are difficult to obtain. This might be done using the same model provided by studies of untreated outpatients off the waiting list, thus comparing matched groups of patients who were offered inpatient treatment, in which the one group did not accept but continued outpatient treatment. Difficulties would then arise from the different attitudes towards acceptance of treatment and the fact that, in those families where the offer of inpatient treatment was refused, the variable of pathogenic family interaction with the child at home might continue to operate in a way which did not apply to the child in hospital. It seems unlikely that a completely satisfactory design would ever be achieved, but this does not lessen the need for more follow-up studies of the outcome of residential treatment along the lines of those carried out by Warren (1965a and b) and Weiss and Burke (1967) in adolescents.

During a three-year period, including nine months during which only half the beds were occupied because of rebuilding, 22 children finally diagnosed as having neurotic disorder were admitted as inpatients to the children's department of the Maudsley Hospital. There were twelve boys and ten girls, age range 5 to 13 years, with a mean age of 10·5 years. Of these, eight children were admitted because of school refusal, five girls and three boys with an age range of 7½ years (mean age 11 years). The period of stay in hospital for the whole group of children (22) ranged from 10 days to 17 months with a mean of three months. The longest period spent in hospital was by a girl with school refusal, with severe food refusal and vomiting which was thought to be incipient anorexia nervosa. Of the whole group, two children were recommended for special education as maladjusted pupils, one at a residential and the other at a day school.

CHAPTER FIVE

Inpatient Treatment of Children with Psychosomatic Disorders

Philip Pinkerton

Throughout the whole field of clinical child psychiatry, no group of cases provides more scope for inter-disciplinary liaison than children with psychosomatic disorder, yet their treatment varies inordinately from one centre to another, especially in respect of inpatient provision. Here, the range extends from a narrowly symptomatic approach, essentially short-term in scope, to fully comprehensive programmes embracing the whole child and his family relationships.

Essentially, within a given unit, the plan of treatment is determined by three main factors: the professional orientation of the therapeutic team; its interpretation of what constitutes a psychosomatic disorder; and the inpatient facilities available to translate that concept into appropriate therapeutic action.

Relevant Diagnostic Categories

Controversy still persists about the designation of psychosomatic disorder. In one sense, all cases might be said to qualify, although this relates more to management approach than to actual nature of the presenting problem (Pinkerton, 1965). In a stricter sense, so relatively few disorders merit the term as seriously to challenge their need for separate consideration at all.

In practice, at the interface of clinical responsibility between paediatrics and child psychiatry a large and commonly occurring group of problems does invite our attention. They share the common factor of physically presenting symptomatology and therefore tend to filter through paediatric channels of referral, yet their aetiology is neither uniform nor necessarily organic. A classifying procedure is therefore needed to permit a rational code of management for this heterogeneous group, and my experience has led me to suggest the following practical divisions (Pinkerton, 1971a; 1972b).

1. *Somatopsychic States*

Cases with a primary organic substrate, nevertheless yielding psychological sequelae. Common examples on the medical side are epilepsy, minimal brain damage, diabetes, cystic fibrosis, congenital cardiac lesions, thyroid dysfunction and various dermatological problems; on the surgical side, head injury, neurogenic megacolon, urogenital anomalies (including poor sex differentiation), meningomyelocoele and various orthopaedic lesions similarly qualify for inclusion.

2. *Primary Psychogenic Disorders with Somatic Presentation – 'Pseudosomatic'*

Cases in which, conversely, no organic lesion is demonstrable, despite the leading symptomatology. Enuresis is perhaps the most commonly occurring example, but others include encopresis, psychogenic megacolon, recurrent non-specific abdominal pain, obesity of the compensatory over-eating type, alopecia, trichotillomania, multiple habit spasm, and disturbance of primary habit formation, such as sleep disorder and feeding difficulty, with anorexia nervosa as potentially the most malignant of this entire group.

3. *Psychosomatic Disorders*

More specifically, those cases in which pathophysiology and psychopathology are so intimately interwoven that both components actively and concurrently contribute to the natural course of the disorder. Prime examples are bronchial asthma, infantile eczema, ulcerative colitis, spastic colon, peptic ulceration, migraine (including so-called abdominal migraine) and, more broadly, the periodic syndrome.

Each of these categories poses a separate therapeutic challenge, but certain principles are common to all three in respect of residential rehabilitation.

Indications for Inpatient Assessment

Admission to hospital where special unit facilities exist serves three interrelated functions, none of which can readily be exercised on an outpatient basis. These are: diagnostic refinement or clarification of the presenting problem; introduction to a therapeutic community setting; and the concrete demonstration of response to that milieu.

Diagnostic Clarification

In the field of psychosomatic disorder the presenting problem is often ill-defined and difficult to evaluate. Indeed, this is commonly the reason for referral from an established paediatric service. Characteristic examples include the child with atypical epileptiform attacks; the patient with bizarre orthopaedic gait; vaguely localised 'rheumatic' pain; so-called 'tension headaches'; recurrent abdominal pain and sickness; subjective complaints of locomotor weakness, vague dysphagia or recurrent episodic dyspnoea; atypical sleep disturbance; cryptic symptoms of urogenital dysfunction; or the unaccountable failure of a well-established syndrome to respond to standard therapeutic practice – a frequent feature of diabetes, asthma, eczema or cystic fibrosis.

Head injury is a notorious example, expecially if the issue of compensation is still unresolved, as in, say, a road traffic accident. Here it may be impossible to assess the contribution of organic cerebral changes as opposed to avowed disturbance of function, without a period of inpatient observation. Additionally, the unit routine may itself exert a stabilising effect on behaviour, allowing the problem to be seen in broader perspective, with reassurance, where appropriate, to both family and referring legal agency.

Unhappily, this is still an area of paediatrics less well charted than most in terms of aetiology and rational treatment, so that too many patients and their parents continue to feel perplexed by the persistence of symptoms, where more unequivocal guidance could well resolve these doubts and vague recriminations. In such cases, there is an authority and finality about assurance based upon 'living with' the child which cannot be matched by outpatient appraisal, however meticulous and exhaustive. 'You've never actually seen him in one of his attacks, doctor', is an accusation otherwise difficult to refute.

The Therapeutic Milieu

Having once witnessed and evaluated 'an attack' at first-hand, and so established its credibility, the unit team can now proceed to study the child in greater depth as a person, not just as a patient, and try to understand the personal significance for him and for his family of his particular illness, i.e. to extend the scope of assessment to include the whole field of psychodynamic interrelationship.

In no circumstances an easy task, this is again more effectively achieved through 'living with' the child than through repeated (and, of necessity, prolonged) outpatient attendance. In the first place, admission often provides a much-needed period of respite from mounting reciprocal tensions within the home, and, secondly, it affords a fresh look at the problem by child and family alike, without critical overtones, in what seems a 'neutral' setting. In practice, however, the unit milieu is more subtly positive than strictly neutral, because it deliberately fosters group support and so invites the patient's confidence, thereby creating the climate for his ultimate rehabilitation.

The Concrete Demonstration

Nevertheless, initially we may have to recognise and overcome unsuspected patterns of resistance derived from previous paediatric encounters. One reason for this is persisting suspicion about 'psychiatric' referral; but the converse also applies, in that psychosomatic cases are still too often referred only when they fail to respond to traditional treatment measures. It follows, therefore, that even when pertinent psychopathology is identified, the individuals concerned may only be induced to shift their orientation after demonstrable therapeutic movement – most convincingly achieved through admission. Of particular value in this context is the boost to personal morale in chronic enuresis, encopresis, neurodermatitis and similarly demoralising disorders when even the smallest break is achieved in previously unremitting symptoms.

A brief extract drawn from each of the three main diagnostic categories should serve to illustrate the principles involved.

> *The somatopsychic model.* David N, aged 13, had an eight-year history of diabetes mellitus, poorly stabilised in the past two years, with frequent hospital admissions to adjust insulin dosage. His widowed mother had remarried three years previously, with mutual difficulties in adjustment between patient, stepfather and younger stepsister. David became aggrieved, rebellious and no longer co-operative in diabetic hygiene. Ultimate stabilisation on much-reduced insulin was only achieved after prolonged inpatient sojourn to permit emotional ventilation and personal reorientation.

> *The pseudosomatic model.* Marie S, aged 11, had six months' history of severe trichotillomania, resulting in marked patchy baldness. Her parents were unable to accept a non-organic, self-induced basis of lesion. The patient is the youngest and least intelligent of three siblings, the older two being both of grammar school status. Despite diligent coaching, Marie had failed the senior school entrance examination the previous year. The parental reaction was carping and unsympathetic.

> *The psychosomatic model.* Martin B, aged 10, had a six-year history of bronchial asthma, involving repeated absence from school, frequent outpatient attendance and increasing short-stay admissions to hospital. There was a background of covert marital disharmony with maternal trend to 'live through' the child, as a substitute for emotional aridity in the marriage. The maternal attitude was over-possessive and over-concerned; the paternal attitude, apathetic and disinterested.

In the case of David, the diabetic, the parents' awareness of their own involvement only emerged when the upward trend of insulin dosage began to be reversed, signifying for them unequivocal improvement. The same held true for David himself – the more successful the unit's regime in controlling his diabetes, the more accessible he became as a person and the greater his willingness to concede and ventilate his personal problems. A critical element in 'opening up' this case may well have been the break from home, the escape from mutual recrimination and the prospect of a fresh start without loss of face. Sometimes the timing of these developments can be crucial.

Similarly, in Marie's case, no breakthrough in rapport would have been even remotely possible with these hostile parents until visible evidence was presented to them of successful regrowth of her hair (significantly without recourse to either drug or local therapy). Marie herself, on the other hand, immediately sensed the unit's non-critical attitude (the therapeutic milieu) and thereupon 'thawed' perceptibly long before the first downy regrowth had begun to grace her bald scalp. No doubt, in her case too, the separation itself contributed to the overall therapeutic benefit by allowing both factions to stand back and view the problem more objectively.

In Martin's case, symptomatic remission had previously been achieved, but never sustained and always associated with vigorous upgrading of treatment. No attempt had been made to link the problem either with prevailing parental attitude or with the patient's self-attitude, nor would this have been practical while continuing to focus on pharmacotherapy alone. Only after a convincing period of inpatient stabilisation, on reduced drug dosage despite an active programme of recreation, did the first glimmerings of maternal insight begin to appear, coincident with early signs of emotional emancipation in Martin himself.

Once again, the unit's success was firmly based upon its function of diagnostic refinement, involving here the routine measurement of ventilatory function so that Martin's pulmonary potential could be accurately assessed and the degree to which he could be safely challenged precisely fixed (Pinkerton, 1972a). Setting these limits breeds confidence within the team, communicated in turn to both patient and parents, thereby initiating a chain reaction of progressive therapeutic response.

This kind of impact, unequivocal and self-evident, is rarely possible with entrenched problems on other than a residential basis because outpatient attendance, even as a daily routine, is too gradual and fragmented a process to achieve the necessary 'break-through' in therapeutic momentum, at least initially. Ultimately, of course, a phased return to outpatient surveillance is the optimum plan of action.

Contra-indications to Admission

Admission to hospital, however, is not without potential hazards. Much depends on the age of the child and upon his level of emotional maturity. As a general rule, admission below the age of four is to be avoided except for very limited periods and specific diagnostic purposes, unless the mother can accompany the child without detriment to other members of her family. Indeed, positive value can accrue from their combined admission, but this requires very careful planning and even more meticulous handling. It is vital, for example, to have suitably furnished accommodation set aside and specifically designated for this purpose, so that the mother is not made to feel an outcast and a nuisance among the professional personnel on the unit.

> Jennifer M, when referred at 20 months, had already required two emergency admissions for status asthmaticus. Her mother, a young divorcee, had previously lost a baby through meningitis and was now feeling a total failure both as wife and mother. It took five months of joint rehabilitation on the unit to restore maternal self-confidence, overcome the mother's fears of asthma and teach her to be more competent in routine nursing management, before Jennifer could safely be discharged to outpatient care; however, the exercise was felt to be potentially life-saving and, as such, to merit the complex arrangements involved.

However, even with the most elaborate precautions, great care must still be exercised to avoid the impression, with children of any age, that they are being 'sent away' by rejecting parents. We are not always fully briefed about what may have been said to the intending patient by way of explanation. It is therefore wise to counter any possible misunderstanding by reviewing in advance, with the child himself, the reasons for his admission, reinforced wherever possible by a preliminary visit to the unit. In this way, unfounded fears are more readily allayed and positive rapport more readily established with which to initiate the therapeutic process.

Aside from general guidelines governing intake procedure, there are certain situations in which it is hazardous to contemplate admission, at least beyond a strictly limited objective. These special 'at risk' circumstances will emerge in the course of more detailed examination of the unit's function (page 162).

Unit Organisation

'He's in and out (of hospital) by the minute, but we're no nearer understanding the problem', is a frequent *cri de cœur* of parents perplexed by the shortcomings of treating the disease rather than the child with the disease.

> 'There is a world of difference between . . . resolving an asthmatic attack, stabilising diabetic imbalance, re-imposing drug control in epilepsy, or checking a bleeding episode in ulcerative colitis, with resulting phasic remission in the short term – and the programme of exploring in depth the complex psychosocial background to each case, so that, over and above symptomatic treatment, we can unravel the factors possibly contributing to relapse and thereby avert rather than resolve further episodes.' (Pinkerton, 1972b).

To achieve this breadth of approach calls for special organisation within the unit and specialised skills on the part of its staff.

Paediatric Orientation

Familiarity with paediatric practice is the first of these prerequisites. If, hitherto, in the quest for a rational treatment approach to psychosomatic disorder, emotional factors have been ignored by the more conservative paediatricians, because they preferred the security of their organic preserves, the psychiatric contribution to some extent has been no less biased through its emphasis upon psychoanalytic symbolism to the preclusion of disordered physiology. Somewhere between these two extremes lies the balanced and broadly-based philosophy on which management, to be effective, must be founded; yet in the early days of the child-guidance movement many clinics were exhorted to 'exclude the organic' as a necessary prelude to orthodox psychotherapy, whereas in fact the exact opposite applies – the need to *include* the 'organic' along with all the other aspects of the child in his school and family setting if we are to arrive at a meaningful formulation of the problem.

This means, in practice, a working knowledge by unit staff of routine paediatric procedures ranging from dietetic and insulin control of the diabetic subject to drug control of his epileptic counter-part; from the pulmonary hygiene of the asthmatic, including postural drainage and routine ventilatory function tests, to the complicated skin hygiene of the eczematous child; from the toilet regimes of children with encopresis, psychogenic megacolon or ulcerative colitis, to the restoration of electrolyte balance in severe abdominal migraine or cyclical vomiting; from the persuasive technique of dietary restriction in obesity, to the equally persuasive skill of dietary supplementation in anorexic children; and from the emergency intravenous therapy of status asthmaticus, to the equal emergency of status epilepticus.

Equipotent with these technical skills is the exercise of clinical acumen with which to recognise the imminence of hypoglycaemia in the uncontrolled diabetic, the cyanotic portent of lowered ventilatory reserve in the severe asthmatic, the sudden pallor of a bleeding episode in peptic or colitic ulceration, or the fleeting alteration in behaviour signifying an atypical ictal attack. Shrewd observation therefore must be coupled with sophisticated knowledge in the paediatric aspects of unit management and, predictably, nurses recruited from the sick children's register find themselves more readily at home in this area than staff trained primarily as mental nurses, who require a preliminary period of in-service orientation for their successful adaptation to psychosomatic work.

Conversely, the psychiatric nurse is usually more practised in the skills of relationship therapy, i.e. the matrix within which these paediatric procedures are carried out. There is therefore scope for both backgrounds of training in the optimum credentials for nursing staff seconded to the unit.

Relationship Therapy

Traditional paediatric policy favours early and direct therapeutic action, whereas the psychosomatic approach stresses the value of extended observation to allow the problem to crystallise before finite intervention. Winnicott (1953) has commented on this fundamental difference between the disciplines of paediatrics and child psychiatry (a shift in orientation calling for equivalent change in outlook by the staff concerned). This means the need henceforth to be involved with the child, to feel part of his world, win his confidence, share his secret fears and fantasies, and thus reach a depth of understanding with him, short of which he cannot be helped to ventilate his problems or see them in the fresh perspective necessary for their resolution.

Unit Structure – Staff/Patient Ratio

All this takes time and tolerance far in excess of standard nursing schedules, to achieve which calls for radical modification both in staffing structure and case complement, in line with every other inpatient unit, whatever the type of child predominantly catered for psychotherapeutically. There must be, for example, a greatly augmented ratio of nursing staff to patients, and of these the more senior grades should be permanently seconded to the unit to form its staffing nucleus and so preserve continuity. Similarly, the case intake must be rigorously restricted to between 20 and 25 children, because beyond this it is impracticable to preserve group cohesion.

Personal Reorientation

Of even greater import, the practice of sympathetic detachment, traditionally enjoined upon the nurse, must yield to a closer empathetic bond, at once more emotionally demanding and more subjectively rewarding through the enhanced quality of the relationship; yet this must be achieved without loss of objectivity or of professional judgement. Understandably, this calls for a searching reappraisal of personal attitudes and values on the part of each staff member, which, though challenging and even threatening, is none the less vital to the corporate identity of the unit. Essentially, this is the difference between 'doing things to' the patient and 'being with' the patient (Wolff, 1971).

To be successful and to be sustained, this degree of personal readjustment by individual nurses must be mutually reinforced through the medium of the therapeutic team approach. There is no place in this system for hierarchical rigidity. On the contrary, the doctor, nurse, social-worker and psychologist, in conjunction with the teaching staff of the affiliated hospital school, must not only pool their respective resources so that all keep abreast of each child's individual progress, but must also ensure that whoever is approached by parent or patient, the briefing is the same and parent counselling is therefore consistent.

Unquestionably, the key to success in such a cohesive ward structure is the unit sister, serving as liaison officer within the team, so that however meticulous the conferencing of cases, however regular the seminars and however rigorous the programme of in-service indoctrination for each new member of staff, it is essentially the departmental sister who collates the information and translates into practice the unit's basic philosophy.

The Unit Philosophy

Central to this philosophy, to paraphrase a Hippocratic aphorism, is the principle that knowing the child who has the disease is as important as knowing the disease the child has; plus, in this field, a knowledge of relationships within that child's family.

Potential Models of Interrelationship

(a) *The somatopsychic sequence.* A primary organic lesion may give rise to disordered behaviour or emotional disturbance, on the basis of three main situations:

(i) The lesion itself may 'release' deviant behaviour, as in head injury, through disinhibition, or as in juvenile hypothyroidism, presenting with depression, or as in post-pubertal hyperthyroidism, masquerading as morbid anxiety. All these indeed may yield cognitive sequelae: in cerebral trauma, through genuine intellectual deficit; in myxoedema, through sluggishness in mental function; in thyrotoxicosis, through restlessness and impaired concentration.

Escape from drug control or excessive drug dosage in epilepsy may equally lead to falling-off in intellectual performance, as may the cryptic effects of unsuspected and untreated petit mal. Whatever the cause of this functional impairment, the child's emotional state tends secondarily to be affected, as does the parental reaction.

The pattern of clinical symptomatology in neuro-epileptic disorder is known to be influenced by the psychosocial setting in which it occurs (Rutter *et al.*, 1971). For example, the product of a 'broken home' situation, with its attendant insecurity and deprivation, often reacts with aggressive 'acting-out' behaviour, which tends to be enhanced and exaggerated by any subsequent intercurrent lesion involving brain damage. Pond (1961) has emphasised substantially the same point, namely, that disinhibiting lesions tend to evoke conduct which caricatures pre-existing personality traits.

However, aside from such determinants of behavioural reaction, more general emotional factors also merit consideration under two further headings – the patient's own responses, and those of his parents.

(ii) Acceptance *v.* non-acceptance: if realistic acceptance by the child of irreducible handicap or disorder is taken as his optimum reaction, pathology of attitude may present in one of two main forms: over-acceptance of the lesion, i.e. 'giving in' or 'caving in' with a trend to invalidism or hypochondriasis (illness-orientation); or non-acceptance of disability (expressed as revolt or rebellion) based on refusal to come to terms with demonstrable inconvenience or limitation. Somewhere between these two extremes there is also the tendency to manipulate handicap for purposes of secondary 'gain'.

Robert S, a sensitive, vulnerable boy, aged 12, illustrates the trend to invalidism. Born with minimal spasticity, only marginally affecting speech and motor co-ordination, he nevertheless failed to withstand robust normal schooling beyond the infant grade, repeatedly opting out of playground games and PE, finding difficulty in mixing, and settling at age 7 only after transfer to day special school. Fresh problems, however, have arisen through lack of open-air school accommodation in the senior grade, so once again, at 11 plus, he is failing to cope because of his over-accepting outlook.

By contrast, Warren T, a pugnacious 13-year-old, plagued with cystic fibrosis, exemplifies the opposite trend of bitter resentment against his condition, erupting into aggressive behaviour, flagrant flouting of authority and deliberate sabotaging of his treatment regime, so that he deteriorates alarmingly until admitted for rehabilitation in personal outlook as well as pulmonary hygiene (Pinkerton, 1969).

(iii) Parental attitude: theoretically a separate issue, this can only be evaluated, in practice, in relation to the patient's viewpoint. In the same way, the most useful criterion of assessment (among many potential parameters) is the degree to which parents can realistically accept their child's disability, and indeed the child himself, because of his handicap.

In Robert's case, his elderly parents were excessively protective of this, their youngest child, although repeatedly assured that his spasticity was not of serious import. Their over-acceptance of his handicap simply reinforced his own excessive dependence, and thus served to perpetuate rather than counteract his ill-adjustment. Conversely, in Warren's case, the parents' attitude, though eminently realistic and justifiably concerned, still clashed with his teenage revolt, in a constant conflict of wills over the management of his cystic fibrosis. In yet a third example, a mild spastic reminiscent of Robert S, the father's attitude in particular was abrasively rejective of this 'biologically inferior specimen' of whom somehow he felt ashamed and whom he instinctively wished to disown. The impact on this child, a boy equally as sensitive as Robert, was quite disastrous emotionally.

In all three cases, a period of inpatient reappraisal proved an essential prerequisite to rehabilitation – first by helping to define and, subsequently, to re-align the attitudes of patient and parents alike, although in each case the therapeutic indications were quite different. Similarly, when children are suspected of manipulating their disability, thereby holding parents to emotional ransom, a short period of inpatient observation often helps to clarify the real extent of handicap, and so expose convincingly any functional overlay as a first step towards promoting parental confidence in future management.

(b) *The pseudosomatic case.* Identical considerations apply when the lesion is primarily psychogenic, but evokes a somatic channel of expression – the converse aetiological sequence. Here, pathology of parental attitude antedates the presenting problem, but similarly ranges from over-involvement on the one hand (excessively positive affect) to rejection, or at the very least non-involvement, on the other (excessively negative affect), with a corresponding spectrum of reaction in the child.

Sheila R, an adopted child aged 9, became withdrawn and morose, relapsed into bed-wetting, and developed patchy, unsightly alopecia fifteen months after her mother gave birth unexpectedly to a baby boy, henceforth over-valued by the entire family circle at Sheila's expense. Her sense of abandonment, though quite unwitting on the parents' part, was none the less acute and overwhelming (non-acceptance of self).

Ian D, on the other hand, the surviving twin of a difficult premature birth, developed a febrile illness at age 6, suspected to be acute rheumatism. Despite full recovery, with no residual carditis, a functional cardiac murmur was recorded at follow-up, involving discreet surveillance for twelve months before reassurance could be offered to his anxious mother. Nevertheless, she remained so oppressively protective that when referred at age 8, Ian showed classical signs of cardiac neurosis – vasovagal attacks, palpitation, excessive sweating and inframammary pain – requiring a further year of inpatient reorientation to resolve.

In each case, the manifest physical presentation was determined by antecedent emotional pathology, to which the child in turn reacted with complementary feeling tone. Once established, these respective attitudes tend to be mutually reinforcing, so that the more dependent and heart-conscious Ian becomes, the greater the degree of maternal over-concern, and, conversely, the more withdrawn and isolated Sheila becomes, the greater the contrast with her animated baby brother and the wider the resulting chasm emotionally with her parents. The process is essentially a circular one, tending to reciprocal perpetuation.

Considerable therapeutic effort is called for to reverse this trend, the crucial first stage frequently necessitating concrete demonstration of improvement in hospital. Complementary to interpretative therapy with the child, both on an individual and group basis, is liaison with parents in order to relate back to them the composite impressions of the unit team and so promote their increasing insight (Abercrombie, 1972).

In practice, and aside from the specialised role of the psychiatric social worker, the senior nurses on the unit, being the most frequently available staff members, are encouraged to liaise with parents during visiting, to compare notes with them about the behaviour of the child at home on leave at weekends, or during school holiday periods, and later to relate these impressions to the weekly staff conference. Parents are regularly invited to join these meetings, to exchange views with the staff, to ask supplementary questions, and thus to help clarify formulation of the problem and be guided in turn by the team's concerted findings.

Ultimately, there emerges from this dialogue an overall concept of the problem, on which a rational strategy of management can be planned and put into effect.

(c) *The psychosomatic case*. This same process of evaluation in depth, involving the same contributory factors, is equally applicable to psychosomatic disorder in its classical form, i.e. where organic and emotional components operate and interact concurrently. The role of inpatient assessment in these cases entails the precise analysis of that interaction.

Common to all truly psychosomatic disorders is the substrate of pathophysiological vulnerability which constitutes the basic lesion and which varies according to the target organ affected. In asthma, this is expressed as excessive lability of the bronchial system (Jones, 1966; Pinkerton, 1967); in migraine, as a neurovascular anomaly of the intracranial microcirculation; in eczema, as atopic hypersensitivity of epidermis; in spastic colon, as neurohumoral hyper-irritability of the large gut (Chaudhary and Truelove, 1961); while in peptic ulcer it is reflected in raised serum pepsinogen levels (Weiner *et al.*, 1957).

It follows, therefore, that no case of psychosomatic disease is ever entirely psychogenic, i.e. there is no such thing as 'psychological asthma' or 'psychogenic migraine'. On the other hand, emotional factors can profoundly influence the natural course, therapeutic responsiveness and prognosis of any disorder in this group, in a way quite different from the sequence in somatopsychic problems, e.g. epilepsy, diabetes or thyroid dysfunction.

Such lesions share an irreducible core of residual pathology irrespective of drug or hormonal control, whereas in, say, asthma, eczema or migraine there is a capricious variability in presentation, i.e. the patient may be asymptomatic for long periods without treatment. It is this mercurial element which complicates management and underlines the importance of psychodynamic exploration.

In this sector, no less than in the others, the parameter of acceptance versus non-acceptance, on the part of both patient and parents, is equally applicable (Pinkerton, 1971a). For example, in the case of Martin, the 10-year-old asthmatic with the background of marital disharmony (page 146), over-acceptance by the mother, prompted by her own emotional needs, is matched by Martin's own over-acceptance, each reinforcing the other to perpetuate an invalid state reversed only by inpatient treatment.

> James G, aged 7, severely handicapped from infancy, profoundly resents his asthma, minimises its effects and protests his fitness even when manifestly dyspnoeic and cyanotic. His father, a professional football coach, shares this non-acceptance as the negation of all his aspirations for the boy. Again, their attitudes reinforce each other in a mutual pact of denial of disability, fraught with danger because both tend to ignore legitimate signs of deterioration in the asthmatic state.

In Martin's case, inpatient reorientation was indicated to promote his emotional emancipation and to curtail his invalid outlook; in James's case, inpatient rehabilitation was equally pressing, but for precisely antithetical reasons, namely, to promote a more realistic attitude to his handicap by teaching him (and his father) to live with the asthma and within the limitations imposed by it.

The unpredictable character of clinical symptomatology in this group makes it imperative to institute a period of observation in as stable a setting as possible in order to permit a valid assessment of baseline function in the target organ. Armed with this data, the team can evaluate the severity of the lesion in physiological terms and so gauge more precisely the significance of psychodynamic factors in the individual case.

In this exercise, Martin emerged as a physiologically 'mild' asthmatic but with gross emotional overlay. Knowledge of his good potential made it possible to encourage more activity without endangering his ventilatory reserve; to reassure him and his mother regarding favourable prognosis; and to promote in both a more positive outlook, with the minimum of maintenance pharmacotherapy. Conversely, in James's case, once the severity of his asthma had been objectively confirmed through tests of ventilatory function, authoritative guidance could be given about management, aimed at curtailing avoidable challenge and maintaining maximum pharmacotherapy.

In both types of case, baseline assessment represents the very cornerstone of comprehensive evaluation; yet, to be valid, it can only be undertaken in an appropriate inpatient setting.

In practice, there are many combinations of pathophysiological status, parental attitude and personal orientation on the part of the patient, not only in asthma, but in other psychosomatic disorders. An over-protective maternal attitude, for example, may be resented by a child robust in outlook, if not in physiology, thereby leading to rebellion and non-co-operation in treatment. Equally, an immature child with invalid tendencies, spurned by an unsympathetic (non-accepting) parent, simply becomes more abjectly self-deprecating.

Alternatively, to be non-accepting, parental attitude need not be *actively* intolerant. For example, overt bronchospasm may just as readily be induced by neglect or denial of legitimate emotional needs in a susceptible subject (Pinkerton, 1971a); nor is this sequence by any means confined to asthma.

To unravel the complexities of each case obviously calls for appraisal in depth through the concerted efforts of a therapeutic team equipped with inpatient facilities. There is, however, no uniformity about this treatment. On the other hand, with increasing experience since the unit's inception in 1957, certain principles have evolved governing length of stay, indications for discharge, reasons for retention, transitional stages in rehabilitation, and alternative avenues of disposal, all of which merit consideration.

The Temporal Factor in Residential Treatment

The relevant nosological syndromes in the age range 5 to 15 accommodated within the unit for investigation and treatment during a representative three-year period (1969–71) are listed in Tables 5.1, 5.2 and 5.3. These also provide some indication of the time-scale involved, which extends from short-term assessment (one to three months), through the medium range of three to six, and six to twelve months, to the longer-stay category retained beyond twelve months. Each of these groups has its particular significance.

The Short-stay Case (one to three months)

The majority of these children are admitted primarily for one of three reasons; diagnostic clarification, the restoration of self-image, or the strictly limited objective. It takes perhaps two to three weeks for the average child to settle and accommodate within the unit before an assessment can be instituted with any validity. Thereafter, within the next month to six weeks, a clinical picture emerges which is progressively more meaningful and less equivocal.

Neuro-epileptic disorders (head injury, epileptic behaviour problems, developmental lag syndrome) head the list of cases to which this principle applies because they, in particular, often pose the need for clearer definition of the presenting problem; thus, among the relevant group of 14 children listed in Table 5.1, 50 per cent had been effectively discharged within the first three months, all of them having achieved an acceptable diagnostic formulation.

The same held true for three of the four orthopaedic lesions (Table 5.1) presenting with bizarre or unaccountable exaggeration of their functional disability. Equally, within the series of primarily psychogenic disorders (Table 5.2), the problem posed by recurrent abdominal pain could be satisfactorily resolved in half the cases within the first three months, and in three of the four cases respectively of 'rheumatic' myalgia and conversion hysteria encountered during this period (one hysterical blindness; two upper limb contractures).

On the other hand, while an encouraging response was also achieved within three months of admission both with enuretics and encopretics (almost 50 per cent in each group), this was attributable not so much to diagnostic clarification as to the undoubted boost to

Table 5.1 Somatopsychic disorders (1969–71)

Diagnostic category		*Boys*	*Girls*	*Duration of stay (months)* 1–3	3–6	6–12	12+	*Total*
Neuro-epileptic lesions including head injury and developmental immaturity	with reactive behaviour disorder	11	3	7	2	2	3	14
Cystic fibrosis	ditto	2	2	—	—	2	2	4
Diabetes mellitus	ditto	2	1	—	—	3	—	3
Urogenital anomalies	ditto	2	—	—	—	2	—	2
Orthopaedic lesions with secondary functional overlay		2	2	3	1	—	—	4
Hirschsprung's disease with secondary soiling		1	1	—	—	1	1	2
Hypothyroidism with associated affective disorder		—	1	—	—	1	—	1

personal morale, so vital in such wretched and disheartening conditions. Nevertheless, diagnostic considerations are still pertinent because not all children so affected respond rapidly in this way.

The rapidly remitting enuretic. Analysis of the enuretic sample in Table 5.2 reveals that the majority of rapid remitters were children (mostly boys) whose wetting pattern was now largely self-perpetuating. The original psychopathology, where it could be traced at all, seemed no longer so obtrusive, but in its place varying degrees of family revulsion had built up in response to the very chronicity of the syndrome and this of course had further undermined the patient's self-image. Breaking into this circular process had thus become a priority therapeutic target and the immediate indication for admission.

The rapidly remitting encopretic. Quite different considerations seem to apply, however, to the encopretic sample. Their number is smaller

Table 5.2 Psychogenic disorders with somatic presentation (1969–71)

Diagnostic category	*Boys*	*Girls*	*Duration of stay (months)* 1–3	3–6	6–12	12+	*Total*
Enuresis (including diurnal)	18	12	14	12	2	2	30
Encopresis (including psychogenic megacolon)	13	6	9	5	4	1	19
Recurrent abdominal pain	3	5	4	3	1	—	8
Obesity	3	4	1	6	—	—	7
Hysteria (motor and special sense)	3	1	3	—	1	—	4
Diffuse 'rheumatic' myalgia	1	3	3	1	—	—	4
Tics	2	1	—	3	—	—	3
Alopecia and trichotillomania	1	2	—	1	2	—	3
Anorexia (including anorexia nervosa)	2	2	—	—	3	1	4
Cardiac neurosis (effort syndrome)	2	—	—	—	2	—	2

but, among the subgroup achieving remission within three months, the pertinent factor was not so much compensation for mechanical chronicity as restoring morale in a particular type – the *regressive* soiler. Characteristically, this is the child who responds to threatening personal stress (divorce, re-marriage of widowed parent, unexpected birth of more favoured sibling, foster-home difficulties) with a regressive pattern of neuro-vegetative breakdown, as distinct from aggressive soiling or overflow incontinence secondary to bowel negativism, both of which take longer to respond (Pinkerton, 1965).

Broadly, these cases equate with at least some of the children in Anthony's group of discontinuous soilers (Anthony, 1957), i.e. the child who is clearly guilt-ridden and in conflict over his soiling. Reflating his ego thus becomes a priority measure in the overall programme of management, provided always that he does not misconstrue his admission as further evidence of parental rejection, and that the family dynamics have positive potential for fairly rapid realignment. In other words, the aura of mutual recrimination at home, with its deflating impact on the child's morale, must be judged sufficiently hostile in the short term as to outweigh the dangers of further alienation of patient from parent, which could result from planned admission.

Nor does this principle apply only to soiling: it is equally applicable to any situation in which parental aura is assessed as actively non-accepting, even critical, perhaps as much of the child as of his disorder, and especially if the patient himself is equally intolerant of his condition. A classical example is the childhood asthmatic, significantly handicapped in pathophysiological terms, yet deliberately disregarding danger signals and even refusing medication (if he can) because he wants to prove that he is not so very different from other children, and because he wants to retain the parental approval he feels himself otherwise in danger of forfeiting through being labelled 'inferior' or 'damaged' biologically (Pinkerton, 1972c).

It is, of course, essential in all such cases to establish in the first instance a stable and monitored routine within the residential setting, as a baseline upon which to assess optimum ventilatory function, optimum insulin needs, basic thyroid medication, or whatever the particular case dictates. This indication is obviously the greater where prior conflict at home has contributed to physiological flux and so inflated insulin requirements, depressed ventilatory function, or, for instance, increased acidity and pepsin production in the child with gastric ulcer.

In any case, removing the child temporarily from the aura of domestic tension provides a beneficial period of mutual respite. But if, in the process, we successfully demonstrate physiological improvement in hospital without increase in medication (perhaps despite reducing medication), we must be careful to ensure that this is not interpreted by already critical parents as a reflection on them, i.e. on their adequacy of home management (Pinkerton, 1971a). While the concrete demonstration is often necessary, both for the patient to experience and for his parents to observe, before any significant shift can be achieved in established pathology of attitude, the exercise should be approached with great caution in order to avoid any implication of challenge. In particular, the situation is to be avoided in which parents can upbraid their child for failing to achieve at home the level of betterment demonstrated in hospital, so prompting him to deny that he is as ill as he really is (perhaps to a dangerous degree), or, alternatively, inducing him to play them off against the hospital as a manipulative manoeuvre, with equally hazardous consequences.

The term 'parentectomy', coined by Peshkin (1930), is often taken to embrace any situation where the child benefits by being away from his parents; but it is a misleading concept because it can be all too readily over-simplified and so applied without the great discrimination it deserves (Pinkerton, 1971b). The lesson to be drawn for the child at risk is that inpatient rehabilitation, where it is indicated,

Table 5.3 Psychosomatic disorders (1969–71)

			Duration of stay (months)				
Diagnostic category	*Boys*	*Girls*	*1–3*	*3–6*	*6–12*	*12+*	*Total*
Asthma	21	11	4	7	8	13	32
Asthma and eczema	4	4	2	3	1	2	8
Periodic syndrome including abdominal migraine and cyclical vomiting	5	1	1	2	2	1	6
Peptic ulcer	1	2	—	—	3	—	3
Ulcerative colitis	2	1	—	—	—	3	3

should be embarked upon with the strictly limited objective in mind, balancing one set of needs (the practical demonstration, the 'breathing space', the clarification of physiological status) against the other – the need to avoid challenge. Among the 40 children with asthma, or with asthma and eczema, listed in Table 5.3, while the great majority merited an extensive sojourn for a variety of reasons yet to be discussed, a significant minority (15 per cent) were by design returned to outpatient or daypatient care within three months, not because they were any the less significantly affected, but because for them it was felt particularly expedient to carry through the policy of limited objective, and especially so for the younger age group of 5 to 7.

Similar considerations apply to diabetic children, but in their case eventual discharge may well be delayed by difficulties encountered in stabilising insulin dosage.

The Medium-term Case (three to twelve months)

Organic considerations. Technical reasons concerned with medical or surgical re-ablement may in fact dictate the length of stay involved and prolong it considerably. This was certainly so (Table 5.1) with the diabetic children under treatment in the unit and also with the fibrocystic cases, the hypothyroid girl, several of the epileptic children and those with neurogenic megacolon or urogenital anomaly. An equivalent situation pertained in peptic ulcer and ulcerative colitis (Table 5.3) and in anorexia nervosa (Table 5.2). In most of these conditions, relatively prolonged periods of inpatient rehabilitation were required, extending to twelve months and even beyond.

Psychopathological considerations. Similarly, within the psychogenic series, certain syndromes stand out as requiring longer than average periods of residential re-ablement. These include cases of alopecia, which seem relatively slow to respond, anorexic problems with a negativistic basis, cases of effort syndrome or cardiac neurosis, and the group of encopretic children in whom soiling represents either an aggressive response, or an overflow phenomenon secondary to negativistic retention of faeces. Cases of bowel negativism seem especially refractory, the more so when they are referred at an already chronic stage, tending then to be associated with loss of tone in the terminal colon tantamount to psychogenic megacolon (Pinkerton, 1958). These, in particular, may well take twelve months, or even longer, to rehabilitate as inpatients.

Physiological v. *psychological factors.* Among the asthmatic and eczematous children, about half qualify as medium-term cases, a proportion achieving discharge within six months, although others require manifestly longer to stabilise within the unit. It should be borne in mind that most of these cases have been referred on the basis of their refractory response to standard treatment procedures (including steroid resistance) and so tend to be both long-standing and seriously handicapped in physiological terms. As such, they cannot be taken as representative of the asthmatic population as a whole.

With this reservation, those relatively more impaired in ventilatory function, or with more resistant skin lesions, will obviously be retained for longer periods, while relatively lesser degrees of pathophysiological involvement will clearly qualify for earlier discharge, provided that relevant psychopathology has been successfully identified and the foundations laid for its rehabilitative treatment.

Hospital ward v. *special unit.* Creak (1971) has referred to the difficulties involved in treating the asthmatic child within the restricted setting of a teaching-hospital ward, where the emphasis must necessarily be focussed on the target organ, with remedial measures in keeping. The value of a unit organised and equipped to offer comprehensive facilities is that over and above a purely medical, physiotherapeutic and pharmaceutical approach, there is physical scope for the child to move around as freely as his condition permits, to go to school on the hospital site, or even to attend an outside school, to test his exercise tolerance by exploring the hospital grounds at will, and yet still to be supervised throughout this range of activities by trained nursing personnel. One inevitable consequence is the shift in emphasis from illness-orientation to fitness-orientation – a curious paradox within a hospital setting, but nevertheless central to the readjustment in outlook being engineered for the child.

With such extended facilities at his disposal, plus regularly organised outside trips and educational visits, any misgivings about mechanical incarceration are rapidly dispelled and even a span of several months passes quickly, the more so in that weekend leave at home is a planned feature of the unit system. This not only permits continuing contact with home and family, but allows the staff to gauge the child's reaction at successive stages to re-exposure on the domestic front, and so to determine the optimum point at which to consider his discharge. From the parents' viewpoint, it provides them with a regular check on progress, which they can assess more realistically within their own home, thus making it easier to convince them in pragmatic terms that improvement, once begun, is actually taking place. This in turn leads on to considering with them *why* it is taking place and how it may be consolidated.

Mean duration of inpatient stay. The whole process of psychotherapeutic rehabilitation with parents and child tends to encompass, on average, two terms of hospital school; each is of approximately ten weeks' duration so that, with a holiday period intervening, the usual time-scale involved is perhaps four to six months. Certainly, this applies to most categories of psychogenic disorder with pertinent psychopathology (Table 5.2), e.g. the obesity cases, the tics, almost

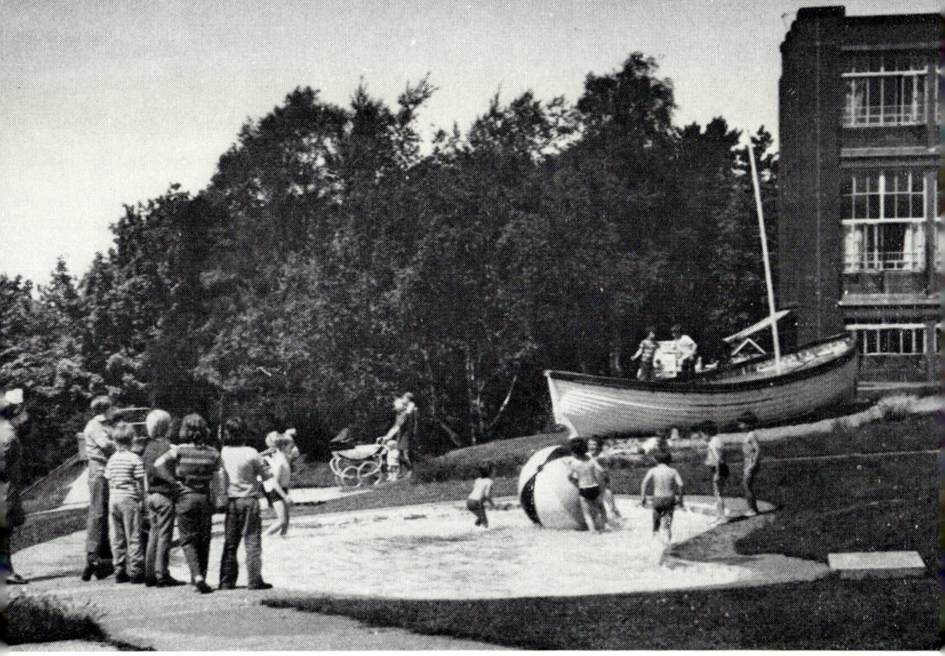

Fig. 5.1

The Royal Liverpool Children's Hospital, Heswall: the psychiatric unit playground

Fig. 5.2

The Royal Liverpool Children's Hospital, Heswall: the psychiatric unit team in conference

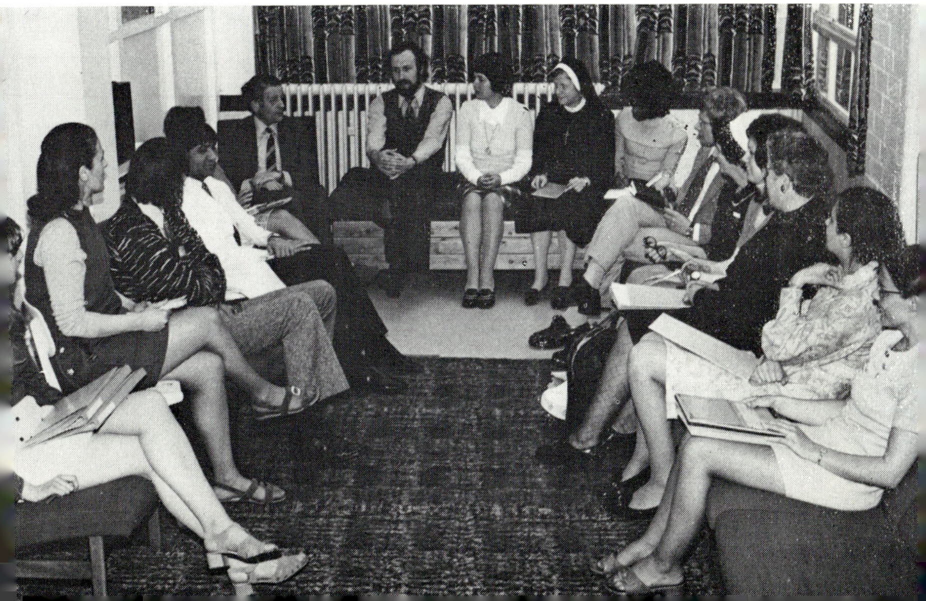

half the children with recurrent abdominal pain and some 40 per cent of the enuretic sample. In fact, for the 'psychosomatic' group as a whole, four to six months represents the statistical mean for inpatient treatment.

Symptomatic v. *'psychosomatic' management.* The efficacy of this approach is difficult to demonstrate convincingly because of the problem of establishing satisfactory controls. Nevertheless, by matching two small groups of asthmatic children for degree of disability and then allotting them alternately to comparable unit regimes, each with meticulous paediatric management, but exposing only *one* of the groups (parents as well as patients) to the rehabilitative team approach, it proved possible to show that, while both groups enjoyed virtual freedom from attacks during their stay in hospital, the children exposed to 'whole patient' therapy held up after discharge for significantly longer periods than their unexposed controls, without recourse to readmission on anything like the same scale. Clearly, therefore, the unit, to be successful, must provide more than standard symptomatic measures, however comprehensive these are in themselves (Pinkerton, 1967). (See Figure 5.3.)

Two considerations emerge from this discussion. The first is the need for continuing supportive therapy with the child and his family, sometimes for considerable periods after discharge in order to consolidate the rehabilitation begun on an inpatient basis. Aside from the pilot experiment described above, experience has shown a discouraging trend towards relapse, especially in psychosomatic disorders, if no such follow-up takes place; conversely, supportive contact does seem to constitute a positive stabilising influence.

The second consideration, the obverse in a sense, is that in certain circumstances this approach does not achieve the desired effect, however meticulously conducted. There are particular reasons for its failure and they call for modifications in the treatment formula. These are in fact the cases which constitute the long-stay group.

The Long-stay Case (over twelve months)

Of all the 'psychosomatic' cases accommodated in the unit during the three-year period under review, one child in six required to be retained for longer than a year, and in some instances considerably longer. Three main reasons could be adduced for this policy: severity

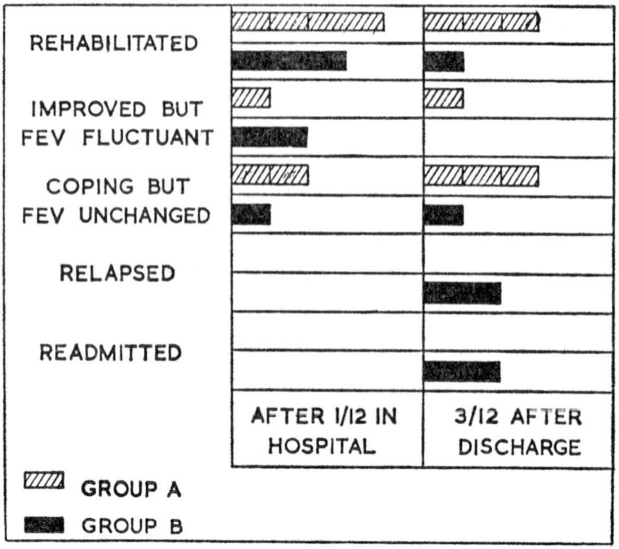

Fig. 5.3
Therapeutic progress of the subgroups
Group A – treated group   Group B – controls
FEV – forced expiratory volume
(Reprinted from the *Journal of Psychosomatic Research*, **11**, 11, 1967)

of pathophysiological state, refractory psychopathology, or adversity of personal life circumstances.

(i) *Pathophysiological involvement.* More than half this important minority were asthmatics, or cases of asthma-eczema syndrome, between them representing the most commonly occurring truly psychosomatic disorder. They also constitute the most tantalising with regard to treatment because, despite vigorous therapeutic measures, a proportion of them simply fail to achieve, or at least to maintain, the level of stabilisation necessary to cope with day-to-day stresses beyond the routine of the unit. They go home at weekends and for short holiday periods but, in essence, they must become reconciled to an inpatient sojourn of two, three, or even more, years.

(ii) *Refractory psychopathology.* In almost every one of these cases, however, serious physiological impairment is not the only factor involved. Closer analysis rarely fails to uncover covert psychopathology either in the patient himself or in the attitude of his parents, militating against stabilisation. So consistently, in fact, does this association occur (Pinkerton, 1972a) that it warrants enunciation as a general principle: in significantly handicapped asthmatic children, persistent failure of response to radical therapy, including generous steroid medication, should always evoke the suspicion of concurrent psychopathology, usually non-accepting in character and more often covert than overt.

It is this combination of pernicious emotional pathology with significant organic pathology which makes for resistant clinical pattern (in ulcerative colitis, eczema or peptic ulcer, no less than in asthma) and so necessitates extended stay in hospital.

On occasion, with persistent psychotherapy, it is possible to reverse pathology of attitude, promote realistic acceptance of irreducible handicap, and re-establish a sufficiently positive outlook to withstand the frustrations, discouragement, apprehension and sense of impotence inseparable from any chronic disorder of uncertain prognosis.

Group therapy with parents, if a suitable nucleus can be established, may provide just the right approach to re-education, but it must be persevered with for long periods and at regular intervals if it is to have a sustained effect. The whole exercise, in fact, should be conducted as a group endeavour, involving family doctor, school doctor, local school staff and hospital team, with the corporate aim of easing the child out of hospital and, thereafter, keeping him out. More often, however, such re-ablement proves impracticable because either the child or his parents remain inaccessible to rehabilitative therapy, so that if retention in hospital is not to be perpetuated some alternative provision must be found.

(iii) *Adversity of personal life circumstances.* A third contingency contributing to prolongation of stay is the eroding of personal security caused by major disruption of family ties. Nothing can be more devastating, especially for the younger child, so that when a case presents in which symptomatic severity seems sharply at variance with the degree of physiological impairment anticipated, adversity of personal life circumstances should be suspected as a possible explanation of the discrepancy. This is taken to include the child disadvantaged through parental alcoholism, psychopathy, frank cruelty, neglect or serious over-crowding; or emotionally deprived through divorce, desertion or separation, without compensatory substitute provision. Asthmatic cases are particularly vulnerable to sociopathology of this kind because of their labile bronchial system (Pinkerton, 1970), but sociopathic stress may equally potentiate other syndromes, notably recurrent non-specific abdominal pain, conversion hysteria and bizarre 'epileptic' patterns, and including enuresis and encopresis and even, on occasion, migraine and ulcerative colitis.

In bronchial asthma, the precise assessment of ventilatory function through the medium of spirometry (not a difficult technical procedure) permits the reliable monitoring of clinical state to an extent unequalled in any comparable disorder. It is relatively simple, therefore, to gauge whether the presenting symptoms are commensurate with, or disproportionate to, the known level of physiological severity.

When, in circumstances of intact ventilatory function, the record of asthmatic 'trouble' is disproportionately high before admission and yet reverts dramatically to a symptom-free state in hospital, without recourse to drugs, sociopathic stress is likely to be a contributory factor. In prognostic terms, the most pernicious combination is that of serious bronchopulmonary involvement, with irremediable sociopathology; whereas, in diagnostic terms, the wider the discrepancy between 'trouble' at home and 'trouble' in the unit, the less significant the likely role of organic pathology and the more significant the contribution of sociopathic stress. Conversely, the more closely home and hospital situations approximate in terms of prevailing clinical pattern, the greater the potential 'organic' import, especially if frank asthmatic attacks persist despite withdrawal from stressful home circumstances (Pinkerton, 1971b).

In the long-stay case, consideration of these various determinants is an essential prerequisite to any review of management, alternative to hospital retention.

Channels of Alternative Provision

Various provisions exist as alternatives to extended stay in hospital; the choice depends on which of the three main determining factors most contributes to delay in discharge, and also on the availability of local resources. The key to subsequent placement lies in the child's potential for maturation, almost irrespective of the kind of stress to which he is reacting. Whether this be sociopathic, or mediated more by interpersonal strife, it is its intractable character which dictates the need for some provision alternative to home.

The Socially Disadvantaged Child

In the experience of the Heswall unit, children handicapped primarily by adversity in their personal life circumstances do ultimately mature to the point of being able to withstand previously intolerable levels of stress operating within their own discordant homes, provided satisfactory alternative provision has been made for them in the interim. This may involve a period of two, three or four years, or even longer, and a choice of programmes ranging from foster home placement, through family group home, or local authority children's home, to special school accommodation of various types, depending on the attendant circumstances. In the absence of significant 'organic' involvement (as in, say, the physiologically 'mild' asthmatic), once initial stability has been procured in hospital, transfer to an appropriate foster home or small family group may be all that is required to consolidate remission on the promise of newfound security.

On the other hand, more serious pathology operating in any organ system (e.g. the gut, as in coeliac disease; the CNS, as in epilepsy; or the metabolic system, as in diabetes) may well prolong the time required for stabilisation in hospital and thereafter pose the need for special school placement in collaboration with the substitute home.

For some cases, the supervision provided by day 'open-air' schools may be sufficient; others may require the more structured routine of the residential school, perhaps on a weekly boarding basis, to supplement fostering; while still others may warrant quite a different boarding placement – the residential maladjusted school. Here, the indication is dictated by a separate set of factors, arising from 'syndrome shift'. A typical example is the child initially handicapped by bronchospasm, atopic eczema or neurodermatitis which repeatedly erupts in face of sociopathic stress at home, but just as rapidly remits in hospital. On occasion, within the unit, such a child may so successfully learn to ventilate his problems as to forego their somatic expression (even under stress) and so enjoy symptomatic relief; the pressures themselves persist, but henceforth they evoke a more forthright response in the form of aggressive behaviour or rebelliousness, sometimes as difficult to contain in the hospital unit as within a tension-ridden home. In these circumstances, the more robust atmosphere of the school for maladjusted children may be just the environment to absorb this new development and direct it into more positive and acceptable channels of expression.

Patients who are products of sociopathology by no means constitute a homogeneous group, so that the placing of individuals calls for careful evaluation of all the relevant factors before the final choice is made from the available alternatives. Throughout this exercise, a recurring problem is the failure of social welfare officers to appreciate the needs of children who react to social stress with physically presenting symptoms. Once labelled as 'physically delicate', these children tend to be relegated to residential schools on a truly long-term basis with no real recognition of their need for continuity in personal relationship. There has been a tendency to shy away from the physical 'label' as if thereby the child no longer qualifies for social rehabilitation, because he constitutes a 'medical' problem.

In fact, physical presentation and emotional deprivation are complementary aspects of the same basic problem, calling for continuing liaison between medical and social casework agencies in jointly promoting the holistic welfare of these disadvantaged children.

Intractable Interpersonal Pathology

Entirely different principles govern the disposal of psychosomatically 'sick' children, drawn from ostensibly 'intact' homes, who have been subject nevertheless to covert interpersonal tensions no less intractable and, therefore, no less inimical to their security.

When pathophysiological impairment is significant enough to prolong such a child's stay in hospital on organic grounds, but his eventual homecoming seems nevertheless unpromising because of insoluble conflict within himself, or with his parents, some compromise is clearly indicated to combat the dangers of chronic hospitalisation and yet maintain adequate surveillance without adding to the parental sense of challenge.

Foster home placement or its equivalent is neither feasible administratively in these circumstances, nor would it be tolerated by parents of this calibre, who might well regard it as a reflection upon their own shortcomings in management. By the same token, suggested transfer to residential special school could be similarly interpreted. Worse still, special boarding placement for a period long enough to prove mechanically successful can set the seal upon parental disengagement and so consolidate the rift in relationship with the child, thereby reinforcing his sense of isolation.

Liaison with local schools. To minimise the risk of such adverse developments and yet safeguard the patient's physical welfare, while still aiming at a more positive outlook, we have introduced over the last few years an experimental link with selected schools in the locality, one primary, two grammar, two secondary, and the sixth a preparatory school with both a day and boarding complement.

At an appropriate stage in the child's physical and emotional rehabilitation, complementary to parallel advances in his educational progress within the hospital school, he has been 'promoted' (usually with one or two others, forming a special little group) to the outside local school in keeping with his age, where he attends daily from the hospital on his own initiative, returning to the unit each evening, and normally going home each weekend.

So far, 20 children have been 'launched' in this way, of whom 13 are asthmatic, one a case of ulcerative colitis, and one cystic fibrosis. In all, the boost to personal morale has itself been highly therapeutic, the more so in that most of these patients had not been able to attend normal school for years; but other benefits have also accrued, including advances both in the academic and social spheres. For example, the curriculum and facilities of the outside school clearly offer more than can the hospital school, especially for the older pupil who is at a particular disadvantage regarding senior studies if he is retained for any length of time. Equally, in terms of social development, there is scope for learning to mix on more equal terms with robust, healthy children without always feeling different. This makes for a positive competitive attitude (the antithesis of the sheltered hospital ethos) and so promotes increased poise and self-confidence.

Success in these areas cannot fail to affect even the most critical of parents and perhaps modify their intolerance to some degree. Moreover, the hospital as a base for continuing surveillance is marginally less challenging than the implications of residential special school.

Ideally, if topographic considerations permit, the outside school should be regarded as a bridge between hospital and home in these difficult cases, with the aim of first encouraging identity with the school and so bolstering personal security to the ultimate point of the child being able to rejoin his family despite the unchanged situation of interpersonal conflict on the home front.

The Problem of Adolescence

As these children reach the age group of 14 to 16, fresh problems of adjustment arise which are inseparable from teenage development. Although in theory the unit caters for the standard age range of 5 to 16, with the occasional admission of a pre-school child (accompanied by his mother) or the retention beyond 16 of an older child completing treatment (e.g. in anorexia nervosa), in practice the senior age groups present by far the greatest difficulty in satisfactory accommodation and adjustment within the unit.

This problem is, of course, by no means confined to units dealing with psychosomatic disorder; it is common to all hospital-based facilities (surgical, medical, psychosomatic) which seek to provide a service for the teenage patient, because these youngsters have largely outgrown their childhood status but have not yet acquired the mature orientation of adults. They are neither one thing nor the other, and as such they merit special consideration, acknowledgement of which remains woefully lacking in the country as a whole. This situation has drawn comment from both the British Paediatric Association (1959) and the Royal College of Psychiatrists.

Within the Heswall unit our main problem has been how best to harness this emerging adolescent awareness without disrupting established protocol and how to foster, rather than stifle, individual expression while preserving corporate identity. We are posed, in fact, with a double problem: how to combat the rising level of anxiety among unit staff generated by the teenage challenge (a particularly difficult position for the traditionally trained nurse); and how to conjure up a programme appropriate to a 15-year-old from a hospital model originally designed for the much younger child.

There is no ideal solution to what is essentially a paradoxical situation – and certainly none without imaginative planning of a purpose-built unit, with perhaps separate hostel-type accommodation for the adolescent in its grounds, and the necessary staffing structure to go with it. Certainly, anything short of this optimum arrangement is bound to meet with recurring crises of adolescent unrest and emotional lability, with adverse repercussions on patient and unit alike. The best that can be said in the present uneasy situation of compromise is that prior awareness of the potential for disturbance goes a long way towards its more effective absorption when a particular eruption occurs.

The Day Hospital

The pre-school or infant school child is not only more vulnerable emotionally, and therefore more susceptible to separation trauma, but is actually at greater risk in 'organic' terms. For example, the danger of side-effects from prolonged steroid dosage is appreciably greater in the younger age groups, and their resistance in general is less well established than in the older child.

In situations judged to be inimical to the younger patient's early restoration to his own home, the risks associated with prolonged retention can sometimes be reduced by converting the case to day-patient status. If distance from home does not preclude it, the child continues to attend the hospital school on a daily basis, thereby enjoying uninterrupted continuity both of staff management and work schedule, plus continued nursing and medical supervision, while establishing his home re-entry. Progressively, as confidence is built up in patient and parents alike with consequent easing of mutual tensions, an increasing proportion of the supervisory programme can be handed back to the family without endangering the progress so far achieved. Because this programme can be modified according to individual needs and continued for varying lengths of time, e.g. one, two or three school terms, or even longer, it has proved in practice a highly efficacious half-way stage in the ultimate rehabilitation of the younger child especially. For the older age group, its value is necessarily curtailed by the limited scope of the hospital school curriculum.

Therapeutic Continuity Through Enhanced Communication

Finally, it is important to think of the inpatient facility as only one part of a continuum of therapeutic rehabilitation, rather than as an end in itself. There are clear-cut indications for adopting this procedure and when to adopt it; and equally finite principles governing optimum duration of stay and when to promote discharge. There is often, for example, a prodromal phase preceding admission (i.e. one can admit at too early a stage to be convincing) and a follow-up phase after discharge to consolidate inpatient progress. Improvement may not have been achieved without this residential interlude, but equally it may not progress without subsequent continuity; and the key to ensuring therapeutic continuity is *successful communication at all levels.*

The first of these is the level of interpersonal communication between the child and his family, assuming disturbance in emotional dynamics to be a contributory factor in most of our referrals. Repairing interpersonal relationship is in fact a fundamental function of the unit and to achieve it involves a campaign – no less – in inter-disciplinary liaison, starting with communication within the hospital itself.

This means reciprocal dialogue between paediatrician and child psychiatrist, with constant feedback to the referring family doctor. If an outside school placement is envisaged, it means extending liaison to the school medical officer, the teaching staff concerned and the administrative personnel who will actually engineer the transaction. Misunderstandings can readily develop in this chain of communication unless the most meticulous care is taken to brief everyone involved. Similarly, if fostering or local authority care is contemplated, it is vital to link up and maintain contact with the child-care staff responsible and to ensure that they clearly understand what is planned for the child.

Prospects for the Future

With increasing emphasis upon community-based medicine, it may well be that future management programmes will successfully concentrate upon a casework approach sufficiently comprehensive to keep the child out of hospital, or at least significantly to curtail current lengths of stay.

But this is a vision for the future, involving a radical increase in community social work provision at present impracticable both numerically and in the specialised experience demanded. For the moment, therefore, and for some time to come, the inpatient facility, properly deployed, must continue to play a definitive role in the treatment of childhood psychosomatic disorder.

I should like to pay tribute here to all members of staff on our unit – nursing, secretarial, para-medical and medical – without whose devoted team approach neither the work of the unit, nor this account of it, could ever have been undertaken. My particular thanks are due to Sister Edith Broughall of our unit for her painstaking compilation of the tables which appear in the text.

CHAPTER SIX

Psychotic Children

George Stroh

Essentially, the subsequent pages are the fruit of fourteen years' experience in charge of an inpatient unit for disturbed children. In that time we cared for over sixty children whom I would describe with varying degrees of confidence as psychotic. This experience thus extends over a fair period of time and includes a sizeable number of children for whose day-to-day life I was largely responsible. This entailed a considerable degree of involvement and therefore familiarity with their daily problems, and those of the staff that looked after them. My concern was not unlike that of a professional parent, the parental aspect allowing a fair degree of mutual involvement and the professional aspect providing what may be termed an objective, scientific or logical check on proceedings. The reason for these opening comments is to make it clear from what vantage-point my views obtained. Some of these views may find ready agreement in those of similar experience.

Diagnosis and Classification

The first, and controversial, issue to be dealt with is that of diagnosis and classification of the childhood psychoses. Though much has been said, unsaid and resaid on this issue, it is still largely a matter of 'controversial floundering' (Kanner, 1958). The common denominator that underlies all psychoses is by some referred to as a break with reality (Despert and Sherwin, 1958; Eisenberg, 1967), by others as a fundamental perceptual disturbance and failure of self–non-self separation (Stroh and Buick, 1964; Mahler, 1965; Ornitz and Ritvo, 1968a). Perceptual disturbance and failure to distinguish the self from the environment (a dangerously loose but important concept) are also breaks from reality; indeed, all mental disturbance is by definition a break from reality and only distinguished, often arbitrarily, from normal breaks by frequency and intensity. This applies, for instance, to fantasies in which the normal child's life is rich, and to fantasies clearly abnormal in content, which may equally appear in neurotic and in psychotic children. Despert and Sherwin (1958) distinguish childhood schizophrenia from obsessional neurosis on the basis of the intensity, that is the fixity, of the 'obsessional' thoughts that may occur in either condition. But can the bizarre compulsive behaviour of the obsessional child or adult be called reality-oriented even though the patient knows, or says he knows, that it is irrational? It may be more correct to say that he has a sort of double awareness in which reality and fantasy are not clearly distinguished. When one of our children said that his nose had legs because it was running, it was the sort of joke many children might make or appreciate. With him it was not a joke but half a question, to be turned into a joke if we threatened him by laughing at him. Our assertion that noses had no legs he accepted readily as our view of things, a view to be incorporated perhaps later into his scheme of thinking.

This brings us to the important problem of the relation of reality to the development of self–object (or self–environment) separation. Inner and outer reality will be in normal balance if there is an optimal discrepancy between the outer reality and its inner representation. If these are much the same then there is little difference between outside and inside – there is no outside and no self. This is a point we have to bear in mind if we aim to impose, with the best of intentions, 'reality' demands on a child which he can absorb and assimilate only in an imitative way. If, on the other hand, the inner representation of the outer world is inadequate – if the discrepancy between inner and outer reality is too large – there will not be, so to speak, enough points of reference to allow the individual to relate meaningfully to the environment. In other words, psychotic manifestations vary in degree rather than in kind from other disorders or from the norm; this accounts for the great variety of psychotic manifestations.

If we postulate the existence of a third area of reality (perhaps in the nature of double awareness mentioned earlier) which is interposed between the inner and outer one and which overlaps and fuses with them, we might then suggest that where the discrepancy between the outer world and its inner representation is small this intermediate area will be large – there will appear to be a fusion between inner and outer reality. Where the discrepancy is large, the intermediate area will be small. Its relative absence prevents a smooth flow between inner and outer reality. The clinical observations that lend some credence to this scheme are the abrupt switches between normal and psychotic behaviour that can be observed in many non-autistic, psychotic children.

Basically, most attempts to classify the childhood psychoses fall into two sometimes overlapping groups (Eisenberg's, 1967, comprehensive classification is on the whole modelled on adult psychiatry): one indicates or implies that psychosis lies towards the end of a continuum (Bender, 1947; Beres, 1956; Stroh, 1962); the other uses age and sometimes manner of onset as the main criteria (Despert, 1938; Mahler, 1952; Kanner, 1949; Anthony, 1958; Rutter, 1967). More recently, Kolvin *et al.* (1971) have investigated childhood psychosis on the basis of age of onset, calling the early-onset type 'infantile psychosis' (IP) and the later one 'late-onset psychosis' (LOP). They found significant differences between these groups in terms of symptomatology and cognitive development, while the differences were not quite so significant, or perhaps less clear-cut, in terms of cerebral dysfunction and parental background, personality and attitude. That the age at which a severely disruptive element strikes a developing organism will be significantly related to, if not largely determine, the ensuing disorganisation can be taken for granted, and it may even have a differential secondary effect on the parents. While such typology is of great interest, it is likely to include among its units types which are in other respects not sufficiently similar to justify inclusion under one umbrella.

Diagnostic Groups

The five sub-groups which we have found useful on clinical grounds are, with two exceptions, much the same as have been variously described in the literature. Such a classification is by no means exhaustive:

it does not, for example, include psychotic depression (which was diagnosed in two children over a period of ten years), nor obsessive-compulsive psychosis (one child), nor does it take account of about half a dozen children who could not be included in any group. Table 6.1 summarises the distribution of boys and girls in the diagnostic categories to be described.

Table 6.1

Diagnostic category	*Total*	*Boys*	*Girls*
Childhood autism	16	13	3
Organic with autistic features	12	7	5
Schizophrenia	5	4	1
Traumatic psychosis	7	4	3
'ESN psychosis'	13	8	5

Of the three 'conventional' categories the first, the autistic group, has been often and clearly defined (Kanner, 1943; Rimland, 1964; Kolvin *et al.*, 1971; etc.). The group comprised sixteen children (thirteen boys, three girls); but even this group did not give the clinical 'feel' of being altogether homogenous. Some autistic children, for instance, are aggressively intrusive (even though they show perceptual avoidance and may or may not have rudiments of speech), while others remain persistently at the periphery of things. Interestingly, Despert (1938), in a paper written before Kanner's epoch-making one, speaks of autism as 'a capital symptom of schizophrenia in the younger children', and describes affect as either completely 'severed' from the environment or in the 'form of impulsive and apparently non-motivated demonstrations'.

Set aside from the first group was a somewhat heterogeneous second which consisted of children with clear indication of cerebral dysfunction in terms of history, EEG findings and epilepsy. This group comprised twelve children of whom four, all boys, showed marked clinical features of brain damage, such as unpredictable and hyperactive behaviour; of these four children, two had frequent grand mal seizures (one died in status epilepticus three years after he had been transferred from High Wick), the other two had marked EEG abnormality (one with evidence of temporal lobe pathology). This group was small because it was the admission policy not, as a rule, to admit children with clear-cut evidence of brain damage. Of the remaining eight children in this group five were girls, and the group as a whole can best be described as consisting of severely subnormal children with autistic features – by now a well-known entity representing patients in whom no significant improvement can be expected. Clinically these patients overlap with the non-assertive autistic type.

The third group, the schizophrenic, was similar to the late-onset psychosis described by Kolvin *et al.*, except that those symptoms which 'have high discriminative value' (perplexity, incongruity of thought and affect, hallucinations, etc.) were more strictly adhered to. We would hesitate to make the diagnosis without a history of schizophrenia or a schizophrenic-like illness in one or the other of the parents (in this very small sample only the mothers were thus affected). Four such children were in that sense clearly identifiable as schizophrenic; a fifth can be included with some doubt. Certainly in one of them, the only girl, abnormal behaviour patterns were recognised within the first year of life.

The last two groups to be described are included among the psychoses by virtue of the intensity and breadth of the disturbance, because of the faulty adjustment to reality, the grossly distorted or diminished relationship to people and the sometimes bizarre symptomatology. They also share with other psychoses the non-discriminative but highly distinctive characteristics of treatment procedures being uncertain or experimental and the outlook in terms of good recovery unfavourable. A clinical example of each of these, and of the schizophrenic syndrome, is given later in this chapter. The first consists of children who have been severely traumatised in early childhood, both physically and mentally, a syndrome we call 'traumatic psychosis'. Our group consisted of seven children (three girls); this relatively small number is probably misleading as the condition merges into other conduct disorders, anti-social behaviour patterns, etc., and the assignment to one or the other group may depend on the nature of one's clinical involvement and preferred frame of reference.

The damaging effect of being exposed to early aggressive influences has been widely described (Helfer and Kempe, 1968; Rutter, 1971; Freud, 1948; Rubinfine, 1962; Rosenfeld, 1972). Clinically, the syndrome fits most closely Dockar-Drysdale's description of the 'frozen child' (Dockar-Drysdale, 1968). In her introductory comments in the paper on frozen children Dockar-Drysdale said that her 'main object – in the first place at all events – was to insist that people would realise what it was like to live and work with such children'. In our experience these children emerged as a group clearly distinguishable from any other by the tensions they produced in the unit, their aggression and the counter-aggression they elicited from the staff, and the way they became at times the centre, the most talked-of, worried-over children at the hospital. The main reason for this is probably the utter confusion produced in the caring adult by the contradictory behaviour of these children. Such a child can be charming and endearing, and then,

> ... in astonishing contrast become suddenly savagely hostile, especially towards a grown-up with whom he has been friendly. He will fly into sudden panic rages for no apparent reason in which he smashes and destroys anything in his vicinity.
>
> It is repeatedly reported that he is improving and hopes are raised; it is claimed that he is making a relationship at last, but each time disaster follows, until finally he becomes intolerable to his environment. (Dockar-Drysdale, 1968)

He (literally, in one of our children) bites the hand that feeds him. The sudden, unforeseen switches from enchanting to aggressive and at times cruel behaviour leave the caretaker bewildered. To this must be added the tendency of such a child to 'befriend' an adult on the fringe of his environment, on whom he makes no demands and to whom he displays all his charm. The 'friend' cannot understand the anger and hostility engendered by the child in his special caretaker (a situation which the child exploits to the full), until he comes closer into the child's orbit, with the inevitable resulting disenchantment, and the search for another fringe person.

Cruelty and aggression is indeed a feature of this condition; sometimes it is directed against the self. One child aged two-and-a-half years had her cot padded because she was so self-destructive, and wore a crash helmet by the time she was admitted to High Wick one-and-a-half years later; another, a boy aged five years, beat up a defenceless autistic girl in the space of two unattended minutes, injuring her badly and causing her admission to a general hospital. What punishment or corrective experience could be devised for this? He was taken the following day to the hospital and shown without reproach, the child's injuries. He looked, unmoved. The apparent absence of remorse, conscience, guilt, super-ego is characteristic of these patients:

it appears to be a psychotically total unawareness of the consequences of their actions – a 'reality blindness' (Redl and Wineman, 1951).

Essentially, then, the traumatised child seems capable of forming a strong bond with the caretaking adult, but suddenly appears to find this good experience unbearable: it turns sour on him, and his behaviour becomes hostile and destructive. At this point he tends to tear the bond he has formed with the adult. When a certain equilibrium is reached he tries again, only to destroy the bond once more. It is likely that by this time the environment will tend to reinforce, in reality, the feelings of threat and hostility which have largely been his own projection. In this way early life experiences are being repeatedly recreated.

Rutter (1972) says in his comprehensive review on maternal deprivation (p. 103) that it 'seemed clear that experiences involving bond disruption do *not* normally lead to an "affectionless character" but there are grounds for suggesting that a failure to form bonds in early childhood may have this outcome'. He suggests further, though this remains to be proven, that there may be a sensitive period from, say, six months to two or three years for the development of normal attachment behaviour, 'after which bond formation becomes increasingly less likely'; and concerning 'affectionless psychopathy' (p. 118) he says, 'The little evidence available suggests that the most tenable hypothesis is that a failure to develop attachments (or bonds) in early childhood is the main factor'. In the case of traumatic psychosis we must add the all-important rider that the faulty development in bond formation is caused by, or at any rate associated with, early experiences of violence which the child has either experienced himself or has witnessed in his intimate environment, or both. One might further conjecture that the normal bodily tensions of infancy were not, or were only inadequately, resolved into pleasurable body feelings and that in addition, and specifically, early experiences of physical aggression widened, perhaps irreversibly, the gap between feelings of bodily tension and their pleasurable resolution. To repeat: failure to develop early bonds is important, but the cause or nature of this failure – early experience of violence – is decisive.

The last group which can, rather lamely, be called 'ESN psychosis' emerged, paradoxically, by not emerging at all: its relative non-descriptiveness was a characteristic feature. These children rarely present a management problem, at any rate in a place like High Wick. Though sometimes aggressive, generally when they are roused, their violence is nothing compared to those of the traumatised group; the oddities of their behaviour are not so extreme as those of the schizophrenic or autistic children. To the staff they rarely produce the rewarding responses of a neurotic or behaviour-disordered child, nor the challenge of an autistic or schizophrenic.

This group consisted of thirteen children (five girls). In twelve cases their cognitive level was in the ESN range,* one was low average. In such children early development is sometimes slow, generally uneventful and, although their slowness and their oddities are described more or less emphatically by the parents, they find their way to nursery or infant school. From there they are usually referred because they do not mix with other children (and for that reason are sometimes labelled autistic) and because they are quite unable to do any work; or because of their 'strange behaviour' (another reason for thinking them autistic, though if anything their oddities are more schizophrenic-like), such as bizarre movements and odd postures, or a flow of words sometimes quite sensible, and often – on closer attention – nonsense, somewhat in the nature of *vorbeireden*. Their fantasy life can be intense and overwhelming, often in relation to childhood sexuality. They masturbate freely, sometimes soil and urinate on the floor; there is a good deal of attempted sex play and much excited and confused talk about all this. Although this may sometimes seem little more than exaggerated, readily out-of-control 'normal' sex play, it often appears in times of stress, such as before holidays, and may then be an expression of anxiety, bringing further anxiety in its wake. Indeed, the overt anxiety of these children is often marked and openly expressed. They are fearful of being left alone without an adult and they tend to be immensely jealous of, or threatened by, other, usually smaller children. Their self-esteem is low, they give up readily or preferably do not start at all; the process of living seems to overwhelm them at times and it is then that the break with reality widens and they become confused and bewildered. They are isolated from other children but make clinging, intensive contact with their caretaking adult.

Equally intense, and intensely ambivalent, is the relationship these children have with their parents, particularly the mother. They desperately wish to go home as often as possible, though it is apparent that the bond with the mother is itself a highly confusing one – a

* ESN (educationly subnormal) refers to children of below average and above severely subnormal intelligence (IQ approximately 55–75) for whom in Britain special educational facilities are provided.

relationship to which the concept of double-bind can be applied with some justification. There was evidence of neurosis, but not psychotic illness, in at least one of the parents of the group described. None of the children came from a broken home and the parents were invariably well-meaning and concerned. For these children, the co-existence of below-average intellectual awareness and emotional problems in the family may perhaps be not fortuitous but significantly relevant to the child's emotional maldevelopment. A child who appears to function normally, or nearly so, or whose defect can readily be denied, particularly in early childhood, has demands made on him which he cannot fulfil. He becomes confused and anxious and his reponse confuses his parents, who, tending to be over-anxious and easily stressed, overreact to this confusion, thus setting up a vicious circle. The growing child will become increasingly aware of the demands of everyday life and of his failure to meet them.

Indications for Inpatient Assessment and Treatment of Psychotic Children

Children are now considered whose disturbance is clinically described as psychotic, irrespective of whether there is an 'associated organic brain disorder or mental subnormality' (Rutter *et al.*, 1969). The existence of an organic factor may tell us something about the aetiology of the condition but it is unlikely to give us any more than a crude outline of the clinical picture; for the details and subtleties we shall have to take recourse, as always, to a behavioural assessment. Nor will our knowledge of the organic aetilogy, with a very few possible exceptions, for example, neoplasm, itself give us any clear indication of the most appropriate management or treatment – here again we shall have to rely largely on our clinical (that is, behavioural) data. The relevance, at least at present, of the search for the causative or significant organic factor lies in the hope that early or prophylactic measures can be taken to prevent the development of a psychosis. Even if the time comes when we discover the structural causes of the functional psychosis, which have not yet been ascertained (Eisenberg, 1967), we shall still need to observe the child in his environment for a fuller understanding of his illness. Some work has been done (Hutt *et al.*, 1965; Ornitz and Ritvo, 1968b) to correlate behavioural characteristics with physiological findings, and here is an area for future research that may eventually prove fruitful.

What, then, is the purpose of inpatient assessment for psychotic children? The purpose essentially is to find the basis for the next step to take, how to help the child and the family by suggesting the relevant form of treatment or assigning an appropriate placement. Assessment itself has no function and it presupposes that there exist proven forms of treatment and readily available facilities. Neither is strictly true but we are not justified in taking a stance of therapeutic nihilism. Indeed, one can widen the meaning of assessment to include a process which in some cases at least will help to create or formulate a plan for treatment. As such a plan will be based on the current interaction of the child and his environment – a mutual testing-out procedure – assessment and treatment will be seen to merge. In as much as this is so, and includes as an essential step the formation of bonds, one could argue that neither structurally nor conceptually is the distinction between assessment and treatment desirable, rather that the two should be seen as a circular process.

Considering evaluation in its broader sense, as largely overlapping with treatment, the indications for using a residential setting will apply largely to both. Firstly, as already indicated, we want the fullest possible picture of the child's reaction patterns over a period of time. One can immediately point out that some of the most important and revealing information, the interaction with his family, will be missing or sketchy; from that point of view the child's assessment could be carried out in his home. There are obstacles to this: the family may feel neither inclined nor able to accommodate another person in their midst and there would be few people who were trained, experienced and willing to carry out such a task. To some extent this gap in our knowledge can be met by information from the parents or by enabling the parents to live in the unit for brief periods. Still, there remains a defect in our evaluating and therapeutic equipment, particularly as treatment started in the unit could be carried on in the home to better advantage if there were available help of an experienced and appropriately trained worker.

Secondly, admission is indicated for those forms of treatment that are, for example, specifically linked to residential care, so-called 'milieu therapy': essentially this implies balancing the needs of an individual child with the demands of the community he is part of. Of the staff it demands that they be flexible, informed and realistic. It is in the nature of childhood psychosis that it is often most difficult to remain realistic for those who are too intimately involved, like parents, while the restraints and limits of flexibility of the normal home can or should be extended in a suitably structured institution. Other forms of treatment, because of their intensity of planning and execution, are best carried out, at least initially, in an inpatient setting; an example of this is given in the last part of this chapter.

Thirdly, there is the positive step of separating the child from his home environment. This may be therapeutic in itself, as in the case of the traumatised child, but also less obviously in other psychotic children whose behaviour produces such tensions and disruptions at home that, far from benefiting from family care, they may be driven further into their psychoses. Too many parents appear to be expected (or expect it of themselves) to look after their psychotic child for too long, with no benefit to the child and great hardship and possibly harm to themselves. The indications for admission of a psychotic child must be understood not only in terms of his own treatment but in relation to the whole family.

For residential staff, too, looking after psychotic children and living with them presents its own problems. Some are similar or more intense forms of what one would find with neurotic, behaviour-disordered or even normal children, others are more specific. The unresponsiveness and the slow progress, if any, of the autistic child, the bizarre behaviour of the schizophrenic, the bewildering turnabouts of the traumatised, the 'sillyness' of the 'ESN' – all may arouse great anxiety in the staff. Associated with this is the sometimes primitive behaviour, the display of raw instincts with little modification into socially tolerable, let alone acceptable, forms: compulsive masturbation, intensive sexual play and sexual exploration of others, staff and children; urinating and soiling into clothes, on the floors, in the garden; swearing; unbridled aggression and destructiveness directed against adults, in whom it may produce feelings of counter-aggression, against children, when it may elicit anger and despair, and against themselves, when the observer's reaction is of shock and utter bewilderment.

The anxiety in the caretaking adult when confronted with such undisguised sexuality and aggression is caused by the threat to his own adaptive structure, the defensive system which he has developed. The extent to which he can cope, or learn to cope, with such behaviour will be a measure of the quality of integration of his own primitive sexual impulses and aggression into his personality. Above all, it is the loss of reality sense in the psychotic child that makes his behaviour more or less incomprehensible and confusing. The tendency of the adult is to cope with incomprehensible behaviour either by detaching himself emotionally from the confusing person, which is clearly an undesirable course for the caring person to take, or by trying to make sense of the non-sense. This carries its own dangers, in that the adult's urgent need for clarification may lead to premature and unhelpful conclusions.

From what has been said so far it will have become clear that the ordinary problems of residential treatment, its planning and its execution, are greatly increased with psychotic children: the planning, because there is no generally accepted or proven form of treatment, but mostly applied general principles of child care (consistency, child-oriented management, formation of attachments), laced with a wide range of treatment procedures ranging from behaviour modification to psychoanalytically-oriented therapy, adjusted largely on an *ad hoc* basis to the prevailing circumstances; the execution, because of the nature and intensity of the children's unsettling influence on the staff, who in the main are either concerned with executing the plan or whose management provides the background against which any other treatment procedures will take place. Indeed, with two such unknowns it is difficult to be sure whether it is the treatment or the 'execution' that does the good, or prevents the good being done. Wenar *et al.* (1967) describe the effectiveness of three milieus to change the behaviour of autistic children. Using Ruttenberg's behaviour-rating scale for autistic children they found that the large, long-established state institution providing custodial care did no worse, and in some ways better, than a modern state hospital offering a therapeutic programme of activities which were 'planned with care but executed with indifference'. Most successful was a small psychoanalytically-oriented day centre with a high staff–child ratio, where emphasis was put on emotional relationship between staff and children and where the 'senior staff devotes a significant amount of time to maintaining their (the child-care staff's) interest and enthusiasm'.

The Structure and Functioning of the Unit

There are eighteen children in residence, ages ranging from four to thirteen years. About one half or a little more are psychotic, while the others can be classified as neurotic or having behaviour disorders.

Severely mentally or physically handicapped children are not admitted as a rule. The length of stay varies with the severity of the disturbance and will be limited if the child reaches the age of about thirteen years or if it is thought that the unit cannot any more be of specific help to the child or the family. No child in further need of residential care is discharged until an alternative placement has been found. Children may remain at the hospital from one year to several years; the annual turnover is six to seven a year.

The children are divided into groups of from three to five, each under the care of two child-care workers who work at opposite shifts with an overlap period during the middle of the day. Within each group, one child-care worker is specially responsible for one or two children. In this way a high degree of consistency and continuity of care is achieved. There is a daily programme of structured activity for which the children are divided into three groups (school, nursery and pre-nursery) which are run by two teachers and a senior child-care worker respectively, assisted by one or two child-care workers. The child-care workers assist in the same teaching group for one year, after which they usually move to one of the other groups. The programmes provide for the individual needs of the child and range from body-awareness training and perceptual learning, through social and habit-training to formal education. Some children have individual psychotherapy and speech therapy. The consultant-in-charge is responsible for the administration of the unit and its planning, which is carried out on the basis of discussions with all the staff. Another consultant (also part-time) is concerned, together with the social worker, for the counselling, support and treatment of the parents (Tischler, 1965 and 1971).

The day-to-day care of the children is undertaken by ten child-care workers (four additional staff provide night cover) of good educational background, who may or may not have had previous experience of work with children. Most of the staff remain for two years, a few stay longer. Many go on from High Wick to take up further education or training, a few stay in the field. An in-service training was instituted in 1958 (Stroh, 1960 and 1968).

A specific feature of the functioning of the unit is the attempt to integrate social, therapeutic and educational aspects of care with the day-to-day care of the child. Two factors help towards achieving this aim: the participation of the child-care workers in the teaching or activity groups, and the structure and function of certain regular meetings. In these groups the child-care worker is concerned largely or altogether with children other than those in her special care and at any rate she will come to know the children in a different context. The discussions of the teaching groups are each attended by all teachers, the consultant-in-charge, the social worker and any other professional staff available, and those child-care workers who assist in that particular group. Similarly, the therapists discuss regularly with individual child-care workers the behaviour and progress of each child in treatment. In this way it is hoped that the everyday care of the child will be sufficiently informed and consistent to provide a sound and essential basis for whatever specific educational or therapeutic measures are being taken.

It has been suggested earlier that much of the inpatient treatment of psychotic children is determined by our knowledge or theories of principles of early child development, modified or expanded by a variety of treatment procedures based on the experience, training or hunches of the planners. The implication of this is that there exists no one clearly successful therapy, but that all have had their successes or, more commonly, failures. The obverse is equally true, namely that we are not yet in a position to exclude any form of treatment because it has not been sufficiently successful. In the following section are described in more detail some of the typical problems presented by the groups of children outlined earlier, with their implications for residential treatment.

The Traumatised Psychotic Child

Lucy came to the unit at the age of four and a half years, barely able to toddle, with practically no language, incontinent of urine and faeces, the size and appearance of a two-year-old and suffering from nutritional anaemia. She demanded constant attention and when left would rock on all fours and wail. She had witnessed endless quarrels and experienced severe deprivation and maltreatment. The mother was fully aware of her antagonism to the child, felt extremely guilty about it but was unable to do anything about it. Indeed, it is often a feature of these situations that the parents, or one of them, are aware of their grossly negative feelings and are asking in a disguised way or quite openly for the child's protection from their own aggression. Within a year Lucy's improvement was dramatic. She talked indistinctly but with a good vocabulary, she walked well and joined in with groups of other children. She no longer required constant attention and played imaginatively with miniature toys.

The improvement was such that it was decided to try her in a normal infant class. This, in retrospect was the first mistake: what became painfully obvious later on was that her progress in learning and acquiring new skills was in no way matched by her emotional development. Any new demand, however small, was likely to bring out her utter need for dependence – and her inability to tolerate this dependence. She was withdrawn from school after one term because of her increasing demandingness and because she had become increasingly aggressive and destructive at High Wick. There was evidence of this before (she had, several months before, suddenly and 'playfully' pulled at the broken finger of her special child-care worker, gleefully laughing at her pain), but now it had become more overt and in the years to come became a matter of constant concern and counter-aggression. In the course of a few days, for instance, she pushed one child down the stairs, trapped another's hand in the door, threw a cup at a third, pulled her curtains down, broke her locker and tore all her summer dresses. She tore the dresses, she explained, because of the 'y' in the name tabs; she didn't like 'y' because the letter was contained both in her name and that of her own child-care worker. It became one of her 'worry words' and she had many of them over a period of time.

Worry words 'got in her mind', making her feel anxious and aggressive. At one time it was 'z' and she drew 'zig-zags' all along the floor, being both fascinated and terrified by her drawings. At times her fantasies, for example pretending to be a cat (walking on all fours, miaowing), became so intense that they seemed to take over her whole personality. At other times she desperately wanted to be a boy. She insisted on wearing shorts, tore them in front to 'make them like boys'' and twisted them to make a bulge because she 'had a penis underneath'. Wearing these shorts made her very excited and aggressive to the little boys so that eventually she was persuaded to revert to wearing dresses. She could be cruel and sadistic, torturing animals to death under the guise of loving them, and once, at home, threw a kitten on the fire. She could be charming, showing apparent concern for the well-being of her child-care worker, or amusingly polite, thanking the cook for 'a lovely meal'; or show an impish sort of nastiness when she went through a prolonged phase of 'wanting to get rid of' her favourite child-care worker, Miss Tilly. She obtained the information that God decided who should live or who should die and then proceeded to plead that Tilly should die. One day when Miss Tilly arrived as usual on duty Lucy exclaimed in mock despair, 'Bloody God. Tilly's here, not dead'. In the end her favourite child-care worker could take no more and asked to be relieved of looking after her – Lucy succeeded in 'killing' the person she liked most.

Lucy had individual psychotherapy for four years, four times a week, by an experienced and understanding therapist. For the first year or so she loved going and spoke fondly of her therapist. There was some real improvement, particularly perhaps in her ability to tolerate frustration. For the last year the sessions became battles of attrition, of incessant whining and nagging and attacks on the therapist, but there was no improvement and treatment was terminated – in the end she 'destroyed' her therapist too. It was then decided to give her complete individual attention divided between two child-care workers. This lasted for six months, after which Lucy was no better and the child-care workers at their wits' end. Her tendency to be preoccupied with bodily sensations and functions had become a prominent feature. She was worried by noises, she croaked and coughed and complained that feelings in her throat made her do this, she rushed to the toilet every five to ten minutes to urinate and to the tap to have a sip of water; eating and sleeping were a constant problem, often she had to be fed by herself and she required heavy night sedation.

Her behaviour reached such a crescendo of destructiveness and all-absorbing, never-ending demandingness, by now rarely confounded by periods of sensibleness and charm, that all the staff felt as though they were being taken over by this eleven-year-old – forever discussing how to cope, what steps to take next. The staff had, it seemed, collectively become the object of her destructiveness and had lost control over her. Her urgent transfer was sought to a subnormality hospital (her IQ was low average) where it was hoped that the no-nonsense attitude and stricter routine might help. She was bright and amusing at the intake interview for the new hospital and soon admitted. For a while she was the darling of the ward, but soon the charm wore off and she became locked in her usual battle. She had to be heavily sedated (various attempts at using drugs had no positive effect on her behaviour but made her at times more tolerable) and eventually she was taken out against advice by a relative, to live in her home. There were no problems for about six months, and she even had some home tuition. She then began to attack the relative dangerously and was admitted to a mental hospital.

This history illustrates the characteristic features of the severely traumatised child: a child under intensive tension and distress which she experiences, expresses and reacts to largely in terms of unpleasurable bodily sensations and functions. In her demands for relief she tries to attach herself to one person, but this person's attempts to help are seen as acts of aggression which she not only rejects but frantically fights against. Lucy succeeded in eliminating this 'threat' again and again, she may even thereby have found some temporary relief, only to be driven once more by her re-emerging tension and distress to seek help from another person. This ever-recurring process also explains why apparent progress or improvement is at best precarious and often misleading.

Some general points of management follow from the preceding description and comments. All one's attention must be directed towards promoting the formation of a bond between the care-taking adult and the child, or perhaps more accurately, to prevent this bond being broken. All the unit's available resources must be mobilised at such a crisis point to provide external control and structure for the child, and support for the staff. If the child once again succeeds in breaking the tie the likelihood is that his destructiveness will increasingly dominate him and the environment, as happened irreversibly with Lucy. A similar result may occur if the bond is broken for external reasons, for instance prolonged illness of the important adult or when the adult eventually leaves. If the disruption of the tie occurs when it is new and only precariously maintained, the trauma to the child may be wholly destructive. If at all possible this break should not occur until the child has had the experience of a loving and secure attachment. In our limited experience at the unit, although the break may even then be intensely distressing, with all-out attention and care by those familiar to the child he may be got through this distressing period. In calmer times it may help to bear in mind two other points: take care not to stimulate, but if anything slow down, cognitive development or acquisitions of new skills, as these may prevent, or interfere with, the development of earliest emotional development; and as a corollary, do not be confused by the child's fluctuations of mood and behaviour, nor hood-winked by precarious or apparent progress.

Of the seven 'traumatised' children treated at High Wick, two did badly (both are in mental hospitals) and two did fairly well – one of these was later working. The results in the remaining three could not, at the time of writing, be assessed, as the follow-up period was too brief; it appeared that the outcome in two was hopeful, in the third poor. A final word about the parents of such children: they are themselves the victims of adverse circumstances, and to blame them is entirely out of place. At the same time, to try to persuade them into a continuance of a relationship of which they are clearly incapable is misguided. Early detection and inpatient care are the first essential and positive steps in the treatment of these children.

The 'ESN Psychotic' Child

Reg was referred from the infant school (all the children described were either in a nursery or infant class before coming to High Wick) because of his isolation and 'bizarre' behaviour. From the age of three-and-a-half to four years he became increasingly difficult at home, in fact he dominated the family: he screamed when the parents talked to each other and would not tolerate their having a meal together – the father had his in the kitchen for the sake of peace. He had many fears concerning buttons and clothes: his mother had to buy him clothes without buttons, he would otherwise tear them off, and she had to wear an apron to cover the buttons on her blouse or cardigan; jumpers had to be without sleeves and for a time he refused to wear a jumper at home, but did wear one in bed when he had a cold. His speech was curious: he never asked questions and became increasingly disinclined to answer. He showed no initiative.

By the time he was five years old he demanded complete attention from his mother, and was apparently jealous of her activities: 'Mummy must not sit down'; 'Mummy must not read the paper'; 'Daddy go away'. If he was thwarted he would let out a piercing, deafening scream. He was six-and-a-half years when he came to High Wick and stayed for six years. His preoccupations and fears expressed themselves in different ways over the years. He was terrified of being hurt, of being 'broken'. When he jumped about with fear he always held his penis. Buttons and clothes continued to be his main preoccupation, but there were many others: drains, chimneys, planes and buses. He removed the wheels of toy buses and he knew the number and destination of all buses in the vicinity. In his aeroplane phase he endlessly looked at aeroplane books and almost seemed to become a plane himself. When he wore a blue jumper he was a 'BOAC jet' and when he had his red jumper on he was a 'BEA jet'. He insisted on being called 'Jet' and screamed his long piercing screams when referred to by his name, but later agreed to be called 'London Airport jet Reg' – another example of the psychotic child's propensity to draw one into his psychotic orbit, and how not to respond to this.

He had an uncanny knack of using apparently meaningless words or phrases to tease other children ('High Wick pyjamas Philip' or 'Put Peter in the field' would drive Philip and Peter to distraction), but the slightest teasing retaliation drove him into a frenzy. His behaviour in school was characteristic and basically remained unchanged: he was listless and apparently disinterested, except in buses, etc., which no doubt helped him to learn to read and write. He found it all 'too difficult' and readily anticipated failure. He was always most eager to go home, generally every weekend, but his behaviour at home did not improve – at any rate the parents found him too difficult to manage and his behaviour irritating beyond toleration, nor were they able to accept our offer to help them by counselling or support in their management of Reg.

From High Wick he went to an ESN boarding-school, then he lived for a while unsuccessfully at home, and then he went on to a hostel. At the age of eighteen years it was possible to have a limited conversation with him. He talked of his life since High Wick and his 'difficult' time at home. He now 'fancied' girls. His great complaint was still that boys were teasing him and there were particular words that made him wild. At the moment it was 'smell'. Sometimes, he said, he felt sad and worried, sometimes happy. When asked what made him most happy, he replied, 'when I see the new buses'. Later he talked of killing himself because he was being teased. Sometimes he threatened one or other of the boys in the hostel – in fact he never physically attacked anybody.

The characteristic features of children with this disturbance, as outlined by the description of Reg and indicated earlier, are the emergence of difficult behaviour by about three years of age; the progress to nursery or infant school where they are out of place; the lack of drive or interest except in certain areas of preoccupation in which they become quite proficient, but their general concern with the problems of initiating or proceeding with a task and fear of failure. Their anxiety is also expressed by many and often varying fears and preoccupations, typical of which are clothing fads present in at least nine of the thirteen children studied; these are almost invariably encouraged and colluded with by parents (usually the mother) and, as seen in retrospect, often by the caring staff.

The difficulty in forming more than a one-person relationship seems to be one of the most significant features with these children. It is shown by their apparent fear or unease of actually being with two important adults at the same time. This was a feature of their behaviour at High Wick in their relationship with their parents, and it extended as a conflict between home and hospital. The tie between child and home is a strong one, albeit largely anxiety-driven, which, though pulling in the same direction as a bond of affection, interferes with the healthy formation of such a bond. Two potential areas of conflict arise from this characteristic: firstly, between the parents, and parents and child, and, secondly, between the home and the hospital – the latter, curiously, often expresses itself in terms of parental complaints about the care of the child's clothes by the hospital.

An essential aspect of the treatment of the child will therefore be to help him towards the acceptance of more than one strong emotional involvement at one time, basically with more than one person, but eventually referring to people and, say, learning. Much of this can be done in school and in everyday life at the hospital – but in the last resort it must include the parents. As the parents come to see themselves and the hospital as allies with the common purpose of helping the child, they will increasingly feel that they, as father and mother, are allies, rather than split forces, *vis-à-vis* their child. To the extent that his disturbance is part of a family problem it will be helped in this way. The intrapsychic reflection of the family problem emerges in the child as a fear of growing up and particularly in his confused gender role. Many of his anxieties bear the stamp of preoccupation with infantile sexuality, which is shown by his confused and worrying body-image; probably it is this which is expressed in the clothing fads. The confusion is enhanced, as suggested earlier, by the particular balance of understanding and non-understanding that is a feature of the ESN child. This is, of course, speculation, but in itself it should not be surprising that a child's cognitive potential plays a significant part in his adjustment to life. Certainly, this 'balance' must be constantly borne in mind when dealing with these children's fantasies and fears and everyday experiences: they need more things explained to them more frequently and more simply.

All the children followed up (eleven out of thirteen) had maintained the same intellectual level irrespective of their adjustment otherwise. Seven of the eleven children were living at home; of those old enough to work (three), all had at one time or another done so in a sheltered environment: two were still working. The others went to ESN schools or special classes in normal schools. Of the eleven, nine families were seen regularly (mother and/or father) for therapy or counselling, never more than once a week. In six of these the child had become well integrated at home, in the three others this was not possible. In at least one of these three this was because of the deterioration of the child; in another, though the child lived at home, this could not be called a healthy integration. Of the remaining two children followed up whose parents were not seen regularly, one child lived at home, the other in a hostel.

The Schizophrenic Child

The clinical picture of chilhood schizophrenia has been well described by Kolvin *et al.* (1971) as 'late-onset psychosis', though in the exceedingly small sample studied (five), compared to theirs (33), we found unusual behaviour in all the children before the age of two years. Thought disorder, incongruity of affect (rather than blunting), perplexity and attitude of suffering are the most prominent features and so is genetic loading: in all five families there was evidence of schizophrenia among the parents. There was never more than presumptive evidence for the existence of hallucinations.

Daniel was a placid baby, so still and silent that he was thought to be deaf. At two years he went through a phase of outbursts of screaming, knocking his head against the wall and throwing things about; to this point he might have been in the early stages of autism. Before he was four he had calmed down again. His speech became bizarre: 'Why doesn't the ceiling talk?' 'Why doesn't the wardrobe walk?' He expressed many strange fears, as of things eating him up and of being swallowed by little insects; he was frightened of trees and grass and the sky and the pictures on the wall.

He came to the unit when he was six-and-a-half years old. He was clearly confused about himself and other people, about the functions of different parts of his body and the difference between people and objects. He said questioningly. 'There are three Daniels', and he referred to himself or part of himself in the third person: 'I don't flap my hands, Daniel flaps his hands.' If his child-care worker was cross with him he might say: 'There are two Miss Bours, I don't want there to be two.' He asked, 'What are my eyes for?' 'Can I talk to my teeth?' 'Can the floor talk?' But soon, by being confronted with 'our' reality (Des Lauriers, 1962) without being denied his own, his strange ideas became less fixed and he tentatively began to accept our reality: 'No, Daniel', he would answer himself in a gruff voice, 'the floor can't talk. The floor is not a person, it's a thing. Things don't talk. Only people.' He would hold long dialogues with a piece of wood or any other object he might be playing with, or mutter to himself, jumping up and down, getting red in the face, shaking his arms and flapping his hands. He got quite angry on these occasions, grumbling and shouting, and this behaviour gave grounds for suspecting hallucinatory experiences. This behaviour later greatly diminished.

Schoolwork is another area of experience to be used in inculcating and sharpening reality testing. In Daniel's case, with his degree of comprehension and sense of fun, the teacher used a series of statements which Daniel copied from the blackboard and to which he had to reply with a single 'yes' or 'no': for instance, 'Grass is green'; 'A cat has five legs'. Gradually these statements became more emotionally loaded and demanded some degree of judgement, and he had to reply with 'true' or 'not true', and later 'true' or 'false': e.g. 'I like swimming'; 'Mark is good at sums'.

Number work, too, in the use of workbooks and apparatus, provided him with an opportunity of experiencing the process of establishing certainties of fact, the existence of which is largely independent of moods and feelings.

In his relationship to his child-care worker he was generally warm and affectionate. He had three changes of child-care worker in five years, which is an unusually large number. He was angry and confused when the first one left him, but two years later he could talk of her with affection and recall many pleasurable experiences he had with her. His next child-care worker told him a month in advance that she was going to leave and he said, 'I might be very sad when you are gone'. Soon he began to withdraw from her. There was a part of the garden in a far corner which he called 'Lean Lane', where he went and talked to himself. He said: 'When you leave I will go to Lean Lane'. The child-care worker asked him to take her to Lean Lane, and there they sat down and she explained as best she could why she was leaving and that there would be a new child-care worker to whom he would be able to talk as he did with her.

At the time of writing he was still with the unit and continuing to improve.

The fact that Daniel and other schizophrenic children, in marked contrast to the autistic and severely traumatised child, have the capacity to form a close attachment to a caring adult may well indicate that they formed a close bond with the mothering person in infancy. Possibly the existence of such a bond covers up or delays the onset of the psychosis, so that it appears as a 'late-onset psychosis'. But while the formation of the early bond may lay the foundation for the child's capacity to form good attachments later, it may also be a contributory factor in the formation of childhood schizophrenia if the mother suffers from schizophrenia or a schizophrenic-like illness at that time.

It was in this group only that the occasional use of drugs was found beneficial. Chlorpromazine tends to reduce anxiety and tension and appears to shorten the periods of inaccessability. More impressive with Daniel was his response to psychotherapy. This added another, all-important, dimension to the 'reality-confrontations' he was faced with in school and in everyday life.

The other four schizophrenic children all showed varying degrees of improvement of their reality orientation, but apparently not enough for it to be maintained in their later environments. All went from High Wick to special schools; two of these, eight and ten years later, were in a subnormality and a mental hospital respectively. The other two remained in special schools. One, after five years, was a friendly and conforming adolescent, but with limited responses; the fourth child was transferred only recently.

The Autistic Child

The group of severely subnormal children with autistic features, or autistic children who are either untestable or who score at the severely subnormal level, and in whom there is evidence of brain pathology, is only briefly mentioned here. Apart from improving their level of socialisation we have been unable to produce any significant or basic changes, nor have we been able to work out a consistent plan of action for these children. Raising the level of social behaviour is, of course, important, just as adequate and proper care is essential – not only for the child's sake but also for the sake of the family.

There seems no point in adding to the descriptions of childhood autism which range from Kanner's original paper in 1943 to, say, Rimland's account in 1964, nor do the results of our efforts appear to differ appreciably from those reported in the literature (Eisenberg, 1957; Rutter, 1966). It may, however, be of interest to report a treatment procedure, originally pioneered by Helen Clancy in Brisbane, which was used with one child in the unit with equivocal and yet encouraging result. It is included here in the belief that it is of practical and theoretical interest, that it has not been described in detail before nor, as far as is known, been attempted in this country, and because the procedure is relevant to our discussion in that it involves the parents and demands, initially at least, the special facilities of a residential unit. This treatment was developed by Clancy and her colleagues (Clancy *et al.*, 1969; Clancy and McBride, 1969) initially for the purpose of correcting the feeding abnormalities so frequently found in the autistic child. They soon noticed that, with improvement in eating, 'significant changes also occur in other facets of behaviour'.

The rationale for this procedure is briefly as follows: a bond is normally formed between the baby and his mother, produced by her caring attention (feeding, bathing, cuddling) and the baby's response to it. This bond forms a basis for the further development of the child. With the emergence of the stranger-response at about five to seven months the bond has become truly reciprocal. In the autistic child, it is further suggested, this bond is absent or abnormal. Why this should be so is uncertain, nor is it necessary to know the original cause or causes to understand the autistic process which, once it is initiated, is seen as self-perpetuating, reinforced by the behaviour of the child and his environment (to begin with, primarily the mother).

An example of this process would be the feeding situation – selected because lazy sucking and feeding problems are common in autistic children and because feeding is of great importance in establishing a bond between mother and child. It is suggested that 'the feeding situation rapidly becomes aversive to both mother and child so that contact between the two becomes minimal'. The treatment attempts to reverse this process by using feeding to establish a new bond between mother and child. This bond is then used secondarily to foster 'the acquisition of behaviour normally developed in the socialisation process'. The treatment procedure to achieve the first aim, is, briefly, as follows: the therapist (feeder) offers the child a slightly unfamiliar food (the same throughout) at each mealtime. The mother is present and becomes the comforter. When the child has accepted the food, 'usually within a week', the mother takes over the feeding and other new foods are gradually introduced. As mealtime becomes increasingly pleasurable it can be used as playtime, and so to influence the child's social development. Within three months the child is expected to return to his family, when a similar programme of social and perceptual learning is continued at home and in a suitable pre-school environment. The authors claimed some measure of success for all twelve children they had treated in this way.

Julie was aged seven years nine months at the commencement of treatment. She had been with us for one-and-a-half years, during which time she became easier to manage (for instance, she had stopped spitting at people) but basically remained unchanged. She 'wafted' through the corridors, apparently oblivious of people and things. In addition to marked perceptual, particularly visual, avoidance, she had most other features of childhood autism: stereotyped activities – in her case primarily tapping; no, or hardly any, verbal communication, in that she used only single words, such as 'tea', 'water', 'fish', etc., in a largely inappropriate context; she rarely ran, but skipped across the room and had a tendency to toe-walking; there was no constructive play and she appeared to prefer to remain alone, tapping. The range of foods she appeared to like was small and there were periods when she refused meals for days. Feeding had been a problem in infancy and her lack of resposiveness had been noted during the first year. She had had several apparently major fits in the past, but the reports of the EEG done aged five years and seven years indicated no significantly abnormality. Both parents had had very difficult childhoods, but had emerged, as adults, with a mature adjustment to work and people. The father had worked as a salesman and was now undergoing teacher's training, the mother worked as a shorthand typist. Both parents were highly intelligent. Julie had a brother three years younger who was bright and healthy.

This particular family was chosen for treatment because, with this symptomatology and her age, Julie's prognosis was felt to be unfavourable; also because the parents were likely to be most co-operative and because practical considerations were reasonably favourable – the plan was to carry out the treatment during the father's long Easter holidays so that he could look after the boy and visit the hospital frequently. The plan was outlined to the parents, including, of course, the fact that this was the first attempt. The difficulties of the procedure were, if anything, magnified in the discussion with the parents, who were none the less keen to start. The mother moved in with Julie to occupy a small self-contained flat in the attic of the residents' quarters. The treatment team consisted of the therapist ('feeder'), child-care workers and the psychiatrist who was mainly concerned with co-ordinating the programme and planning it with the help of the other members, and giving support to the family, particularly the mother.

The feeding programme began one day after Julie and her mother had moved in. The slightly unfamiliar food consisted of a 'preferred' food, cereal, camouflaged a little by adding minced meat. The therapist offered it on a spoon to Julie either silently or with such words as 'Tea, Julie' or 'Dinner, Julie'. Throughout the treatment no attempt was made to persuade or cajole, the feeder remained throughout relaxed and friendly, uninvolved but not aloof. After offering the food for about a quarter of an hour the feeder removed it until the next meal. There were three 'meals' a day and the child had no food in between, but water or diluted juice when she wanted it – the fluid intake and output was charted.

The mother spent practically all meals with Julie and got her up and bathed her and put her to bed most days. She spent at least five hours with her every day either by herself or with a child-care worker – and days with a non-communicating, non-comprehending, non-playing child can appear endless and endlessly frustrating. However, already after two days her mother became aware of signals from Julie that immediately released her maternal feelings. At the last feed of the second day the mother describes how 'Julie sat on her chair and then straight onto my lap . . . she was cuddling me and looking into my eyes all the time; I felt she was so close to me and needed me, it brought tears to my eyes and she wiped them away for me, a thing she would never have done before . . .'.

> Immediately after tea (she had not accepted any food) the mother was keen to bath Julie, to continue looking after her with the feeling of closeness between them, but Julie had become unresponsive again and just cried angrily and splashed the water furiously. Her mother felt doubly hurt and despondent, but later the presence of the child-care worker acted as a catalyst and brought mother and child together again. Julie picked up a puppet and licked its face; her mother turned this into a game, and made the puppet clap hands, Julie holding on to her mother's fingers, smiling and laughing whenever her mother laughed. She held on to the puppet and seemed to copy her mother's facial expression of laughter, surprise or expectation. That night Julie slept peacefully from 7.30 p.m. to 6.20 a.m. – most unusual for her.

This episode appears to illustrate the vicissitudes of the early relationship between the mother and her autistic child. Possibly the extent to which the mother can tolerate rejection by the baby is one determining factor in the self-perpetuating autistic process. Another is the extent to which the environment unwittingly reinforces the child's cutting-off behaviour.

> During the treatment period we were sometimes diverted from the prime aim of enabling her to take the offered food by following her cues that led away from this aim – joining her, as it were, on the autistic side of the fence. One example was her use of cutting-off words. She seemed to become increasingly verbal at one stage during the feeding sessions, using her usual words, 'tea', 'Pat', 'train', etc., again and again. Her mother responded willingly as though entering into a kind of conversation: 'No, Julie, tea later', or 'We'll see Pat soon', or 'Julie went by car, not train', and so on. This interchange went on increasingly over two sessions until we realised that her mother had become a partner in Julie's stereotyped behaviour which in effect became a diversion from the treatment process.
>
> Julie refused food for eight days. The first day or two she would barely look at food offered on a spoon by the feeder, but simply push her hand away, careful never to touch the spoon or the food. Sometimes the push was hesitant, sometimes emphatic; sometimes she pushed with her fingers, sometimes the back of her hand. Gradually she began to look at the food intently and for longer periods. The tension in some of these sessions is difficult to describe: the spoon was brought slowly and gently towards her mouth; if it came too close or was moved too quickly she would inevitably jerk her head back as if stung, then she moved forward, coming quite close to the spoon, her lips moving then remaining absolutely still for endless seconds, as though transfixed; but in the end she

could not overcome whatever it was she had to overcome. On the fourth day, at tea-time, she touched the spoon with her finger, tasted a little food, spat it out, smeared some on the table and tasted a little, picking it up from the table. But then she said 'No' to the feeder and emphatically pushed her hand away. Sometimes she would scream, and bite and scratch her mother, but never the feeder. At times she tapped the table hard, tapping close all round the plate, but never touching it.

Of the tea-time feed on the eighth day the mother wrote in her own notes: 'I led Julie to her chair; she didn't want to sit on it at first, so I sat on her chair with her on my lap. She calmed down a lot so I gently persuaded her to sit on her own chair. She was very quiet then. I stroked her fingers and reminded her now and then of her nice tea. She tried to side-track me again a few times by saying 'Walk', 'Pat', etc., but I just smiled and nodded. She accepted this. She never tapped once or scratched me, but looked into my eyes a lot and touched my fingers and played with them – she seemed so different. Mrs S (the feeder) never said a word at all to Julie, and Julie often looked at Mrs S as if wondering whether to take the food or not. It was entirely up to her to take the food. She dipped her fingers into the bowl first, wiped it onto the table and tasted it twice; then she wanted more off the spoon with her fingers, then eventually she used the spoon with Mrs S. We were all so relieved.' To the observer the bond between mother and child before the acceptance of food seemed complete – the way they held hands and Julie gently touched and stroked her mother's hand gave one the feeling of deep love and trust between the two. Even so, before Julie could actually touch the food the conflict and distress on her face was painful to watch. The uncertainty about the 'goodness' of the food emerged clearly when several times after accepting it she spat it out and cried, as if suddenly the food or the process of eating had turned 'bad' or 'dangerous' again.

But this unfortunately was not the end of the story. She refused the first two meals the next day. I saw her shortly before the evening meal and was impressed by her awareness and eagerness I had not seen in her before. She ran into the eating room, immediately sat down expectantly, at once grabbed the spoon with food on it, held by the feeder, put it to her mouth, touched it, and then jerked away as if struck and refused any food from then on. For the next day or two there were still moments when she seemed torn and sometimes close to accepting it, but the twelfth day came and with it, I felt, the limit of our tolerance. As it was feared that the situation had by now become insuperably threatening to her, the feeding procedure was modified. Whether, by giving in, we had collectively become the victim of the autistic process, that is, colluded with it, will never be known. The next feed took place in the kitchen – feeder and mother busying themselves in the background and Julie sitting at the table with her bowl of food in front of her. She soon touched the food, ate some, spat some out. At the next meal in the same situation she accepted the spoon after a little while from the feeder, then from her mother who took over the feeding from then on. During the first two weeks or so she ate greedily, always wanting more, but she also got angry and often spat some of the food out.

Soon a more normal feeding pattern was established and she never reverted to the former uncertain feeding pattern. At the time of writing she was living at home and coming daily to High Wick, where her mother spent four days a week helping in the programme of perceptual learning that is part of our activities in the group of which Julie had been part since her admission.

In the four-and-a-half months after Julie began to feed, the changes in her behaviour can be summed up as follows. Visual avoidance as a pathological phenomenon virtually disappeared. Her whole behaviour, markedly so for the first few weeks, showed a social responsiveness that was noted even by people who knew nothing of her treatment. Her language remained extremely limited, but an outstanding new feature was her occasional spontaneous babbling (also reported by Clancy) and the equally spontaneous putting together of two and three word sentences, appropriate to the situation: 'Daddy come'; 'Daddy car'; 'Mummy cook toast'. There were the occasional 'monologues' in the presence of her mother, continuing for many minutes: 'Mummy cook, Mummy apple garden, Mummy egg cook toast', and so on. There was considerably more inflection in her voice and the use of cutting-off words greatly diminished. There was the beginning of meaningful play with miniature toys. Above all, her mother had become demonstrably the most important person in her life.*

Julie's undoubted initial improvement was not altogether maintained – a feature all too common in the treatment of autism and other severe disturbances in childhood. Whether this shows up the fault in the treatment procedure or is an inherent feature of the psychotic illness, is not known, but it does seem to indicate the possibility that successful treatment must encompass two essentially different procedures: one powerfully intense and relatively brief, the other building on the results of the first slowly and painstakingly. The changes described above are significant, but the total gains remain small. This may be due to the inefficacy of the procedure, which would be contrary to the reports by Clancy and her colleagues; or due to inexperi-

* I wish to acknowledge the central and most taxing role of the 'feeder', Katrin Stroh; and I would also like to thank Julie's parents, who read and approved the report of the treatment, and whose devotion was an inspiration to us all.

ence in the method – a possible factor; or to the fact that the child was older than the children hitherto treated.

Whatever the shortcomings of the treatment or the application of it, some interesting questions are raised: what is this powerful force that prevented Julie from accepting food for eight days (twenty-four meals)? What enabled her to overcome it on the eighth day? What happened three feeds later when she eagerly anticipated the food and, after the first touch on her mouth, completely rejected it? Was her taking in and spitting out an example, albeit a most important one, of the autistic process: acceptance and rejection and finally total rejection? Freud (1925) suggested that, initially, in the development of judgement, 'the attribute to be decided about may originally have been good or bad, useful or harmful. Expressed in the language of the oldest – the oral – instinctual impulses, the judgement is: "I should like to eat this" or "I should like to spit it out".' Does Julie's behaviour indicate a basic fault of judgement on what is good or bad, useful or harmful?

Conclusion: The Evaluation of Inpatient Care

The results of treatment at High Wick are hard to evaluate because of the large number of variables involved. To assess any unit of this kind requires painstaking work by specialised staff over a long period of time. On the question of the treatment of the children alone, such investigation would have to deal with a variety of controversial issues. One would have to decide, for instance, what constitutes desirable change in, say, an autistic child for whom only limited improvement can be expected; when comparing the efficacy of different methods of treatment one must be reasonably certain that they are carried out with a comparable level of competence; one would have to recognise, and act on such recognition, that childhood psychosis does not just comprise childhood autism and 'the rest' – whether 'the rest' is called schizophrenia, late-onset psychosis or something else.

The function of an inpatient unit may include treatment of the parents, and the separation of the child from his home becomes the first important step in this process. With the traumatised psychotic child, for instance, this separation is as much for the sake of the parents as of the child. After admission, the extent and timing of the continued contact between parent and child requires constant reappraisal and may be a decisive factor for the child's progress. When the psychosis is an intrinsic part of a wider family problem this must clearly be given the fullest attention. One can hardly speak of a successful treatment outcome if such children, greatly improved, return to an unchanged home environment. Nor need one's work of necessity be considered a failure even if there is little or no improvement in the psychotic child. The very fact of having him cared for in a residential unit where no thought nor effort is spared to help can bring relief to the parents. We know something of the stresses and tensions that become part of the life of the parents who look after a psychotic child, and the social limitations which such care entails (we know nothing of the possible long-term effects on the siblings), and it must surely be part of the function of a residential unit to help the parents to regain their stability and enable them to lead a fuller life, without losing their concern for the ill child.

These are some of the points to be considered in an evaluation of the work of an inpatient unit, in addition to other functions such as training, teaching and research – anything less than a complete assessment may not only be inadequate but, indeed, distort our understanding of the needs and the complexity of residential care for psychotic children.

CHAPTER SEVEN

Assessment and Treatment of Language-Disordered Children

H. M. N. Rees

It is said that a medieval king with true scientific objectivity confined the rearing of infants, over a period of ten years, to deaf-mute nurses on an inaccessible island. The results of these regal 'experiments', ostensibly to discover the 'language of heaven', are not reported. We can be in little doubt, however, that only primitive, non-verbal vocal behaviour developed in these children, so that the regal thesis was disproved.

Such folklore dramatically illustrates something which behavioural scientists have subsequently slowly and painfully learned: that the human infant is a biosocial organism whose development can be impaired by social as well as by inherent or acquired biological defects. The more complex and phylogenetically late the acquisition of biosocial skills, the more vulnerable they are to bio-social insults. Language, man's latest phylogenetic acquisition, is the most vulnerable. Recent work with chimpanzees only confirms that by and large language is possible only in the human species (Premack, 1971).

Independent life in our modern technological society is scarcely possible without language, no matter what intelligent visuo-spatial ability the individual has. Language is mediated via the dominant cerebral hemisphere and visuo-spatial abilities by the non-dominant hemisphere. Language is normally acquired by auditory-vocal means by the listening and speaking infant. A child whose auditory-vocal mechanisms are damaged can, however, acquire language at a less complex level, by visuo-motor skills such as reading and writing, finger-spelling, lip-reading or a systematic gesture language.

A normal child's thinking is initially talking instructions to himself, and a fundamental task of early childhood is to learn to integrate such increasingly internalised talking and doing. Thinking and reasoning depend on being able to code internal and external realities, past, present and future, in the manageable symbols of language, which may not necessarily be verbal. Thus the individual is free from bondage to current environmental stimuli, and so can solve problems one at a time by the process of the internal dialogue we call thought. The clarifying of both internal and external environments is mediated through language schemata, by means of which order is imposed on a child's view of the world and of himself.

Only thus can cognitive experience be communicated to others. The fabric of human intercourse, whether in social exchanges or in the conveyance of emotions by the arousal of feelings of any kind, depends upon the possession of language. Through language persons and things are anchored to reality by being given a word-label. Thus a child can acquire the knowledge that people and things in the environment, such as parents and home, have a permanence even when temporarily absent.

Language mediates an appreciation of self and non-self, and body image. Thus a child can control powerful feelings by the insightful, externalising effect of putting such feelings into words. The growth of ego-functioning is facilitated by the acquisition of language, which helps the child 'programme' his emotional reactions and behaviour and allows him to distinguish between reality and fantasy (de Hirsch, 1970).

Finally, *play* is not possible for a child who has no inner language, and play development is vital to the development of a child. It has been shown that the complexity of play is highly correlated with language development, play developing in form and complexity from sensori-motor exploration to imitation of adults' actions with common objects (whereby a child defines their use before naming), and then to playing with miniatures (cars, animal models, dolls-houses, etc.). Next comes inventive and imaginative play, and finally playing by rule (e.g. dolls-house play, ludo, etc.). Deaf children with little or no verbal speech play imaginatively and demonstrate that they have inner language. Thus much can be learnt about a child's level of acquisition of an inner language in the clinical situation by careful observation of his play.

Life without internal language and its external communication in some form is life without our greatest human asset, and is almost certain to result in a highly restricted, often institutionalised existence.

Planning for Language-disordered Children

It is an unfortunate fact that often the economic argument appears to be the most effective in administrative planning. Children with language disorders in institutions often live out their allotted 'three score years and ten'. This costs the community, at current rates, around £75,000 per person, with little return. The cost to an individual, in terms of the loss of the basic human inheritance of communication and a happy and constructive life, is incalculable. At the same time, the techniques of evaluating language potential and of a methodology for treatment of language-disorderd children are engaging a number of professions. The individual skills of these can be augmented when they work as part of a multidisciplinary team in a specialised, hospital-based unit for children with language disorders.

The main theme of this chapter will be to outline the method of isolating those children with the potential to acquire language from the larger number of children whose language defect is irremediable. Medical and neuropsychological indications of which children are those with a potential for language development are beginning to reach diagnostic usefulness. A teaching-diagnostic treatment regime is, however, necessary; this implies the existence of a skilled staff in an efficient language unit.

The total number of children with language disorders, excluding those due to secondary conditions such as mental subnormality or congenital deafness, is greater than the available resources, medical and educational, can deal with. Meanwhile the selection of cases and the precise delineation of treatment methods are necessary. Methods are needed which can be replicated elsewhere and can, if possible, be used by parents, teachers and speech therapists as well as by medical personnel who have learnt the basic skills involved. In a time of shortage this approach is of paramount importance in this hitherto neglected area of treatment. It implies an experimental approach such as that advocated by Tizard (1966) which defines, in operational terms, the child, the means of assessment, the method of treatment used, and the indices of change.

A description of an approach to this ideal in the design of a particular regional language unit, where a treatment programme catering for these goals is being evolved, will follow.

Normal Development of Language and Speech

Pre-language Development

The various abnormalities of language and speech can only be understood in the framework of normal language development. Most observers agree on the importance of the first year of life, when the very basis of language and communication develops. Comprehension and utterance develop roughly in parallel, to their mutual advantage. For the sake of coherence it is useful to describe separately what is a reciprocal interaction. Imitation and comprehension normally precede language, but since vocalisation occurs first, the development of language utterances will first be described. Nevertheless both utterance and comprehension are preceded by the loving interaction which characterises the normal mother–child relationship, when the mother responds non-verbally as well as verbally to all sorts of emotion-laden activities of the infant. This can be seen in the continual interaction between mother and young infant, her adjustment to the baby's posture, or her reactions to her baby's discomfort and so on. The infant comes to regard his mother's vocalisations in the feeding, bathing, comforting nurturance as part of this love relationship out of which eventually mutual verbal communication naturally emerges.

In early infancy vocalisation is simply a means of communicating needs. Crying to indicate various discomforts predominates, but the gurgling and cooing of bodily satisfaction are also heard, reinforced by the mother making similar comforting vocalisations in the nursing situation.

Babbling, usually from four or five months on, is the next stage. It accompanies the baby's delight in making and hearing his own sounds, for example while playing with his toes. Around seven months the babbling increasingly gets nearer and nearer to the sounds of his own language environment, whereas earlier on the primitive sound-making in babies is similar throughout the world. Babbling gradually stops if its pleasurable content is not appreciated by the baby: thus the congenitally deaf baby around this age ceases to babble.

The first primitive bi-syllabic babble words of the 'mama', 'dada', 'baba' variety are the product of a near approximation of simple words in the language environment, and are reinforced by delighted parental response. What has happened is that over these crucial early months of babbling, the child has performed the fantastic feat of so ordering the complex reflexes of expiration, vocal cords, and peripheral vocal mechanisms as to produce a consistent sound which is appreciated as consistent by his own auditory system. A complex feedback of musculo-kinaesthetic movement of the vocal mechanisms, monitored by the increasingly discriminating auditory apparatus, is being established. This is the very basis of the phonological or sound-producing system, and it depends upon the integrity of the nervous system.

Even in some children with severe sensori-neural deafness, with provision of suitable amplification and deaf education techniques the establishment of the essential vocal-auditory feedback loop can be maintained and verbal ability established (Fry and Whetnall, 1954).

The development of speech proceeds in almost geometrical fashion, from two or three words at twelve months to thirty words at eighteen months, 200–300 at two years, and increasing dramatically to around 2,000 words at age four to four-and-a-half years. Such rapid comprehension and utterance of this large number of meaningful word labels, without conscious teaching by the parents, is a remarkable achievement. It is done simply by the normal imitation processes of the young child.

The Acquisition of Grammar in a Normal Child

Even more remarkable than this rapid acquisition of so large a vocabulary from eighteen months to four years is the rapid acquisition of grammar. It requires an imaginative effort for adults to realise that in the brief course of two years or so, following a child's first words, he has succeeded in mastering the exceedingly complicated grammatical rules of his own language, again without conscious teaching by his parents. The child is simply exposed to a 'corpus' of spoken language, often with incomplete sentences such as are usual in the average home. From such a 'language corpus' the child infers and utters syntactic and semantic rules, but these are preceded by imitation of intonation, the prosodic qualities of spoken language.

Furthermore, different children exposed to differing samples of language, not only in our culture, but in all the known language cultures studied, achieve by around five years of age this remarkable ability to utter and comprehend an infinite number of correct and original sentences, never previously heard by the child. These basic processes of language acquisition follow a significantly similar development in children belonging to all the languages so far studied. The only tenable hypothesis is that potential language acquisition is inbuilt biologically in the human brain (Lenneberg, 1967; Slobin, 1972). It is only vaguely shown in the higher apes, where a simplified visual language analogue has recently been taught by skilled and painstaking research workers (Premack, 1971).

As stated earlier, this phylogenetically late-acquired function is highly complex and therefore comparatively readily broken down by various adverse factors, usually biological. Such damaging biological agents operate during foetal development, during the paranatal crisis and in early childhood. If the damage to those brain structures subserving language is the causative factor, then such damage must be bilateral or centre-encephalic. Unilateral destruction of the dominant cerebral cortex which subserves language in early or mid-childhood only temporarily disrupts language, with transference of function to the uninjured hemisphere. Similarly, gross environmental deprivation may produce a language defect, but here evidence is accumulating that until mid-childhood or later a radically improved and enriching environment may produce a delayed but dramatic language acquisition (Clarke, 1968).

The psycholinguistic theories of language development will not be discussed; indeed, a stage has not been reached at which psycholinguistics can be other than a tentative aid in the development of a more exact therapy (Crystal, 1972). Nor is it proposed to describe the acrimonious dialogue between the proponents of the psycholinguistic school led by Chomsky and the followers of the behaviouristic school founded by Skinner.

In brief, the breakthrough into early grammatical language, rather than simple word labelling, occurs around the age of eighteen months. The child combines two words grammatically by using a limited number of 'pivot' words with the larger number of word labels or 'open class' word labels. Thus utterances such as 'all-gone milk', 'all-gone dada', are examples of a first pivot word: 'all-gone'. From such pivot words many adult grammatical parts of speech are later derived.

The remarkable thing is that similar early speech patterns occur in all languages, and in no way could they have been derived from adult speech forms. There is merely a handful of such early basic grammatical rules, and these are used in various combinations with the finite number of words which a young child uses to produce an infinite number of grammatically correct sentences, which are original in the sense that they have never been heard or uttered previously by the child.

The fact that rules are inferred and subsequently adhered to tenaciously, and this in spite of attempts by adults to make the child revert to an early correct but simply imitative speech, can be seen when the incorrect inflection, by over-generalising the rule, is used in the irregular forms of plural nouns and past tense verbs. Thus, for months a child will insist upon giving the plural form of 'sheep' as 'sheeps', and 'foot' as 'foots' or 'footses', or inflecting the past tense of irregular verbs, e.g. 'I bringed it', or 'I throwed it', 'breaked it', etc.

The Behavioural Side-effects of Language Delay

Most complex early bio-social human activities depend upon an underlying neuropsychological intactness, which in such a phylogenetically late acquisition may rapidly break down. Even in normal development the stages in a child's complex language are acquired within a wide time limitation and yet may be quite normal. Such a delay may sometimes be a family characteristic. Thus there is a good chance that an otherwise normal three-and-a-half-year-old, who can comprehend well but can say only the odd word, will speak normally by six-and-a-half. Reassurance to the anxious parents is therefore justified, provided the cardinal rule of follow-up is not omitted. However, children with severe receptive language disorders have a poorer prognosis.

In children with pathological conditions meriting therapy, the incidence of behaviour and emotional difficulties is quite high, and the acquisition of social training is very often delayed. The overt behaviour disturbance depends on the basic temperamental type of the child, or on a possible reciprocal relationship between paranatal brain damage and the behavioural reinforcement received from the environment. At opposite ends of a continuum, two different behavioural types occur: the hyperactive, distractible, extroverted child who reacts with severe tantrums to the frustration of his inability to communicate; and, in contrast, the readily-withdrawing, introverted child who avoids the frustration of his communication difficulty or else sticks to non-verbal, usually pre-symbolic means; for instance, taking a parent by the hand to fetch a desired object. Such a child usually avoids play with other children particularly. These children may fit into the not uncommon group of children who present a behavioural syndrome in between childhood aphasia and childhood autism, but these clinical entities will be described later.

Prevalence of Language Disorders

Minor speech and language disorders in early childhood are quite common, but if one takes the more severe disabling disorders in which language development will probably not occur without treatment, the prevalence far exceeds present provision made under the health and education services, especially outside London and the south-east of England. Thus the incidence of the severe disorders which have been surveyed by epidemiological means, such as early infantile autism, severe disabling dysarthria, articulatory deviancy and receptive and executive aphasia, amounts to around ten per 10,000 live births, and the optimum time for therapy is between the ages of three and seven years (Herbert and Wedell, 1970; MacKeith and Rutter, 1972). From this the incidence and prevalence in a particular regional catchment area can be calculated. There are other conditions, such as primary severe subnormality, cerebral palsy and deafness, which are not included in this prevalence estimate.

Diagnostic Classification of Speech and Language Disorders

A simple clinical classification can only be an imperfect model, particularly as in any child there may be several interacting conditions. However, for the sake of coherence and for its pragmatic clinical use, the following classification has been adopted, modified from Ingram (1972).

Primary disorders of speech development

Stammering } These will not be considered here
Aphonia }
Articulation disorders
Dysarthria

Disorders of language development

1. Disorders secondary to other defects
    - Brain damage (cerebral palsy)
    - Deafness
    - Severe subnormality
    - Severe social deprivation
2. Developmental disorders
    - Early infantile autism
    - The aphasias (receptive and executive)
3. Psychogenic disorders
    - Elective mutism

It is proposed here to consider only those language disorders which necessitate inpatient or daypatient treatment in a specialised language unit. Thus most of the speech disorders are excluded, and the main consideration is given to speech defects which are secondary to an underlying language disorder.

Primary Disorders of Speech Development

Articulatory Disorders

Functional disorders in articulation range from the common consonantal substitution and omissions of word endings, as in immature speech patterns normal in early childhood, to gross, rigidly-maintained deviancy in articulation which makes speech incomprehensible to peers and adults. Such severe deviant speech disorders may require a linguist to reveal the abnormal general rules underlying the misarticulation. Whereas the common minor misarticulations are invariably self-correcting with maturation, the latter deviant misarticulations require very skilled speech therapy, preferably several times weekly.

Articulatory disorders are almost invariable secondary handicaps in recovering executive aphasic patients, presumably as the result of the poor development of the auditory-vocal feedback system.

Dysarthria

This term is restricted to the articulation defects which are the result of structural abnormalities of the vocal mechanisms: such abnormalities as malocclusion of jaws, harelip, cleft palate, paresis of tongue or palate; a congenitally short palate which inadequately closes nasal from oral cavities, resulting in highly nasal speech; or neurological damage. Some of these disorders can be corrected by plastic surgery followed by intensive speech re-education by a skilled speech therapist.

Disorders of Language Development

1. *Disorders Secondary to Other Defects*

The brain-damaged child, typically a spastic child, has other handicaps. His motor disability, with its attendant early failure to explore the world and to interact in a reciprocal manner with normal parents' expectations, usually results in parents drastically lowering their expectations, often sometimes encouraging a regressive dependence. The child may have difficulty in hand and eye control, also difficulty in integrating the complex movements of lips, tongue and other vocal mechanisms in order to stimulate his family by the usual increasingly speech-like babble of late infancy. Almost invariably perceptual disorders are present. Thus vocal and especially verbal play increasingly become a losing battle. Since his gross motor attainment would appear to be particularly depressed in comparison with language and social interaction, the child's family may, paradoxically, cease to stimulate him, particularly by verbal means, mainly to prevent frustration. At the same time he becomes impoverished in social interchange as compared with his normal siblings and peers, and often he becomes over-protected and confined to the house in an ambience of caring but non-verbal attendance. His difficulties in speaking are compounded by any dysarthric or aphasic result of brain damage. Meanwhile, because of his impoverished physical environment, he has literally nothing to talk about, and language development suffers.

Such a spastic child should have his world of new experience brought to him. Parents, ideally, should try to undertake the admittedly most difficult task of describing colourful and stimulating play objects with repeated and abundant talk, since the spastic child cannot discover the richness of perceptual experiences on his own. However, the family despair to be tackled was expressed by a mother who remarked, in apparently reasonable terms, 'We talked to him for a long time, as we did to our other (normal) children, and when we didn't get anything back, we stopped' (Berry, 1969).

The reasons why language, particularly, would be expected to be long delayed should be explained in common-sense terms, together with practical advice as to how to stimulate the child with size, colour, shape, texture of attractive toys, or everyday real objects, including their 'definition by use' before word-labelling. Also realistically helpful are frequent car or coach trips to see real hills, wild and farm animals, beaches, 'pomp and ceremony' and so on. Specific speech therapy may be indicated for muscular defects in the peripheral vocal organs.

However, as in all other disorders, an accurate functional diagnosis of a child's deficits is the only rational means to providing a specific therapy, and it always has to be recognised that some cerebrally damaged children (with bilateral or centre-encephalic lesions) may never acquire language.

The deaf child. A child who is *profoundly* or *sub-totally* deaf has very little hearing for any sound and no useful hearing for speech, even when it is amplified through a hearing aid. The *severely* deaf child can hear voice when it is amplified, but cannot distinguish consonants, even when speech is amplified. Both of these groups of children rely on speech-reading for all communication and are educated in schools for the deaf. About 80 per cent of profoundly and severely deaf children have no serious learning disabilities. Their handicap is that they cannot hear speech: until they receive special instruction they do not know that people use words. A hearing aid is almost useless to profoundly deaf children.

These children learn receptive language only under optimal conditions: directly facing the speaker, who has his face towards the light, and speaks slowly and distinctly in simple, straightforward English. They can see clearly the movement of the lips, but for the most part have to guess what the tongue is doing. They hear none of the intonation or stress patterns which add meaning to speech. Speech reading has been called 'intelligent guesswork'. For every word the child learns he is wholly dependent on other people to speak directly to him and make the meaning clear.

The profoundly sensori-neural deaf child is deaf to his own speech He has no auditory feedback of his own attempts to speak, and his vocal tactile-kinaesthetic monitoring control must be slowly developed by associating it with his teacher's opinion of his efforts to imitate her speech via his visual appreciation of her facial expressions, or gestures, of approval.

The high tone hearing loss of the *partially hearing* child is a much less severe handicap. Speech filtered through his imperfect auditory perception is distorted. A hearing aid amplifies the distortion, but does not correct it. However, since the distortion is constant he learns to interpret what he hears. The effect of the distortion is to make similar sounds sound alike, and he cannot distinguish *p*, *t*, *k*, *s*, *sh*, *f*, *th*, or such words as *pat* and *cat*, *dog* and *talk*, *eleven*, *elephant* and *telephone*, without visual clues from speech-reading. With this help, however, partially hearing children learn to comprehend and to use normal language and, according to their general ability, can be educated in partially hearing units or classes in normal schools. These children often show emotional disturbances from which most totally deaf children are free. Special hearing aids that amplify, differentially, high frequencies may be useful.

In cases in which the onset of profound sensori-neural deafness is acquired after the acquisition of spoken language, especially if it occurs between the ages of three and possibly as late as ten years, vocal language may be lost. The younger children are the more vulnerable. With special teaching, which trains the child to rely on speech-reading, spoken language is recoverable, but intonation and meaningful sentence stress are not often recovered. Again, the listener's facial responses or lip-read replies are the only way such a child can monitor or correct linguistic slips, for instance saying 'seventy' for 'seventeen'.

Adequate audiological diagnosis of partial acquired deafness should differentiate two types: high tone deafness, which is a distortion of all input of sound, and conductive deafness, which causes all sound to be perceived as attenuated. A child with normal articulation and normal intonation, but a constantly quiet voice, may have a conductive deafness since his own auditory feedback is abnormally loud at the particular time of deafness. His deafness may, confusingly, vary periodically in severity, and is usually worse in winter months concurrent with upper respiratory tract infections. Antibiotic treatment may replace a middle ear infection with a gelatinous fluid clinically silent apart from an increased conductive deafness. Specialised otological diagnostic and therapeutic techniques will not be considered here.

Mental subnormality. The principal difficulty here is making the correct differential diagnosis, since severely disordered, but potentially intelligent, young children with no language may function at subnormal level, and they are often not amenable to psychological testing in the early stages of diagnostic assessment. Language delay, of course, is often the major presenting symptom of a subnormal child, but he is also delayed in other skills.

As Tizard (1966) and others have demonstrated, considerable increases of general cognitive levels may sometimes be obtained by the placement of subnormal children in optimal conditions with a high staff–patient ratio, and there is little doubt that children so placed achieve a higher level of functioning if they can be kept in their own home.

A reasonable approach after a period of optimal social stimulation would be to regard the moderately retarded child as equal in attainment to a normal child of the same mental age. Nevertheless, such highly integrated mental functioning as would be required in language development may never be achieved, presumably because of a deficit in the neurological basis for language. Added to this there is the usual lack of curiosity, and also often disturbed behaviour, which increase the child's inability to cope with the environment. Conversely, apathy from lack of curiosity is the usual correlate of living in unstimulating or rigidly institutionalised surroundings, where speech is rarely used between staff and patients.

Severe social deprivation. The evidence that gross sensory and emotional deprivation in early childhood have fixed and immutable effects, particularly on such highly complex functions as language, has gained credence from dramatic case reports, as of children confined for years in attics and so on, and the phenomenon of the rare feral child (such as that of Itard). Research into deprivation in infancy, such as that of Bowlby (1964) who invoked 'sensitive periods' in early infancy as an explanatory device, has been severely criticised by O'Connor (1956), Yarrow (1961) and Clarke (1968).

Clarke compared the evidence regarding the outcome in two separate cases of grossly deprived children, each of whom had been kept locked up in an attic for about six years. The more deprived of the two had a subnormal mother and received no subsequent treatment. The other, who had been imprisoned in a similar dark attic with her deaf-mute mother, subsequently received highly skilled and intensive help. When these children were discovered, in their sixth year, both functioned at an imbecile level, were unable to comprehend or utter speech, were grossly underdeveloped physically, mentally and socially, and had rickets. The child of the deaf-mute mother learnt to speak in sentences within two months; was reading and writing in nine months; trebled her IQ in 18 months; and had a two-thousand word count after 16 months. At 14 years she was regarded as a normal girl. The other girl's lack of progress may have been due to her subsequent lack of intensive help, or to her genetic constitution derived from her subnormal mother.

Clarke's conclusion from his evidence is that, in many individuals, only long-enduring experience leads to inflexibility in personality and cognitive structures in the face of dramatic enriching environmental changes. In the field of language development, this conclusion has to be qualified by the probable fact that language learning cannot become normal unless begun under the age of about ten years, particularly if cognition is at a subnormal level in other areas. But, in general, too facile an extrapolation of the critical periods for learning seen in lower animals to human infants, and a too ready generalisation from the occasional dramatic case report, is to be deprecated. The physical, intellectual and emotional handicaps associated with multiple handicaps are often seen in children committed to local authority care after having suffered multiple deprivation over many years. Mapstone's (1969) and Rees and Morley's (to be published) studies illustrate the impossibility of disentangling genetic and environmental factors in such cases.

2. *Developmental Language Disorders*

Under this heading will be considered *early infantile autism* and *developmental receptive* and *executive dysphasia*. It has been decided to consider these three syndromes together for several reasons. Although autistic children are handicapped in several other ways, they often have the same types of language disorder as have children with receptive or executive aphasias. In autistic children, however, the deficit of inner language is more profound.

Autistic children can have the same auditory perceptual difficulties as children with receptive aphasia. Wing (1969), in her study of the handicaps of autistic children compared with other groups, found, that both autistics and childhood aphasics are multiply handicapped combining the problems of comprehension and use of speech, and also right/left, up/down, back/front disorientation, as well as perceptual and some, but not all, of the characteristic behaviour anomalies.

Furthermore, there are children whose clinical features reveal them to be in the hinterland between autism and aphasia and there are aphasic children who, under stress, temporarily preoccupy themselves with the same obsessive rituals while avoiding interpersonal relationships, exactly as do autistic children. Aphasic children shed these habits on removal from stressful conditions, unlike autistic children who have more long-lasting and rigidly fixed, though similar, patterns of behaviour.

Finally, both the autistic and aphasic syndromes have clinical features generally considered to be the result of brain dysfunction or even overt brain damage, and almost never simply due to perverted hearing.

However, the main reason for classifying them together is that they can best be helped by the same type of diagnostic teaching method which identifies their perceptual and cognitive difficulties for possible remedial help. The main aim should be directed towards teaching language, using the most intact sensory system, either auditory-vocal or visuo-motor.

Autism in early childhood. The terms 'autism', 'the autistic child' will here be used to refer to the various psychotic conditions of early childhood. The disorders occur either from birth or with an onset before the age of three years. The symptoms, modified from Creak's points (Creak, 1964) include:

(i) Gross disorder of understanding or uttering language, often with a failure to gesture, or to signify emotional communication. Instead an aloof, unchanging facial expression is maintained.

(ii) Poor ability to make interpersonal relationships, or even an active or panicky withdrawal, often with tantrums, from contact with others.

(iii) Visual and auditory avoidance: that is to say, a failure to make eye contact and a lack of response to a parent's voice, together with perceptual defects in vision or hearing.

(iv) A fierce resistance to any change, or 'obsession with sameness', may show itself either by severe distress if any article of furniture is moved from its accustomed place in the home, or if a different car route is followed to a familiar place. The child may restrict his food intake to a few similar articles (and the similarity may even be in shape, for example cylindrical shapes, such as sausages, fishsticks or chips only).

(v) Almost invariably there are severe emotional upsets, as when the syndrome's onset is marked by tumultuous emotional distress, or the primitive fear–rage reaction when the child's preoccupations are interfered with. There is an inability to empathise with others, and an equal inability to appreciate humour.

(vi) The syndrome may occur in children who show test results on visuo-spatial intelligence tests from high average to severely subnormal level. Nevertheless, even with superior ability on visuo-spatial tests, the child's functioning is not related to his adaptation with environmental reality.

(vii) Often the autistic child is devoid of inner language to such a degree that his play is entirely of a primitive sensori-motor kind, interspaced with his meaningless preoccupations.

Receptive aphasia in childhood. This may vary in degree and in its severe form is a rare condition. A child may present either a complete inattention to all sounds, being 'deafer than deaf', although auditory evoked responses measured by computerised EEG techniques usually show that there is no peripheral or cochlear hearing loss. Less severely affected receptive aphasics may respond to cruder sounds, but are incapable of localising the sound or processing the complex seriation of language. Again, such a child may have an inability to deal with symbolisation in visual as well as in auditory language presented. Such a child may respond to the sense of a simple command, using only key words and situational cues gained from past experience. The condition may occur in early childhood following or preceding a series of epileptic attacks.

As previously described, there are usually other handicaps in common with autistic children, mainly perceptual and behavioural.

Executive aphasia in childhood. A normal developmental language-delay syndrome shades into executive aphasia when there is usually evidence of perceptual difficulties indicative of brain damage. Comprehension may be normal or relatively less impaired than the ability to utter speech. Executive language-delay in a normally learning child with normal comprehension, having normal emotional status and average intelligence, is fairly common and benign. Thus, a child not speaking at three-and-a-half years will have normal speech and language at six years, statistically speaking. But the necessary medical reassurance to anxious parents is always to be complemented by three-monthly reviews.

Most severely executive-aphasic children under five years old, provided they have near average intelligence in the rest of their functioning and have normal comprehension, recover at least to some degree. Word labelling of familiar objects may be taught by special techniques, and they later even learn original utterances. Grammatically correct language sequences finally may occur. Such language development delay is frequently associated with left/right, up/down, back/front disorientation, and reading disability occurs at school, becoming obvious by seven or eight years. There is sometimes a family history of language delay.

The treatment of severely handicapped autistic and aphasic children, especially those with complicated behavioural problems, should ideally be undertaken in special language units, and Ingram (1972) has estimated that about ten are necessary in Great Britain.

The long-term management of such children consists of a graduated series of teaching-diagnostic measures, geared individually towards the particular child's functional handicap: correcting perceptual difficulties when possible and using a child's cognitive strengths to learn language either by the usual auditory-vocal means or, if necessary, by means of visual language-learning or a systematic sign language, eventually passing on to reading and writing.

3. *Psychogenic Disorders*

Elective mutism. This is probably a neurotic condition, usually occurring in early or mid-childhood. The child is known to speak perfectly normally with some people, often the immediate family, or only mother and siblings, while maintaining an invariable silence with other people. Sometimes the condition is associated with an articulatory defect or a minor executive language disorder. It occurs more frequently in girls than boys. The syndrome is an exaggeration of the silence certain young children maintain on entry to school, which usually disappears within a year of school entry.

There tend to be characteristic temperamental traits, such as introversion, a dominant negative mood and a dislike of change. Communication channels, for instance in school, are usually maintained by establishing a special relationship with another child, who interprets the subject's needs and mediates between her and the teacher. The whole situation may be reinforced, either by parents' or teachers' threats or bribes, or by allowing the child to manipulate her environment by evoking anxiety and sympathy in older children and adults, who become excessively over-protective and solicitous. In terms of adult reaction, if the child is negatively reinforced for social adaptation, she will resist behaviour change, because of the secondary gains such as the over-protection and pampering she solicits.

Treatment is usually by psychotherapy or behaviour therapy at a child psychiatric unit, but the parental reinforcing behaviour towards the symptom has to be corrected, by promoting insight into the psychological mechanisms involved.

Some Basic Neuropsychological Correlates of Language-learning

As with all highly-developed human skills, language-learning in children depends upon the possession of simpler neuropsychological functions which become integrated in hierarchical fashion during maturation. A diagnostic teaching programme should detect children who cannot, under optimal conditions, achieve the fundamental skills necessary for language acquisition at that particular time. It may mean changing from teaching an auditory-vocal language to a visuo-motor one, if there is an irremediable deficit in auditory processing.

For the sake of coherence the following neuropsychological functions will be described individually although, of course, to do so is an artificial abstraction.

Attention is the basis of intellectual development, and interfering behaviour patterns such as hyperkinesis and distractibility have to be corrected by management techniques, in order that a child may be enabled to 'learn to learn' (see below).

Perceptual hierarchial development: language is dependent upon a child developing from his early infantile dependence upon 'near' receptors, such as touch and taste, to efficient use of 'distance' receptors, especially vision and hearing.

Perceptual discrimination in either visual or auditory modalities, or both, must have attained, and increased beyond, a basic minimum; this has been shown by the work of Hermelin and O'Connor (1970) in visual perception and McReynolds (1966) in auditory discrimination. The ability to integrate two sensory inputs by a sensory trans-modal coding is also necessary for language development. Sensory input, be it visual, auditory or tactile, must be appreciated in a sequential perceptual pattern. The sequence must be retained in short- and long-term sequential memory stores. These memory stores, and present input, are then compared.

Also present must be the ability to *cue-match* arbitrary visual or auditory symbols with a constant referent stimulus, for example an arbitrary symbol with a colour, and later an auditory or visual word label with its reference. Thus the child becomes able to assign meaning to identified perceptual patterns.

Rule-attaining behaviour and meaningful generalisations are essential if each incoming stimulus is not to be regarded as a novel perception; any internal representational system would otherwise become an intolerable burden on a child's memory system. Rule-making is not only essential in syntax and semantics but even in perception of phonemic patterns. This is not only because different speakers have different intonations, but also because the same phonemes differ as auditory stimuli, according to which other phonemes follow them. Thus, all English children learn to categorise 't' even though it is perceptually different, as shown for example on an oscilloscope, in such words as 'table', 'tom', 'lettuce', 'touch', etc.

Principles of Therapy

The principles underlying the practical treatment of young children with severe language disorders may best be understood if they are divided into their two aspects – general and specific.

General Principles of Management

(i) A structured environment is indicated because of the gross defects shown by these children. They have a tendency to revert to primitive states of organisation, as in autistic children whose activity may have little bearing on reality activities. Such children therefore initially need a 1 : 1 staff : patient ratio, the staff member having a rewarding interaction with each child and striving to keep him occupied with a task related to his language disorder.

(ii) In a multi-disciplinary team it is important that all staff members have an agreed immediate and long-term goal for each child, each using his or her professional techniques. Thus, the psychologist working with a child at the early word-labelling stage would teach the same words, using operant techniques, as were being generalised in day-to-day living.

(iii) A high level of reward (positive reinforcement) for both language learning and socialising behaviour should be the rule, and negative reinforcements (withdrawal of attention, a sharp 'NO', or even a short time-out procedure) confined strictly to defined deviant behaviour.

(iv) Young patients should be admitted as daypatients if the home is within reasonable distance, unless there is undue stress at home or the home is marked by irremediable inconsistency or other psychopathology.

(v) It is vital that, whatever method of management a child is receiving in the language unit, the parents are given specific instructions in generalising this while the child is at home, mainly in terms of attention-maintaining and socialising behaviour, as well as the level of language.

Selection of Patients

It is obvious that some sort of selection procedure has to be adopted for children who are to occupy the small number of places available. At the Charles Burns unit children are therefore initially assessed as outpatients, then by a daypatient or inpatient four-week assessment period, and later during a continued treatment programme on re-admission. Admission and readmissions are selected after exclusion of subnormality and specific syndromes such as histidinaemia and deafness, but principally on positive grounds, namely evidence of an aptitude for learning. Children are discharged if possible to educational establishments.

Specific Methods of Therapy

The Physical Infra-structure of a Language Unit

The language unit of the Charles Burns Clinic includes a series of hutted accommodation units attached to the parent regional inpatient and outpatient child psychiatric clinic (see Figure 7.1). The structure has been designed so that the electronic logic and other apparatus is confined to a central room (see Figure 7.2).

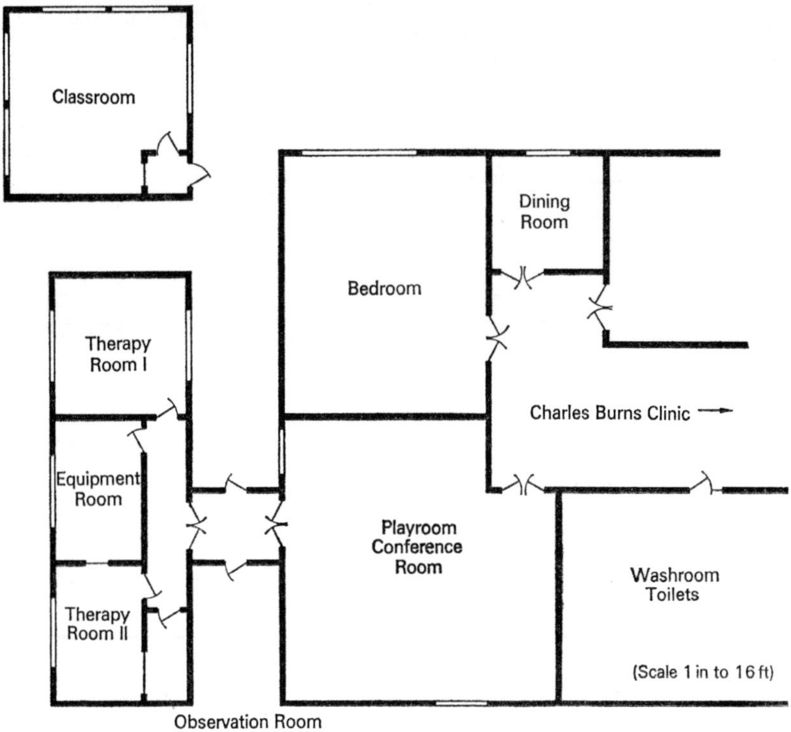

Fig. 7.1

Layout of the Language Unit of the Charles Burns Clinic

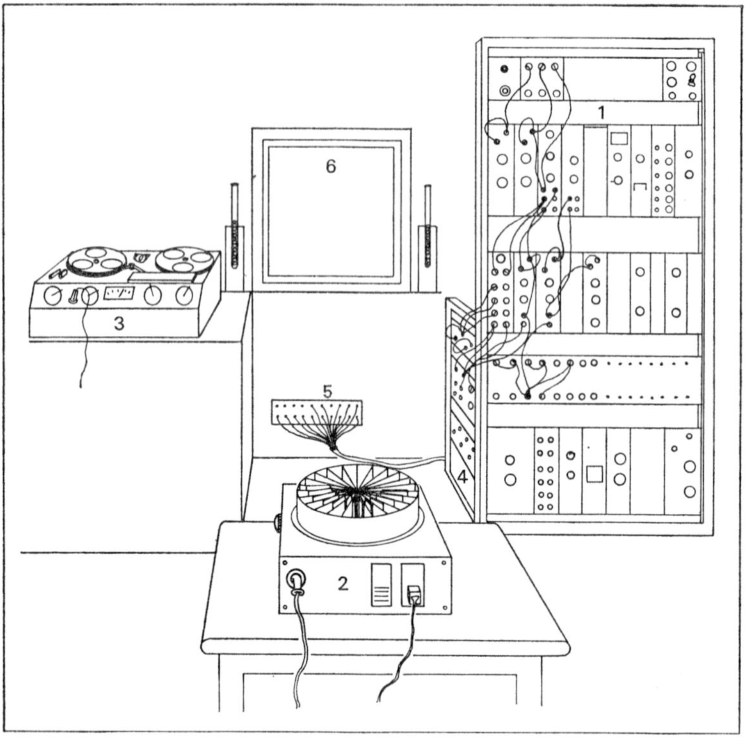

Fig. 7.2

1 Post Office rack with various electronic modules
2 Projector
3 Tape recorder
4 Terminal panel
5 Interconnecting board
6 Back projection screen

The application of electronic learning-devices as aids in the study and efficient teaching of deviant children has hitherto had very little clinical acceptance. One reason is that such commercial learning-devices are inordinately expensive and usually so constructed that only a specific and rigid programme is available. The modular teaching unit in use at our language unit was originally constructed at the Belmont Hospital and described by Evans (1970). The modules which are part of the system can be assembled in different ways to suit the individual child.

The basic plan is that clear pictures of common interesting objects are back-projected onto a screen above the console (Figures 7.3 and 7.4). The therapist helps the child by operant conditioning techniques: increasingly accurate approximations of the child's utterances to those of the therapist are rewarded. The advantage of back-projection is that the child and therapist are in a lighted room and the child can see and imitate the therapist's lip and frontal tongue movements. This brings help with difficult phonemes by means of visual and kinaes-

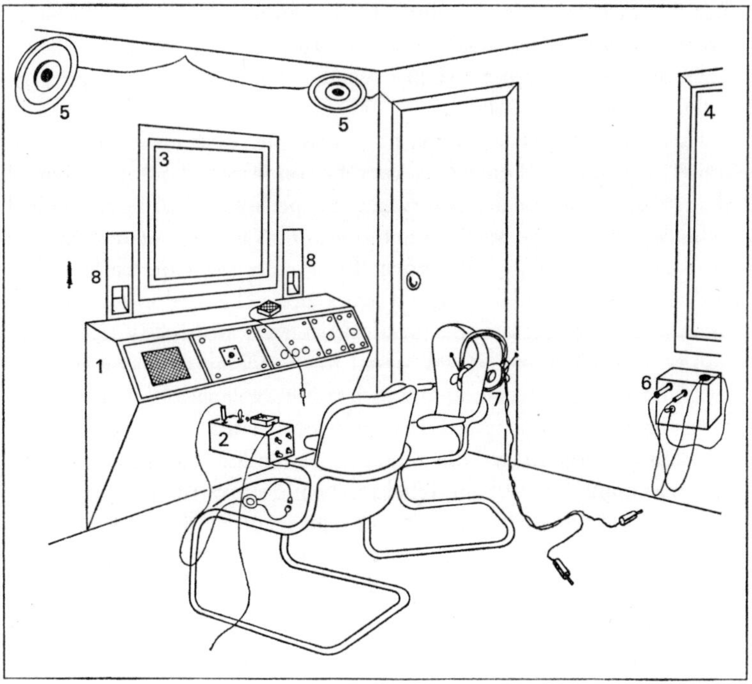

Fig. 7.3

1 Console (including microphone and interchangeable modules)
2 Therapist's control box
3 Interchangeable projection screens
4 One-way screen
5 Loudspeakers
6 Jackplug box for two-way communication with observation room and for audiometric testing
7 Patient's audiometric earphones
8 Reinforcement cups

thetic cues (Nelson and Evans, 1968). Each near approximation is rewarded, while incorrect responses are not. The apparatus is controlled by a master switch in the therapist's control box.

A variety of other teaching techniques can be used to stimulate visual and auditory memory and sequencing as well as auditory/visual transmodal coding and cue-matching.

Initially the rewards are the satisfaction of infantile needs such as a drink or food (jelly is useful) and later sweets or counters dispensed according to a predetermined schedule of reward. As quickly as possible such rewards are substituted by enthusiastic approval ('Good boy!' and similar remarks) by the therapist, and the reward of being able to press a convenient switch which changes the picture and indicates success (Lovaas, 1966).

However, the generalisation of success must be achieved in the ten hours of waking life outside laboratory conditions. Thus it is essential that other professional workers can see and hear what the individual child is achieving in special conditions. This is also essential for the instruction of parents, who normally interact with the child before and after day attendance and at weekends. This is done by having them observe a teaching diagnostic session via a one-way screen (see Figure 7.5). They can at will signal to the therapist or else query a specific therapeutic technique which needs explanation. Thus a two-way communication system has been constructed; a signal light on the control box draws the therapist's attention to the observer's desire to comment and also blocks the child's reward and progress to the next picture. By using a good tape recorder deck, checks of a child's speech twice a week can be recorded in order that an independent investigator (such as a linguist) can check upon a child's progress for research purposes.

Audiology

There are many advantages in the arrangement whereby a pure tone and speech audiometer and the other equipment are in the observation room, while the child responds by operating one of several manipulanda to achieve a reward by correct response (see Figures 7.1 and 7.2).

(i) Pure tones, voice or speech may be relayed via loudspeakers, while the therapist is able to signal her requirements to the audiometrician in the observation room.

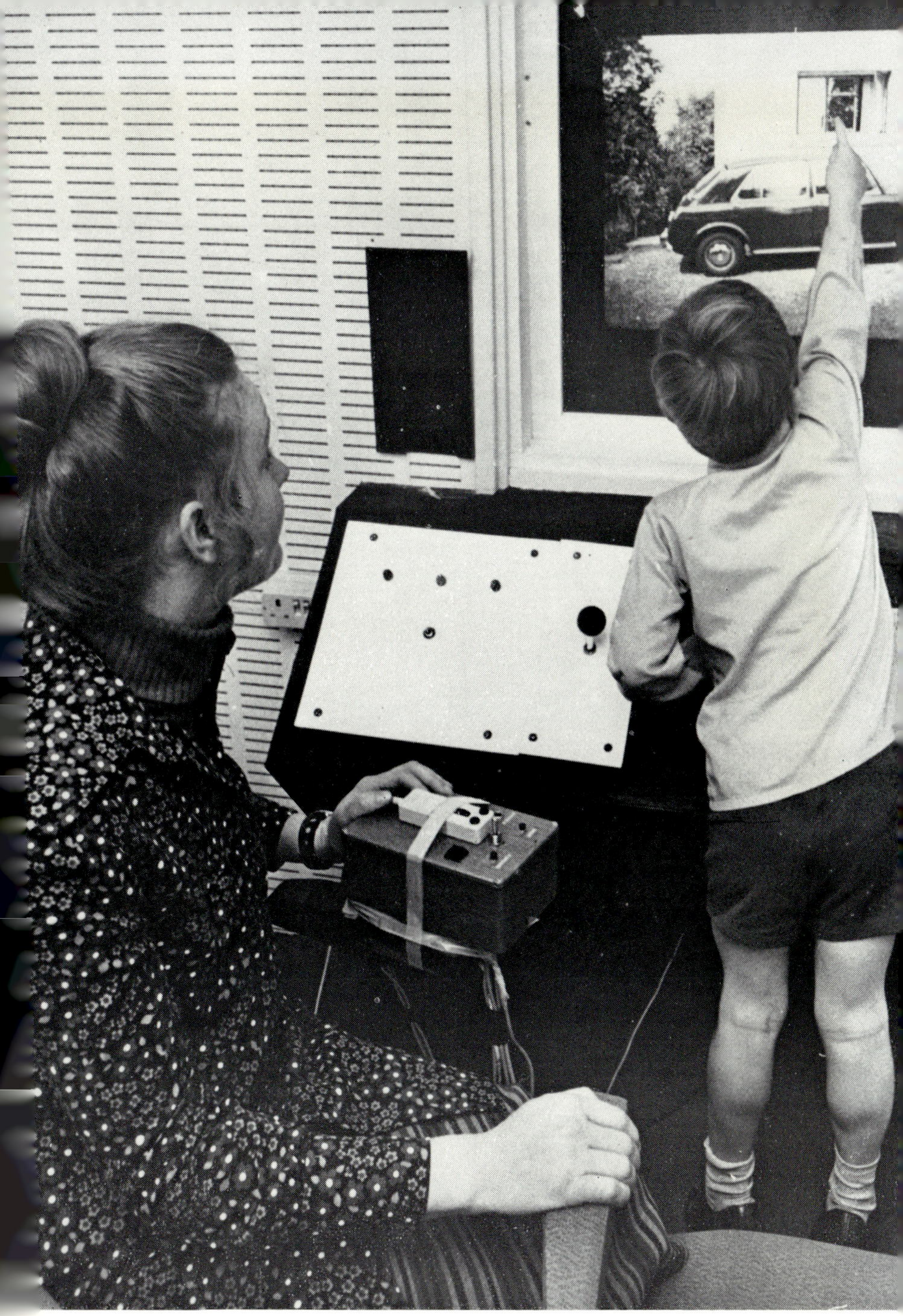

Fig. 7.4

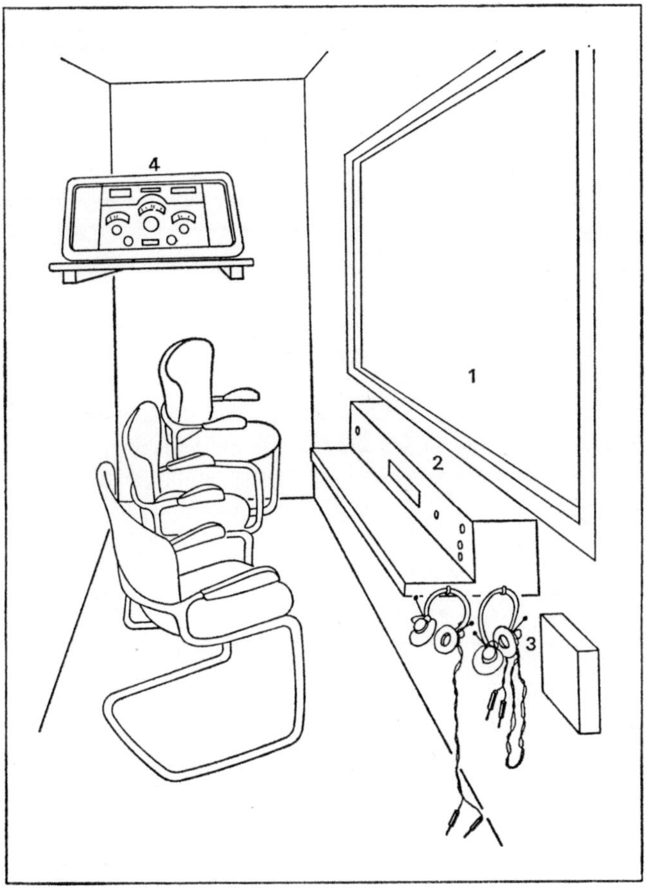

Fig. 7.5

1 One-way screen
2 Intercommunication module
3 Jackplug box with observers' earphones
4 Speech and pure tone audiometer

(ii) The sound is de-personalised, dissociated from the adult; some children (for example elective mutes or autistic children) who have difficulty in responding to people may respond to a de-personalised voice, via the loudspeaker.
(iii) The child is not distressed by having to wear headphones.
(iv) A variety of situations may be used: the child may either be

placed in a fixed position before the console and back projection screen, changing the picture for a correct response, or he may move with some freedom about the room.

(v) The therapist is freed from having to manipulate a machine and can give her whole attention to the child.

(vi) The recording by the audiometrician of the child's responses is done in the observation room, and thus does not distract the child.

(vii) Various techniques can be used, both conditioning and direct teaching methods. These will elicit from the children various responses: involuntary head-turning or cessation of intercurrent activity; conditional or intelligent responses.

A continuing programme of auditory perception activities similar to the visual perception games has a dual purpose: (a) continual reassessment of learning as a previously non-attending child improves; and (b) improvement of the child's responses to auditory input, as a result of the teaching-diagnostic process for auditory recall, auditory memory, auditory sequencing, and transmodal association between auditory and visual stimuli.

In the last analysis the differential diagnosis between auditory imperception and peripheral deafness may, however, be decided by referring such a child for auditory evoked responses, recorded by the EEG with an on-line computer.

Teaching-diagnostic Programme

The language unit includes a specially designed classroom staffed by a teacher of the deaf. This teacher has had special experience in developing a method of teaching individually geared to the often unique difficulties, both perceptual and behavioural, of particular children. Like the speech therapy and operant conditioning programme, the teaching can be observed via one-way screens by nurse-therapists and parents and the teaching experience can be generalised to the day-to-day living experiences in both hospital and home situations. The teaching is geared into the work of the other specialists so that the main elements, whether the aim be to teach language by auditory-vocal or visuo-motor means, become an integrated whole (Rees and Taylor, to be published).

The overall aim is to teach a child by carefully graduated steps an inner symbol system. At first a representational symbolic means of communication is taught to promote concept formation. This leads on later to the discursive symbolic communication system of human language, whether this be auditory-vocal or visuo-motor (a speaking/listening or a reading/writing system) or, failing both, a systematic sign language.

The visuo-motor mode is obviously easier initially, since visual representation of discursive language does not involve the fast analysis of time-sequenced input and output, as does the auditory-vocal mode. This is the more important because the vast majority of language-disordered children have a defect in auditory processing and the other neuro-psychological perceptual functions previously described. However, if possible a combination of auditory-vocal and visuo-motor communication systems proceed together. The teaching approach geared to a particular child is intuitively felt by an experienced, sensitive teacher: recent work by ethologists has underlined this. 'What makes the child avoid you?' 'What makes him upset?' 'What attracts his attention?' 'Will he approach me if I remain perfectly still . . . if I sing quietly and rhythmically . . . if I play with bright coloured objects?' The essential thing is to start. Parents can often help this, by giving of their experience. Does a child enjoy rocking? Then rock him. Singing in one particular rhythm? Even enjoying the noise and movement of a car ride? Then drive with him; and so on.

It is not possible to give a detailed account of the mass of language teaching games in this short chapter, particularly as the material is mainly designed for particular children's needs. However, attention-alerting games, visual and auditory perceptual games, categorising games, sequencing, cue-matching and rule-inducing games are used in a graduated series according to a child's needs and progress.

Finally, there are discursive language games, bringing out of a child the capacity for grammar which he still inherently possesses. Such a detailed diagnostic teaching programme is later to be published by Rees and Taylor.

Staff Structure and Roles

The staffing of units for children with language disorders reflects the basic philosophy of the professional person in overall charge. In this section a personal view of a hospital inpatient/daypatient unit will be described as a somewhat idealised model which the present unit has yet to achieve. It will be seen that most of the professional workers fill at least two roles.

The *nurse-therapists*, usually nursery nurses, are the basic mothering figures, each allocated to one or two children. They work together as a team on a shift system, so that there is a 1:2 staff:patient ratio at any one time. The unit is self-contained, and run as nearly as possible as a home. Meals are taken by staff and children together, and the nurturing and socialising care continues alongside attempts to generalise into everyday life the language programmes individually suited to each child's needs.

The role of the nurse-therapist is of prime importance in providing a warm, affectionate, homelike atmosphere where in the optimal arrangement of environmental variables for effective learning can take place.

The *teacher*, a teacher of the deaf, serves three important functions: (i) that of an audiometrician, using a formal pure tone or voice audiometry technique, as previously described; (ii) she carries out skilled diagnostic teaching techniques using a graded series of attention, perception and cognitive organising tasks, individually exploring each child's ability and providing invaluable information to other team members. The invention of *ad hoc* tests to discover the limits of a particular child's multi-faceted disabilities requires a very skilled and experienced person; (iii) she provides a model of a learning environment, rewarding a child by social approval, and drawing him out of a stereotyped repetitive existence until learning becomes a joy and not defeat.

The *speech therapist* likewise has two functions. The first is diagnostic assessment, using standardised speech and language tests, notably the Reynell tests of comprehension and expression, and the Edinburgh articulation tests, but also observations about a child's ability to use early phrase-structure and grammar. The second function is to provide speech and language therapy. The therapist's specialised professional skills are adapted to this work.

The *clinical psychologist/behaviour-therapist* acts both as a psychometrician, using such tests as the Merrill-Palmer, Wechsler infants' scale, Illinois Test of Psycho-linguistic Abilities, and Vineland social maturity scale, to explore the child's cognitive and linguistic capacity; and, even more, as a therapist and developer of therapeutic methods.

It is necessary to measure abilities and define indices of change in perceptual, behavioural and language development. Primarily, however, the psychologist is a therapist using modern learning techniques such as operant conditioning to shape word labelling, and other behaviour modification techniques to alter deviant behaviour. Operant methods are mainly of value in the early stages of treatment and are used to increase attention and to help children develop phonologically correct word labelling.

From then on, the psychologist working with the team devises methods which facilitate original language development, or else may show that an individual child cannot currently infer grammatical rules. It may be that auditory processing has been so damaged or poorly developed that language learning can only proceed by visual means, for example, using visual symbols similar to those of Premack to facilitate the acquisition of reading and writing.

The *family worker*. The fundamental importance of helping a child's parents and later his special school-teachers, to understand and apply the specific techniques used in the unit has been stressed by several writers. The eventual success or failure of a unit's method of language development for each child stands or falls according to how far the family worker of the unit can generate enthusiasm and put over the specific techniques involved. Too often has the role of a social worker in such units been simply to support a family which has known the bombshell upheaval of having a language disordered, and particularly an autistic, child.

To involve parents as active participants in their child's progress towards his greatest potential, by means of definite techniques used together with those of the unit workers, is to return to a family their basic inheritance of helping in the rearing of a damaged child. The family worker must be sensitive enough to realise when very aberrant need-systems in family members militate against a child's recovery, and will work to change such need-systems, or produce vital information which would favour inpatient rather than day patient status.

The *clinician*, as consultant in charge of hospital inpatients, has overall responsibility in a National Health Service unit. His other functions are:

(i) to determine unit policy, in conjunction with specialised advice from other professional colleagues;
(ii) to select and to promote a thorough medical, psychiatric, psychological, neurological and developmental diagnostic assessment of a referred child, using when appropriate EEG, X-ray and biochemical services, and to refer special problems

to other colleagues, as when auditory evoked responses are required;

(iii) to help to create a unit in which knowledge of therapeutic techniques and research are gently integrated with the nurturant care of these very handicapped children, who have potentially the most to gain of any neuro-psychiatric treatment groups;

(iv) to be able to act therapeutically with a child by knowledge and practice of definitive techniques, and with the family, in concert with the other members of the team.

Summary and Conclusions

Speech and language disorders can present as the most difficult child neurological or child psychiatric problems. The multiple aetiologic possibilities span a wide range of medical and para-medical areas. Ideally, the severely language-handicapped children should be referred to a specialised language unit in a regional centre where a group from differing professions have learnt to work together, each bringing his contribution from his own specialised area, whether this be paediatrics, neurology, child psychiatry, audiology, psychometrics, behaviour therapy, speech therapy, or education of the deaf. Each of these professions can make a unique contribution to an intensive diagnostic process, both in terms of clinical diagnosis and in terms of the discovery and remedying, if possible, of the relevant neuropsychological cause. Such a unit should be in a hospital, with access to the full range of specialised neurophysiological and biochemical investigations. A high staff complement of specially trained nursery nurses should be part of each language unit, so that specialised techniques of management can be re-deployed through these mother-equivalents during the periods away from concentrated therapeutic sessions with the professional people mentioned above. Finally, the child's family members should be taught the specific teaching skills, so that the child is exposed to the same general therapeutic programme, both in language development and in the training of as near normal social behaviour as possible, whether at the hospital or at home.

My thanks are due to Miss Joan Taylor, whe has worked with me with language-disordered children for some years, and who also produced the sketches on which the illustrations were based. I am also grateful to the staff of our unit, from whom I have learned a great deal.

CHAPTER EIGHT

Residential Psychiatric Treatment of Children with Epilepsy and Brain Damage

D. A. Pond

Epilepsy is a common symptom in children, especially the short grand mal or major seizure related to fever, usually between the ages of one-and-a-half and three years. Attacks at all ages may be caused by conditions varying from the trivial to the serious. There are also a great variety of seizure patterns in childhood. Some forms are much commoner than in adults: for example, typical petit mal absences, or minor attacks with prominent myoclonic features. The primary investigations of children with epilepsy and their treatment are for the most part carried out by paediatricians, and less often by neurologists, unless the latter have a special interest in paediatric neurology. Child psychiatrists are usually involved only if there are problems of differential diagnosis and/or associated psychological disorders. The latter may be so severe that investigations are impossible on a paediatric or neurological ward but urgently need to be done if the child's condition is to be treated properly.

Children whose chief presenting problem is mental subnormality quite often have epilepsy as well (up to 50 per cent in low-grade patients). These attacks may be overlooked or perfunctorily treated without adequate investigations, which cannot usually be carried out in most hospitals for the mentally handicapped. In passing it should be noted, however, that control of epileptic attacks in subnormal patients rarely results in any dramatic improvement in their intellectual level. The majority of children who have psychological disorders as well as attacks suffer from epilepsy that is the result of some brain damage: for example, the sequel of a head injury or a cerebral infection. However, though such acquired damage may be presumed from tests, the exact cause is often unknown owing to the inadequacy of existing methods of investigation.

Recent epidemiological studies in the Isle of Wight (Rutter, Graham and Yule, 1970) and elsewhere, have given us a good idea of the prevalence of psychiatric disorder in children suffering from epilepsy. At best, it is at least twice as common (about 15 per cent) as in the random child population. At worst, that is when associated with severe brain damage, and often other multiple handicaps, the majority of such children will show psychiatric disorder. Assuming an average prevalence of epilepsy in children of 7 per 1,000 total population, then a children's inpatient unit for half a million population (i.e. about 100,000 children) could expect to have about 200 psychiatrically disturbed and epileptic children at risk, though at any one time only a tiny proportion of them would need admission.

The prevalence of brain damage without epilepsy is much more difficult to determine since the diagnostic criteria are less clear-cut. Such children present as clinical problems less often than brain-damaged children with epilepsy as well, but as they frequently cause problems of differential diagnosis they are discussed in this chapter.

The phrase 'brain-damaged child' is a convenient shorthand term under which to include a ragbag of children whose disorders do not seem able to be explained in terms of the common environmental and genetic factors used in general child psychiatry, and in whom there is more or less reliable evidence, from history, physical examinations or special tests, of damage to the central nervous system. The term has also been used somewhat misleadingly to describe a particular syndrome or collection of symptoms, on the unwarranted assumptions that only this particular group of symptoms is indicative of brain damage and that they are caused only by brain damage. The subject has been discussed by Birch (1964), Pond (1961) and many others, and only the diagnostic and treatment aspects need mentioning in the appropriate parts of this chapter.

Functions of an Inpatient Unit

These functions may be considered under the headings of assessment and management. As regards *assessment*, admission to a unit is sometimes necessary in order to sort out the nature of attacks from which a child may be suffering. Descriptions of observations by parents, teachers and other non-medicals may not be sufficient to decide whether the attacks are epileptic or not. There are particular difficulties in the differential diagnosis of temporal lobe epilepsy. Children are asked less often than they might be for evidence of an aura, which many of them can describe as well as an adult can, if asked. Indefinable but often unpleasant somatic sensations, distortions of special senses, and emotional states like panic, are not uncommonly experienced as auras by children suffering from temporal lobe epilepsy, but may be missed through lack of questioning. The temporal lobe attack is commonly stereotyped in any one patient, though the pattern varies greatly from patient to patient. Disturbance, if not total loss, of consciousness is almost universal, but it may be brief and not noticed by an untrained observer. Autonomic features, such as pallor, sweating, drooling, are also often not clearly described but obvious when looked for. Children with epilepsy may also have temper tantrums, nightmares, enuresis, and the common syndrome of recurrent abdominal pain with stress – to mention but a few episodic disorders of childhood. Some of these disorders are often thought to have an organic basis, at least in part, but the psychophysiological mechanisms are so far virtually unknown except in general terms, and almost certainly have little connection with the neurophysiological disturbances leading to epilepsy.

To a lay person, all such attacks can easily get lumped together as epileptic once the child has received this diagnosis, but the sorting out of one sort of attack from another is of great importance, especially as regards treatment. There is no substitute for accurate observation by trained staff in this regard. Laboratory investigations are also essential, but serve slightly different purposes that will be described below.

The psychological assessment of epileptic children requires the full programme of comprehensive investigation used in child psychiatry. The same attention must be paid to getting a detailed family history and attempting to understand the family dynamics surrounding any particular child. The problems are intensified, not simplified, by the addition of epilepsy, and it is most important that all those concerned with the care of such children avoid using the diagnosis of epilepsy as an excuse for every episodic form of misbehaviour.

The psychiatric social worker carries out essentially the same functions with the families of children handicapped with epilepsy as with others, but in addition she may have particular roles with regard to the attacks. The epilepsy may have become the focus of a vast amount of family tension. It is still not uncommon to find parents regarding epilepsy as an hereditary degenerative stigma causing its victims to be liable to insanity, crime, perversion, and every other form of anti-social behaviour. There is often an anxious searching of family and personal pedigrees for evidence of disorders that might be related to epilepsy. Attacks may be seen as just retribution for thoughts or actions that might have been harmful to the child from conception onwards: for example, an attempted abortion, or a minor head injury through carelessness in nursing the baby, etc. It follows that the psychiatric social worker involved in such a family must have some clear information, not only about epilepsy in general, but also about the particular form of attack disorder from which the child suffers so that she can reinforce the advice about treatment and prognosis that the doctor will have given.

The assessment of the intellectual functioning of epileptic children poses particular difficulties, as their work capacity and concentration may vary, seemingly capriciously, from moment to moment. Only some of the variable concentration can be directly related to minor epileptic attacks observable either clinically or on the EEG. If attempts are made to control the epileptic discharges by anti-convulsant drugs, this in turn adds a further complication, since these drugs may also slow up intellectual functioning, though probably to a lesser extent than many parents and teachers believe. Different patterns of sub-test scores in intelligence tests are less clearly related to brain damage in children than in adults. Much depends on the time of damage, since in the very young child's brain the surviving cortex has the capacity to learn functions usually carried out by damaged areas. The most striking example of this 'vicarious functioning' is the absence of aphasic disorders in children whose speech area on the dominant side has been destroyed under the age of three years. Aphasic symptoms, more typical of adult syndromes, begin to appear, however, when the damage occurs from about the age of seven years and later.

Projection tests have not lived up to their claims to provide diagnostic indices of 'brain damage', which is hardly surprising since the syndrome does not exist. Nevertheless, the tests may be of value in filling in the general picture of the disturbed child's personality, and give leads to psychiatric intervention, even though the diagnostic question remains unanswered. Much the same considerations apply to other tests of special functions; for example, the Oseretzky test of motor development is a helpful study of psychomotor activities at a higher and more complex level than the conventional neurological level, but the test is not yet sufficiently standardised to have great diagnostic significance. The so-called 'soft' neurological signs need the same cautious interpretation and evaluation in any particular child as part of the total clinical picture. A clinical or educational psychologist experienced in the testing of handicapped children is an essential member of the team of any child psychiatry unit, but especially if many children with epilepsy and brain damage are admitted.

It is important to realise that the psychological pictures associated with childhood epilepsy are very varied, perhaps even more so than in adults. Although several stereotypes have been described, for example the young hyperkinetic epileptic, any idea that there is a typical syndrome of the epileptic child is even further from the truth than is the stereotype of the adult epileptic personality. All forms of psychiatric disorder can be seen with epilepsy, and probably roughly in the same proportion as in the non-epileptic population. Clearly, an enormous epidemiological survey would have to be carried out to settle this question, but the figures from the Isle of Wight survey support this general view. Disorders such as autism, which are rare anyway, are rare in the broad mass of children with epilepsy, though the two disorders are probably associated together more commonly than by chance. In particular, Rutter and Lockyer (1967) have shown that autism sometimes precedes a few epileptic attacks by several years. In most of these cases it is fairly clear that the epilepsy is related to the brain damage which is associated with autism in many such cases.

So far, considerable stress has been laid on the proper use of the ordinary psychosocial methods of investigation found in any good child psychiatric inpatient unit. These facilities are relatively more important than facilities for the physical investigation of children with epilepsy. However, the last must be easily and quickly available, if not to be found in the hospital complex to which the children's unit is attached. Of course, many cases will not come to the child psychiatrist until all the necessary physical investigations have been done, such as neuro-radiology, electro-encephalography, and such newer techniques as brain scan and echogram. Occasionally, however, the electro-encephalogram may have to be repeated on a number of occasions, especially if the patient is having fluctuating disorders of consciousness or apparently uncontrollable attacks.

The EEG is useful in sorting out one form of epileptic attack from another; it is less useful in deciding whether the patient is having epilepsy at all, since interictal EEGs can sometimes be normal in children with clinical epilepsy (though less often in adults). More rarely, specific epileptic features, such as spikes, and spikes and waves, can be found in patients without clinical evidence of epilepsy. The EEG is particularly useful in helping to sort the effects of too many drugs from too many attacks in producing slowness of behaviour and even disturbance of consciousness. The extent to which the child psychiatrist interests himself in the complexities of the EEG varies from person to person, but a few experts around the country are certainly needed, as is explicitly recognised in the *Reid Report on the Medical and Social Care of Persons with Epilepsy* (Reid, 1969). These few special centres will deal with the particularly complicated diagnostic problems and those in whom treatment is so far of no avail, especially as regards the associated psychological disorders (see below).

The methods of referral of patients with epilepsy to child psychiatric units are various and depend on the local circumstances. Paediatricians, school medical officers and general practitioners will send most, but admissions from special schools, especially from the existing hospital schools for epileptics, occasionally occur. A steady stream of patients can also be expected from the various branches of the services for the mentally handicapped, in view of the high proportion of such children having some sort of epilepsy as well.

Some further discussion of the diagnostic problem of brain damage without epilepsy is needed. Patients are not uncommonly referred from many sources for the investigation of possible organic factors in the genesis of certain behaviour disorders: for example, hyperkinesis, especially in young children; violent temper tantrums, and other episodic disturbances, such as peculiar dreamy states; and 'focal' disorders, usually of a cognitive variety, such as specific reading difficulty. They may also be referred with a definite history of brain injury from, perhaps, a road traffic accident after which chronic behaviour disorders have occurred.

In general, and at the risk of dogmatic over-simplification, one can say that brain damage is usually diagnosed too often rather than not enough. A degree of general subnormality greater than would be expected from the genetic endowment of the parents is one of the most suggestive signs of brain damage (the severely subnormal always have such damage). All other symptoms taken in isolation are of less diagnostic value, and the chances of brain damage rise as separate lines of evidence converge; for example, subnormality plus a history of birth difficulties, plus some 'hard' neurological signs, definitely indicates a child with a damaged nervous system, whereas a vague history of birth anoxia in a fidgety, hyperkinetic child with no abnormal physical signs does not carry much significance as regards possible organic factors contributing to the behaviour disorder. Even in the clear-cut cases, care should be taken not to over-emphasise the continuing organic effect of even a severe head injury. As Harrington and Letemendia (1958) showed years ago, long continuing sequelae of such an injury relate more to continuing environmental disturbances and the psychological significance of the injury (for example, parental guilt over their allowing the accident to happen). The evaluation of the importance of brain damage thus depends more on clinical psychiatric skill than on any sophisticated neurological or psychological tests.

The Role of the Inpatient Unit in the Management of Children with Epilepsy

Although, of course, assessment and management frequently go hand in hand, it is nevertheless true that the management of attacks and any possible associated psychological difficulties may be a lengthy business. There will be some children in whom the period of stabilisation will be relatively short and straightforward, but epileptic children with multiple handicaps, such as subnormality or physical disablement like hemiplegia, as well as psychiatric disorder, can form the hard core of the most long-term and disturbed children with which an inpatient unit ever has to deal.

The anti-convulsant control of attacks has changed little in the last ten years. For major seizures, the drugs of choice are phenytoin and phenobarbitone, though it is important to remember that younger children, particularly, sometimes react badly to phenobarbitone, with irritability, depression or other quite serious psychological disorders that may be more serious and disabling than the attacks themselves. There are a number of other drugs which can be considered for uncontrolled major epilepsy; for details, standard works such as Laurence (1973) should be consulted. It is important not to change drugs every time the child has another attack, and the changeover should in most cases be slow, with some overlapping of new and old. Fit control may be a lengthy business occupying months rather than weeks or days. Adequate fit charts are essential and should be meticulously kept by the nursing staff.

The control of minor seizures is often more difficult than that of major attacks. Classical petit mal usually responds fairly well to succinimides or troxidone, though occasionally no drug is of any avail and the child is actually better off all drugs, even though the attacks may continue. It is important to remember that about 50 per cent of children with petit mal go on to major seizures in adult life, though the petit mal attacks diminish. Such children, in fact, rarely come into a psychiatric unit and many authors have commented on their fundamentally good personality. What little disorder may be seen is usually of a neurotic character rather than a behaviour disorder.

The most difficult attacks to control are the focal cortical attacks originating in the deep temporal areas. Primidone and phenytoin often make an effective combination, but on occasions rarer drugs such as sulthiame may be required. The value of temporal lobectomy is stressed by Falconer (1972), but only after full investigation and a long period of treatment under close observation. Other focal cortical epilepsies occasionally occur in childhood, for example attacks in children with infantile hemiplegia; but in these cases epilepsy is only a minor part of the total pattern of disorder, and it is usually easily controlled. Various combinations of anti-convulsant drugs may be needed if the patient has more than one type of attack.

The particular and serious form of epilepsy known in Britain as infantile spasms is treated in the early stages by paediatricians. The children usually come into the hands of child psychiatrists when the attacks are more or less at an end, but the patients have become subnormal and often emotionally disturbed. Severely subnormal hyperkinetic children almost always require some drugs to try and relieve the formidable nursing problem they present. Amphetamine in large doses (up to 40 mg a day) is only occasionally effective, but it is worth a trial. Chlorpromazine can certainly be used, or other phenothiazines if necessary. Although these drugs, especially chlorpromazine, are said occasionally to increase the tendency to attacks, they are quite safe to give in moderate doses provided that the children continue with their anti-convulsants. In very severe cases, haloperidol (Serenace) may be needed. These drugs may have to be continued for months, even after the patient has been discharged from the ward. However, these children show the limited therapeutic value of drugs alone in the management of behaviour disorders.

Over and above the drug control of attacks and behaviour disorders it is of the utmost importance to pay close attention to the child in its family setting. The diagnosis of epilepsy can sometimes be a considerable relief to parents who may have been torturing themselves with guilt that all the disturbances their child shows are due to their own mismanagement. Simple explanations of the physical origins of epilepsy can help parents to come to terms with their handicapped child. Parents should realise that epilepsy has a clear organic basis, most often as a result of acquired brain damage, but occasionally the result of some constitutional instability which, as far as we know, has no clear relationship to any particular form of psychological disorder. That granted, however, it is important to recognise in the management of these cases that the timing and frequency of seizures is very strongly influenced by anxiety and psychological tension. Certain children develop quite characteristic patterns of attacks with particular forms of stress. Others get attacks when the stress is over and they are in a more relaxed state.

The most difficult symptoms to treat are unfortunately those which are also the most socially disruptive, namely, irritability and temper tantrums, poor concentration on any task with a brief attention span, and hyperkinesis. These same symptoms also occur in brain-damaged children without epilepsy and form the hard core of their problems, too. None of these symptoms is, of course, unique only to such handicapped children. Many researchers have shown that the differences from normal are essentially quantitative not qualitative (most parents find that their darling two-year-olds are often irritable, hyperkinetic and concentrating poorly!) Various descriptions of the poor ego-functions of such children have been given which help formulate some aspects of their ward management. For instance, their 'figure-ground' differentiation is poor and in a crowded, busy ward full of competing stimuli from other children in parallel activities they cannot settle to their particular task or game. Small quiet rooms with little distracting decoration, even a high window admitting light but looking onto nothing more exciting than the sky, are a help in aiding concentration. Irritability and tantrums are also significantly diminished if the child spends some time alone with an adult or with not more than one or two other children as well.

A single nurse to whom the child can relate for as long as possible in the 24 hours as is compatible with his or her duty hours, and for as much of the child's stay as possible, can contribute much to building up fragile ego-defences. Such a nurse is particularly useful if she can be taught to collaborate in behaviour therapy training schedules devised by the clinical psychologist. Such schedules are described in detail elsewhere in the book and need no great elaboration here. They need most careful tailoring to the child's own assets and disabilities. Localised sensory or motor disorders may dictate the use of only certain types of signal or response. Epileptic attacks may be precipitated by the stress of difficult learning-situations and thus the schedule would have to be lengthened and graded less steeply. Schedules to teach simple responses to signals (e.g. press a lever to a buzzer) can be effective in low-grade subnormals. Limiting factors are more likely to be in the area of motivation and thus depend on the same personality and environmental factors as do all other behaviour therapy programmes.

In general, a child with epilepsy needs to remain within the unit only as long as is necessary for diagnosis and preliminary stabilisation, and this may mean no more than a few days. Occasionally, however, residence may be prolonged for months if the child needs subsequent special residential placement. In most cases there will be a multitude of practical problems which will come into the province of the child psychiatrist looking after the case. There may be special problems connected with schooling, depending on the child's intellectual level and the type or the severity of behaviour disorder. Older children will need advice about possible careers. The transition between school and employment is particularly difficult for handicapped children. Since this period coincides with adolescence, which is a period of storm and stress anyway, there is a steady demand for urgent admission of adolescents with epilepsy, who can prove very destructive in a children's ward.

Only occasionally will any formal psychotherapy of a child be needed, but of course the psychodynamic understanding of what is going on in the family is a *sine qua non* for proper management of the whole situation.

The contribution of an inpatient psychiatric unit to the management of epileptic children has also to take into account the other residential facilities for the care of such children, especially the hospital schools, formerly called colonies, such as that at Lingfield. Such units provide most of the long-term education and medical care that is needed for the very small proportion of children with epilepsy that cannot be managed in day special schools. Neurological and psychiatric surveys of the children in one of these residential schools have shown a high prevalence of multiple handicaps. More than half had evidence of frank ('hard') neurological signs and/or gross psychiatric disturbance, as well as epilepsy that was difficult to control.

The prognosis in children with epilepsy and behaviour disorder severe enough to need admission to a children's unit must always be guarded. The actual period of inpatient treatment depends on the facilities available as well as the nature of the child's disorder and the parents' view of the situation. A proportion of such children will need longer-term residential care, such as is provided by the existing hospital schools or other special residential schools which will occasionally take one or two children with epilepsy. Such latter places are satisfactory provided adequate medical cover can be assured so that any drugs prescribed will be given regularly. Associated handicaps, such as subnormality or cerebral palsy, may be more important in determining subsequent placement than the attacks themselves. Identifying the best possible treatment for severely disturbed epileptic children entails familiarity with a multitude of agencies for handicapped children.

The prognosis of such children is frequently poor. It is well known, for example, that children with cerebral palsy who have epilepsy as well (and this is at least one-third of them) tend to be of lower intelligence than the others and to pose special problems of management. Children with known brain damage, for example from a traffic accident, who do not develop epilepsy, usually recover faster and more completely than the others.

Only comparatively rarely is there any specific drug treatment for the brain-damaged child without epilepsy. Hyperkinesis without epilepsy responds to the same drugs as with epilepsy. There have been several reports suggesting that carbamazepine ('Tegretol') is of value for a wide variety of 'organic' symptoms, as well as overt attacks, but adequate controlled trials are lacking.

Siting and Staffing

A few remarks should be made about the siting and the staffing of child psychiatry units which have to deal with any number of patients with epilepsy. On one side, such units should clearly have a close working relationship with paediatricians, neurologists and neurosurgeons. The psychiatrist-in-charge should have a particular interest in neuropsychiatry and be prepared to train his staff in the problems arising from the observation and handling of such children. As those who will be admitted are likely to be severely disturbed, at any rate for a while, the concentration of well-trained staff needed is high. There must always be one person capable of fulfilling the ordinary nursing functions, such as seeing that drugs are taken as prescribed and the necessary physical observations carried out regularly.

On the other side, these units will function well only if they are closely associated with the other residential services for handicapped children. Not only will children be sent to and received from the special hospital schools for epileptics and schools for the maladjusted, to their mutual benefit, but the unit will also have an important training function for the staff of these other places.

The Reid report suggested that the majority of epileptics of all ages would be cared for in special epilepsy clinics that should be set up in most district general hospitals. Such multi-disciplinary clinics were conceived as being organised for the most part out of existing medical and paramedical staff. They were not envisaged as needing wholly new staff and buildings, and in many places little more would be needed than the energy and enthusiasm of one person (usually a consultant) to co-ordinate existing activities. However, in the case of children as opposed to adults, the team would need the close collaboration of staff representing the educational services (usually an educational psychologist and the school medical officer) and the paediatric service.

The report also recommended the setting up of a very few special centres to deal with particularly difficult problems. These centres would need residential units for the carrying out of assessment and rehabilitation that could be lengthy. Certain child psychiatric units would be appropriately used in this way when they were closely integrated with the full range of neurological as well as psychiatric services. Newcastle, the Maudsley Hospital and Oxford may be cited as examples of places where there are special units which closely resemble the Reid Committee's plans, though even these places are not ideal in some respects. It was also hoped that there would be an acceleration of the plans of some of the hospital schools (colonies) to admit some children for short-term assessment rather than only for long-term care. Staff increases and better training for them in psychological handling, especially in groups, together with closer liaison with local child psychiatrists, paediatricians and neurologists, should enable better use to be made of their own skills than at present.

Summary and Conclusion

In summary, it can be stated that any good children's inpatient unit in charge of a broadly-trained child psychiatrist should be able to cope with most of the epileptic and brain-damaged children referred to it. There needs to be easy access to the whole range of diagnostic facilities needed for neurological and psychological investigations. The psychiatrist may need to call upon a paediatrician or a neurologist for advice about anti-convulsants and possible drugs to control behaviour, but will need to use his own clinical judgement as to the value of that advice in the light of the total situation. The ward management should be along the same general lines as for any disturbed child, with full use being made of all forms of psychological treatment appropriate to the particular problems shown. For further help and treatment, most of the social agencies, such as special education, will be used from time to time. There will also be occasional need for places at the epileptic hospital schools as they are at present organised. It is to be hoped, however, that children are not sent long distances from their homes for special residential schooling as this makes difficult the continued involvement of the family in the long-term management of the child.

CHAPTER NINE

Three Years' Work in a Regional Unit

Philip Barker

Preceding chapters have looked at the treatment of particular syndromes and types of problem. In an attempt to put the earlier chapters into perspective this one will give a general description of the work of a regional inpatient unit over a three-year period.

The Unit

The Charles Burns Clinic, named after Dr Charles Burns, Birmingham's first child psychiatrist, is situated in a residential district of South Birmingham. It was opened in January 1968 after about ten years of planning, preparation and building. It was intended to fill a gap in the psychiatric services in the area served by the Birmingham Regional Hospital Board. This large area comprised the City of Birmingham itself, the surrounding boroughs of Dudley, Solihull, Sutton Coldfield, Warley, Walsall, West Bromwich and Wolverhampton, and the counties of Herefordshire, Shropshire, Staffordshire, Warwickshire and Worcestershire. The total population served was about five million.

Most, though not all, of the areas mentioned had a child guidance service of some sort, but in only a few was this well developed. The only hospital child psychiatry service with inpatient beds was situated at the Birmingham Children's Hospital. The inpatient unit at this hospital shared a paediatric ward (in which it had half the beds) and operated on a five-day week basis. In a few parts of the region paediatric beds were sometimes used for the treatment of children with emotional disorders.

The Charles Burns Clinic building is in the same grounds as the Uffculme Clinic, a regional centre for the treatment of adults with neurotic disorders and a centre for the postgraduate training of psychiatrists in psychotherapy. The Uffculme Clinic building is a late nineteenth-century residence which originally belonged to members of the Cadbury family. They gave it, before the First World War, to the City of Birmingham which subsequently used it as an annexe to the City Mental Hospital, the name of which was later changed to All Saints' Hospital. Thus it was that with the implementation of the National Health Service Act in 1948 the Uffculme building and extensive grounds came into state ownership.

Uffculme Clinic continued as an annexe to All Saints' Hospital for a time but gradually evolved to become a separate neurosis unit. In the grounds was a 'bungalow' building, said originally to have been a 'summer house' for the use of the Cadbury children who lived at Uffculme. This building housed, for many years, chronic, long-stay psychiatric patients. It was after they left it that it was used as the basis for the new children's unit, the inside being entirely re-designed and a large additional building being provided.

The Charles Burns building is about 300 metres from the Uffculme building, at a lower level and virtually out of sight. Each clinic has its own extensive grounds. There is a large public park next door to which the children have access through a gate. The park contains gardens, a duck-pond, a wooded area and large areas of grass which are kept mowed.

From within the clinic grounds there is scarcely a house in view and the scene is predominantly rural, yet King's Heath, a district of Birmingham, is within a few hundred metres (10–15 minutes' walk) and Moseley village, another district of the city, is only a little further away. King's Heath and Moseley each contain a wide variety of shops and a swimming bath. King's Heath baths are the more readily accessible, being about 15 minutes' walk from the clinic.

The city centre is 2–3 miles distant and is readily accessible by bus, the journey taking 10–20 minutes.

The Building

The building is on two levels, since the site slopes. The children's bedrooms are on the lower floor, as are five rooms intended for the admission of mothers. Unfortunately it proved necessary to turn these into consulting rooms in view of the acute shortage of space for outpatient work, so mothers have not been admitted with their children.

The upper floor contains a large dayroom and an even larger dining-room, three classrooms, an occupational therapy room, various offices and the small, original outpatient area which contains rooms for medical staff, psychologists, social workers, secretaries and receptionist. The children's rooms are mostly large and 'institutional'. There is one single bedroom and one double one.

The grounds around the clinic, and especially those to the south, have been landscaped and laid out to provide a playground with swings, see-saw and roundabout, and also less formal play areas more suitable for 'adventure' play. Three old air-raid shelters are available for the children's use. One has been converted into a playroom suitable for messy activities and sand and water play.

The First Three Years

The first three years of the Charles Burns Clinic saw a gradual build-up of the work. The ultimate aim was to have 29 inpatient and 10 day patient places. But this total of 39 children under treatment was only reached gradually over the three-year period. At first 15 places were available. As funds, and therefore staff, subsequently became available the total rose, reaching the full 39 in 1970.

The period covered by the analysis of work that follows saw the gradual building up of a staff team and the establishment of a ward culture. The clinic had also to establish itself within the hospital group. Staff of other units regarded the clinic sometimes with suspicion, sometimes with resentment (they felt we were getting more than our fair share of resources, while we felt like poor relations, often forgotten) and occasionally with pride. This process was complicated by the merger, in April 1969, of the All Saints' Hospital Management Committee (by which we were originally administered) with the Birmingham (Dudley Road) HMC to form the Dudley Road (Birmingham) HMC.

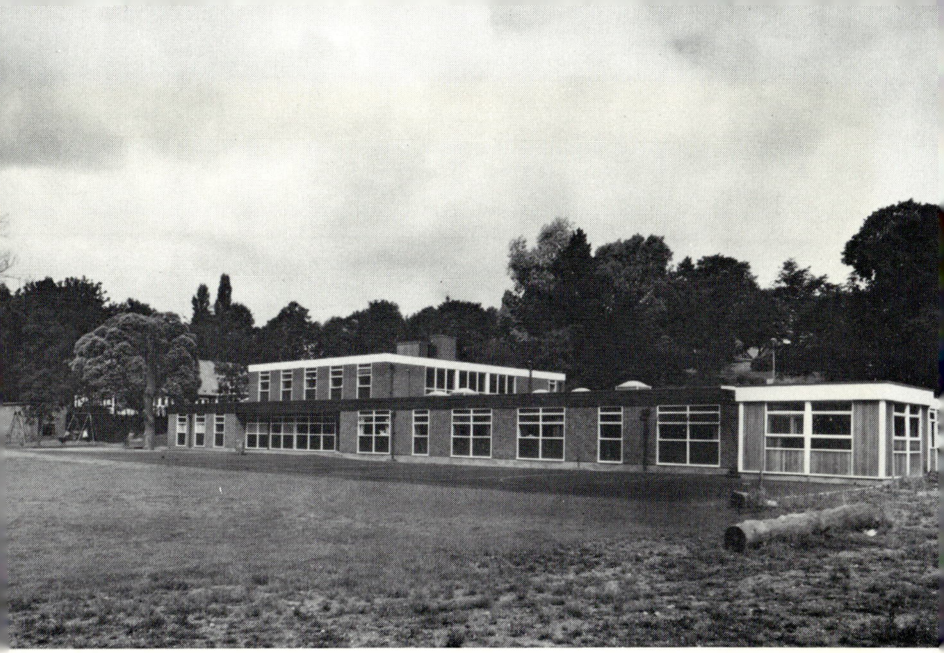

Fig. 9.1

The Charles Burns Clinic

Fig. 9.2

Lunchtime at the Charles Burns Clinic

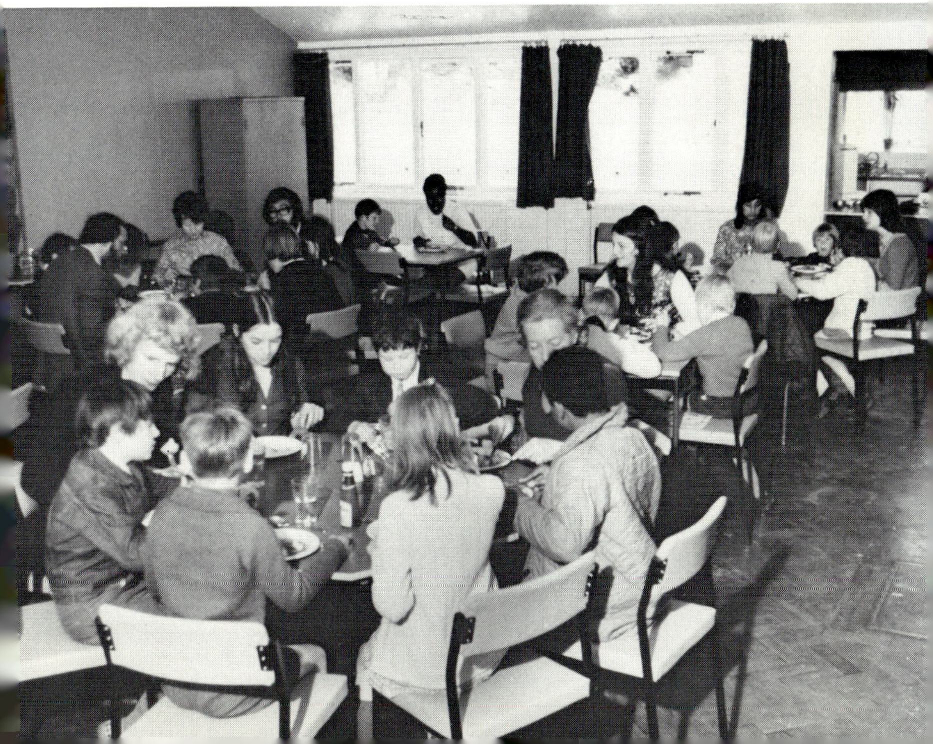

Referral to the Clinic

Initially most of our patients were referred to us from the various child guidance clinics within the region. As the clinic's outpatient service has developed an increasing number of admissions have arisen out of the work with children referred directly to us, chiefly by general medical practitioners. During the period under review, however, the great majority of inpatients came to our clinic as referrals from other psychiatrists. Our policy has been to see all referrals initially as outpatients, however obviously admission is needed. This enables the child and his parents to meet the clinic staff and discuss their problems, and the question of admission, before a firm decision is made about admission. It is also an opportunity to establish a treatment contract with the family.

Experience has shown that the process of admission requires to be carefully planned and carried out. Our present procedure has evolved gradually over the years. It has proved useful to set it out in writing for the information of new staff. The document they are given appears as Appendix A. The essence of the procedure is that admissions are kept under review by a multidisciplinary panel. This aims to keep the clinic's places full and to maintain a satisfactory balance of patients in the clinical groups and in the clinic as a whole. Each child is allocated a nurse-therapist who pays a preliminary visit to the home in company with the social worker. Admission is then arranged for a time when the nurse-therapist will be on duty, and the precise roles of the various staff concerned with the process of admission are defined. Since such a clearly laid down procedure has been followed admissions have been accompanied by noticeably less upset to the children and their parents.

The Treatment Milieu

The environment of the clinic as a whole is regarded as the most important factor in the treatment. A central feature of it is the child's relationship with his own nurse. Early in 1969 it was agreed that the term 'nurse-therapist' should be used, and a schedule of duties was prepared. Parts of this are now mainly of historical interest, as various developments have caused them to become out-of-date, but since it applied during much of the period under review and it still conveys the spirit of the nurse-therapists' duties, it is reproduced below:

1. To take individual responsibility for the care of one or two children in the unit.
2. To act as 'deputy nurse-therapist' to one or two other children: these to be children whose own nurse-therapist is on the other shift.
3. To be the person through whom all information imparted to the child is channelled, and to be the person to whom the child goes to make requests or impart information. 'Information' will include items such as discussion of weekends at home, going outside the unit, spending pocket-money, changes of medication, visits by parents, telephone calls to and from parents, etc. Only if the child's own nurse-therapist, and her deputy, are absent from the unit, should the child's 'contact' be the sister or charge nurse.
4. To spend as much time as possible in conversation and/or play with her own child(ren). This should be at least 1–2 hours per week, often more.
5. To write regular, detailed reports on the one or two children for whom she is specially responsible. These should be at least weekly and may include information passed on by other nurses.
6. To assist generally in the care of the children in the unit, under the supervision of the sisters/charge nurses. In particular it may be necessary to help with the handling of acutely disturbed children who are allocated to other nurse-therapists.
7. To greet the child on admission, show him his bedroom and the unit as a whole and introduce him to the other children and staff.
8. To give the child such help as he requires in the care of his clothes and personal possessions.
9. To visit the child at home if this becomes necessary during his inpatient or daypatient care, for example if he fails to return after a weekend at home.
10. To have only minimal contact with parents, and to refer these, for any discussion of the child's problems, to the social worker, sister/charge nurse or doctor (in that order).
11. To discuss treatment and progress of her child(ren) at least weekly with the doctor, normally in group meetings to be arranged for the purpose.
12. To attend staff meetings and to ensure that all relevant information about her child(ren) is mentioned.
13. On taking over from the night staff or a previous shift, to ascer-

tain whether there have been any significant developments in respect of her child(ren).

14. To report to the sister/charge nurse any apparent change in a child's physical condition: it will normally be the sister/charge nurse who takes any appropriate action in the case of physical illness.
15. To discuss with the sister/charge nurse any acute problem in the management of her child(ren), such as cannot be left to the next group meeting.

The 'nurse-therapists' are mainly 'nursing assistants', that is, members of the nursing staff who come to the clinic without previous training for the work. Despite the modest pay, there has been a steady flow of applicants of high calibre for these posts. Nurse-therapists have been selected on the basis of their personality, intellectual ability and motivation. They have included some remarkable young men and women. Their educational level has been higher than that of nursing assistants in the NHS generally. A few have been university graduates wanting the sort of experience which the clinic can provide before going on to train in fields such as social work, teaching or child psychotherapy. Others have been awaiting admission to institutes of further education. Many left school with good academic records and have tried other jobs without obtaining satisfaction from them. In some cases at least they seem to have found satisfaction at the clinic. Most, if not all, have had at least a little of the idealism which inclines many young people to undertake work with the troubled or underprivileged. In addition to the younger nurse-therapists, who are usually in their early twenties and have included some men, we have also appointed some older women, often people returning to work after bringing up a family. The latter provide a useful balance, with their greater maturity and experience of life and of child-rearing, to the younger staff. For all, a programme of in-service training is provided, together with close supervision of each nurse-therapist's work with his or her child or children.

The nurse-therapists work under the supervision of trained nurses. They too are selected primarily on the basis of their personalities, which are considered more important than the particular course of training they have undergone. At first the clinic was organised as one big group, but as numbers increased this proved unsatisfactory. The children, and the nursing staff, were therefore divided into three groups. Each usually contains 10–12 children (a mixture of inpatients and daypatients) and about six or seven nursing staff. The latter normally include a sister or charge nurse, a staff nurse and four or five nurse-therapists. Nurse-therapists do not normally take primary responsibility for more than two patients, but each may be 'shadow nurse-therapists' (as the 'deputy nurse-therapists' have come to be known) to up to two others. Staff nurses usually act as nurse-therapists for one or two children; sisters and charge nurses sometimes do.

More recently a fourth, smaller group, the 'language group', has been added. This contains up to eight children, mostly (often entirely) daypatients. It is described in Chapter 7. This group did not exist as a separate entity during the period covered by the review of admissions later in this chapter.

Each group has its own doctor and social worker. The doctor, either a registrar or a senior registrar, is in day-to-day psychiatric charge of the group under the supervision of the consultant concerned. He meets the staff regularly, sees the children individually (at least once a week, more often if indicated) and arranges any necessary medical investigation and treatment.

The group's social worker takes responsibility for the investigation of each child's family background and for the necessary casework. This is usually done by the group social worker personally, but sometimes, where a social worker from another agency is already involved, the clinic social worker acts primarily as a liaison link with the 'outside' worker.

Daily Programme

During school terms each child has a programme of activities during school hours, which are 9.30 a.m. to 3 p.m., with mid-morning and lunch breaks. This programme is not usually confined to school but includes periods of occupational therapy and also periods out of school during which the child takes part in activities in company with his nurse-therapist. Each child's programme is individualised and reviewed weekly.

As children progress they often go to outside schools in the neighbourhood while still living in the clinic. This can be a valuable preparation for discharge.

Occupational therapy in the clinic operates along the lines previously described by Barker and Muir (1969) and Barker (1971b). The main functions may be summarised as follows:

(a) Assessment and observation of:
Motor function, including abnormal motor behaviour
Sensory capacities
Capacity to work in a small group, and to share attention, tools and activities with others
Particular interests and aptitudes
Speech and vocabulary
Persistence and ability to concentrate
Relationship capacity
Frustration tolerance
Mood
Fantasy life

(b) Promotion of:
Constructive and creative work, to the benefit of the child's self-assurance and view of himself.
The release of tension and aggression, which can be expressed in joinery, modelling, dressing up and acting, puppetry, percussion and so on.
A helpful relationship between therapist and child, the therapist being a person with confidence in the child's capacity to achieve creative ends, and also one willing to accept the child's limitations and sometimes negative behaviour.

There is considerable overlap between the functions of school and occupational therapy, and many of the above functions are carried out in school also. Generally, however, the teachers concentrate on the basic school subjects, especially reading and number work, in which many of our patients are seriously retarded. Because of the emotional resistance to learning which many of our patients show, a specialised approach to teaching is necessary with, initially, strong positive rewards for even slight achievement.

The school and occupational therapy groups are different from the clinical groups described above. Once school is over, however, and at other times, the group nursing staff take primary responsibility for the children and activities are organised on a clinical group basis. The groups also have their own bedrooms and tables in the dining-room.

Treatment Methods

The general aim is to create a relaxed, informal atmosphere in the context of which necessary limits can be set to the children's behaviour. Children and their nurses call each other by their first names, nurses wear ordinary clothes, not uniform, and nursing staff and children take their meals together. At the same time we aim as far as possible to make the milieu provided for each child suit his current clinical needs. Thus, each child's needs are discussed at group meetings held at least once weekly. The child's relationship with his nurse-therapist is a central feature of the treatment.

Behaviour therapy techniques are increasingly being incorporated into the day-to-day management of particular children. This seems to be in no way incompatible with the therapeutic use of an accepting, caring environment and the application of psychotherapy. In any event, whatever other treatment may be given, the staff must react (or fail to do so) in some way or other when children display various behaviours, adaptive or maladaptive. We therefore attempt to ensure that the reaction of all staff is such as to be therapeutic, believing that the future behaviour of a child depends on the reaction his past behaviour has elicited. Sometimes the treatment goes beyond simply reacting in a particular way to certain behaviours, and additional *ad hoc* arrangements are made. The following examples illustrate this:

Vincent, aged 8, was born in England of West Indian parents. He was admitted to the clinic after he had been found unmanageable in a residential school for maladjusted children. His family background was difficult. His mother had recently returned to Jamaica in order, we were told, to obtain treatment for her 'arthritis'. She was expected to be there for at least two years. The father had arranged for two of Vincent's siblings to live with relatives, one in London, one in the Midlands. The third sibling had been taken into the care of the local authority and was in a children's home. The father did not appear to have the capacity to look after the children on his own. This certainly seemed to apply to his care of Vincent, who had a long history of difficult behaviour.

Following admission, the behaviour which the residential school had found troublesome soon became apparent. Vincent was an extremely aggressive boy, both verbally and physically. He had frequent temper tantrums, some of them precipitated by minor frustrations, but some of them without any apparent immediate cause. He broke many windows in temper and was generally reluctant to accept limits to his behaviour.

He was seriously retarded in his school work and was a non-reader. He also had a mild difficulty with language, due partly to his extensive use of West Indian idiom, and a stammer. There was also a warm and likeable side to Vincent, and at times he could be most pleasant and companionable. He was a physically fit and strong boy with a great sense of rhythm, and he was easily the best dancer in the clinic.

Vincent appeared an insecure, anxious boy who felt rejected by both parents and by the residential school he had attended. Although he had the capacity to relate warmly to people, he had not, it seemed, been able to establish satisfactory relationships with adults upon whom he had found he could rely. He had a need for acceptance and for help with his feelings and with his educational difficulties. We anticipated that in due course, as he came to feel more secure in the clinic, and in his relationships with his nurse-therapist, his doctor and other staff, his behaviour would improve. In the meantime, however, he was an exceedingly difficult child to handle. The problem had to be faced of what to do about his window-breaking and general violence.

This led to an analysis, based on a detailed written record of Vincent's behaviour by the staff, of the precise behaviours he showed. A programme to reduce the more difficult of these was then started. Two 'smiley badges' (circular yellow badges with a drawing of a smiling face on them) were provided. These, it was explained to Vincent, were to be a mark of his progress. When making good progress he would wear two, so that all staff would know how well he was doing. When making less good progress he would wear one; and if serious difficulties arose he might have none. When wearing both badges Vincent had full 'privileges', that is, he could do everything the other children did, go on outings with his group and so on. When he had only one badge the activities available were restricted somewhat (in a way which was explained to Vincent) and if he had none he would be confined to the building under close supervision. This was so that staff could help him start, once again, to progress. Badges were removed for limited, specified lengths of time (of three hours or more, depending on the circumstances). Vincent accepted the plan, the working of which was discussed with him in detail. The staff of the clinic as a whole were asked to give Vincent as much approving attention as possible when he was wearing two badges, less when he had one and to leave his care to the nurse supervising him when he had none.

Initially the criteria for loss of badges were: One badge lost, for three hours – 'milder' misbehaviour, such as aggression to others, throwing things about in anger, temper tantrums. If this behaviour was repeated during the three hours, another hour was added to the period. Both badges lost – 'serious' misdemeanours, such as breaking windows (on purpose), setting fire to things, serious damage to people or property.

Initially such episodes resulted in 24 hours' loss of the badges, but in the light of experience this period was later shortened.

After a while, both in response to our experience of how this programme was working and as a result of improvement in Vincent's behaviour, the plan was modified. Indeed, regular review of these programmes is essential, both to detect any snags in their practical application and to adapt them to changes in the child's clinical state. It is also necessary to keep all the staff informed of what is happening.

So that Vincent should not be the only child with 'smiley' badges, a programme employing them was started with another child at the same time.

This treatment seemed to help, though it is impossible to define precisely how great its part was in the progress Vincent made, since he was also experiencing relationships of a type we thought would be helpful, was receiving help and encouragement from his teachers in learning to read (and was himself very pleased by the progress he made) and was having tranquillising medication.

Maureen, aged 6, was referred from a child guidance service in the region as suffering from an autistic condition. She was an only child who had been conceived after her mother had been sterile for nine years. Although the mother had thought she wanted a baby, when Maureen was born she suddenly felt anxious, worried and inadequate. She wanted Maureen to grow up very quickly and so be out of her hands. The mother's sense of helplessness and of not really wanting her baby seemed to have been compounded by Maureen's lack of response to her; she was said to have been difficult to cuddle and to have shown no affection to her mother.

It was apparent that the relationship between Maureen and her parents had never been close or warm. Maureen had always been overactive and prone to grab things and scream when thwarted. Her relationships were distant and she was a generally withdrawn child who showed little interest in people. She preferred repetitive play, often rather bizarre, accompanied by inappropriate, stereotyped talk. Her mother was quite unable to control her, and her father coped no better, nor could he provide the support mother needed. Maureen was also difficult in school and was excluded after nine months there. At about this time her mother became depressed and made a suicidal attempt. She was admitted to hospital and was still there when Maureen was referred. Maureen had been looked after by the maternal grandmother while her mother was in hospital.

On admission, among the main problems which Maureen presented were persistent screaming (often in response to minor frustrations), hitting other children, repeating phrases (often irrelevant ones) in a stereotyped way, hitting herself, and very slow and messy eating at mealtimes.

After due observation and discussion a programme to deal with these problems was worked out as follows:

Behaviour	*Action*
Persistent screaming, or hitting other children	'Time-out' for two minutes
Irrelevant or repeated phrases	Give adequate reply first time, then ignore completely, possibly walking away
Hitting herself	Hold Maureen's hands and talk of other things
Very slow eating	Remove her plate when everyone else has finished

This programme, too, was reviewed regularly and modified as necessary. It was seen as complementing the milieu and in particular the relationship which we hoped would develop between Maureen and her nurse. It seemed to be of value.

The use of 'time-out' merits further comment. A 'time-out' room has been constructed in which children can be placed for specific purposes. The room contains a minimum of fittings; the walls are of high-density hardboard fixed on battens, the windows are of 'unbreakable' perspex and there is a one-way observation panel in the door. It is situated in the daytime living area of the clinic. Children are only put into this room under specific, clearly defined conditions:

1. The treatment is only to be used for particular, named children. (There are seldom more than one or two children for whom it is being used, sometimes there are none.)
2. The treatment is discussed with the parents and is only to be used with their agreement. The purpose of the procedure is explained to them and they are invited to look at the 'time-out' room first.
3. The specific behaviour for which the treatment is to be used is defined in writing.
4. Each time a child is placed in the room the exact circumstances are recorded in writing, as is the child's behaviour in the room and the time he spends in it.
5. The time to be spent in the room is specified, it often being one or two minutes longer than it takes for the behaviour (for

example, a temper tantrum) to subside. Children seldom spend more than 5–7 minutes in it, and a maximum time (perhaps 8 or 10 minutes) is also specified. It is unusual for the behaviour not to have subsided in this time, but if it does not the whole treatment programme is reconsidered.

6. No child is left in the 'time-out' room on his own unless he is under constant observation through the one-way window.
7. Any child who is programmed to receive 'time-out' *must* do so whenever he shows the specified behaviour in the clinic.

The 'time-out' treatment is based on the principles set out by Brown and Tyler (1968). It appears to be a useful adjunct in the treatment of a few of our children, but is used sparingly. It was available, for example, when Vincent was under treatment but was not considered appropriate in a boy as insecure and rejected as this; another point was that this boy's violence was impulsive and quite brief, unlike Maureen's tempers which were more prolonged.

The use of behaviour therapy techniques (and many other *ad hoc* programmes have been devised) within the milieu has been described in greater detail than have some other aspects of the treatment provided in the Charles Burns Clinic because it is not much emphasised in the literature on inpatient units. But it is only one of many approaches used, including psychotherapy, occupational therapy, remedial education, drug therapy and relationship therapy – the latter being a feature of the living environment.

Three Years' Admissions

From the opening of the Charles Burns Clinic in January 1968 up to the end of December 1970 there had been a total of 193 inpatient and day patient admissions. These involved 164 children. This review covers these admissions. Many of the children continued to receive inpatient or daypatient treatment well into 1970; these periods are covered if they followed an admission during the three years under review. Readmissions after 31 December 1970 are ignored, though they will be considered when the admissions for the period 1971–73 are reviewed in a later publication.

Table 9.1 summarises the treatment given to the children. A majority (127) were treated by a single period of inpatient care.

Table 9.1 Three years' admissions

		%
Admitted first as inpatient		
Inpatient once only	127	77
Inpatient more than once	10	6
Inpatient once, then daypatient	6	4
Inpatient more than once then day-patient	2	1
Admitted first as daypatient		
Daypatient	16	10
Daypatient once, inpatient later	3	2
	164	100

Another ten had multiple inpatient care. In a further eight instances a period of daypatient treatment followed inpatient care. During these first three years only 19 children were treated initially as daypatients and, of these, three later received a period of inpatient care.

The admissions are 'administrative' ones. Thus, if a child is transferred to another hospital (as a few were, for example because of intercurrent disease such as acute appendicitis or for such special investigations as air encephalography) he is 'discharged', even though he returns from the other hospital for continued psychiatric treatment. A few children were also discharged by their parents after a few days or weeks of treatment, only to be readmitted shortly afterwards. A typical case is that of Quentin.

Quentin was admitted at age 10. He was adopted and the only child in the family. He had originally been fostered in infancy with the couple who eventually adopted him when he was four. From about that time on he had become increasingly antisocial, disobedient and aggressive. A particular problem was his running away from home. After a long period of child guidance treatment he was referred for admission. He ran away from the clinic repeatedly during his first few days there. He always went home, and had no difficulty getting there by bus despite usually having no money on him. On arriving home on one occasion he promised his adoptive parents that in future he would behave well so that there was no need for him to return to the clinic. Against the advice we gave the parents in the course of a telephone conversation they decided to 'give him a chance' and to keep him at home.

The 'chance' did not work, and within a week or so it was apparent to the adoptive parents that Quentin was no better. They therefore requested a further admission; we agreed to this on the understanding that they would not again discharge Quentin against our advice. This marked a turning-point in the relationship between the clinic staff and the family, a relationship which has continued, through various vicissitudes the family has experienced, up to the time of writing. This boy appears in our figures as a multiple admission, though in reality his running away, discharge and readmission was all part of a continuing process. Indeed, this sequence of events – discharge against advice, followed by persistence or worsening of the presenting problem, followed by a request for readmission which is agreed to on the basis of a new treatment 'contract' – seems to occur several times a year in a clinic the size of the Charles Burns. It can apparently be a process it is necessary to go through in some cases. The good progress that can follow it has been remarked on before (Barker, 1968).

The children admitted more than once included one who was admitted four times and another who was an inpatient five times. These multiple admissions were not due to relapse but were designed to provide continuing support for those caring for certain difficult children. This use of inpatient care can sometimes, it seems, be valuable. It is illustrated by the case of the boy who was admitted a total of five times.

Michael, aged 11, was referred to the clinic by the psychiatrist at a residential school for maladjusted children. He had been having violent temper tantrums at school and the staff there found his behaviour unmanageable. It improved during his stay in the clinic, but after his return to the school it seemed advisable to provide continuing support. The parents were separated and Michael lived with his father, who also found him difficult to control. Because of Michael's rather insecure place in both his residential school and his home, some short holiday and weekend admissions were arranged. These seemed to relieve the tension Michael created in both home and school, and were also symbolic of the clinic's continuing interest and support.

The *diagnostic categories* into which the children seemed most appropriately placed are shown in Table 9.2. The diagnoses have been made using the first axis of the tri-axial classification described by Rutter *et al.* (1969). The definitions in this paper have been adhered to with two exceptions. One concerns the category of 'mental subnormality'. Rutter *et al.* state that the category 'manifestations of mental subnormality only' should be used in the first axis when this is the only abnormality the child shows – since it appears also in the second axis.

For the purposes of this review of admissions, however, this category has been used also when mental subnormality has appeared to be the *main* abnormality even though some other behavioural or emotional disorder (usually mild) has also been present. The other exception is the use of a category of 'mixed neurotic and conduct disorder'. Five children had disorders in which neurotic symptoms and antisocial behaviour were so evenly mixed that it was considered unrealistic to include them in either of the first two categories listed in the table.

Table 9.2 Three years' admissions

	Boys	*Girls*	*Total*	%
Conduct disorders	52	16	68	42
Neurotic disorders	16	17	33	20
Mixed neurotic and conduct disorders	4	1	5	3
Developmental disorders	20	4	24	15
Psychosis	9	3	12	7
Personality disorders	7	2	9	6
Mental subnormality	4	1	5	3
Adaptation reaction	1	1	2	
Anorexia nervosa	1	1	2	
Normal variation	0	2	2	
Dementia	0	1	1	
Other syndrome (emotional dwarfism)	1	0	1	
	115	49	164	

The children with conduct disorders constituted much the largest single group. In this group boys outnumbered girls by more than three to one. This sex ratio is similar to that found in an epidemiological survey of 10- and 11-year-old children in the Isle of Wight (Rutter *et al.*, 1970). Our admission rates also reflect the relative prevalence of these disorders in the community, as shown by the Isle of Wight survey, in that there also conduct disorders were commonest with neurotic disorders in second place. The proportions of children with developmental disorders, psychoses and personality disorders were, however, all higher than among the disturbed 10- and 11-year-olds studied in the Isle of Wight. This is presumably a result partly of the different, and predominantly younger, age range of the clinic cases, and partly of their selection as children needing inpatient or day-patient care.

Twenty-seven (82 per cent) of the thirty-three neurotic children presented with school refusal (Table 9.3). Only a handful of other neurotic children were admitted for inpatient or daypatient treatment. All the children with school refusal were initially admitted as inpatients.

Table 9.3 Presentation of neurotic disorders

	Boys	*Girls*	*Total*	
School refusal	13	14	27	(82%)
Depression	1	1	2	(18%)
Elective mutism	1	1	2	
Obsessive-compulsive disorder	1	0	1	
Chronic anxiety state	0	1	1	
	16	17	33	

Table 9.4 shows the disorders from which the children classed as having developmental disorders suffered. During the period under review the clinic staff began to take a particular interest in children

Table 9.4 Developmental disorders

	Boys	*Girls*	*Total*	
Language disorder	10	2	12	(50%)
Encopresis	8	0	8	(33%)
Hyperkinetic syndrome	1	2	3	(17%)
Tics	1	0	1	
	20	4	24	

with language disorders, though the language unit (see Chapter 7) had not yet opened. This probably explains why, among developmental disorders, the biggest single group consisted of children with language problems.

Table 9.5 subdivides the psychotic group of children according to the type of disorder they displayed. Three-quarters of the children

Table 9.5 Psychotic children

	Boys	*Girls*	*Total*
Infantile psychosis	8	1	9
'Schizophrenia' (Late-onset psychosis)	1	1	2
Other psychosis	0	1	1
	9	3	12

suffered from infantile psychoses, that is, disorders starting before age $2\frac{1}{2}$.

The *reasons for admission* have been considered by means of a careful examination of each child's case notes. They are difficult to classify, not only because they are often not clearly stated in the notes, but also because they were sometimes multiple. It has, however, been possible to subdivide children into those admitted primarily for assessment and those for whom the clinic attempted to provide treatment designed to help alleviate the disorder. Some children admitted in the first place for assessment were retained for treatment: these have been classified as 'treatment' cases. The distinction is nevertheless somewhat artificial since assessment can only be done in a setting orientated towards treatment; indeed, one of the chief things to assess is how far a child may respond to treatment. Children who had multiple admissions are considered to be 'treatment' cases if at least one of the admissions was for this purpose. Table 9.6 shows the reasons for admission, classified in this way. At one extreme only 9 per cent of the neurotic children came in for assessment; on the other hand, 33 per cent of the psychotic children were in for assessment only. This may be because the psychotic children, as a group, offer less good prospects for treatment. Their numbers are small, however, so too much should not be read into this finding. In the group as a whole just over three-quarters were seen as receiving treatment designed to help alleviate the problems for which they were admitted. The proportion of 'treatment' cases in the clinic at any one time was always bigger than this, however, since the children receiving treatment stayed longer than those only being assessed.

The *mean period of inpatient care* received by the main groups of children is shown in Table 9.7. In calculating these means the total

Table 9.6 Reason for admission – all patients

	Assessment	*Treatment*	*Total*	
Conduct disorders				
boys	14	38	52	68
girls	2	14	16	
Neurotic disorders				
boys	1	15	16	33
girls	2	15	17	
Mixed N.D. and C.D.				
boys	1	3	4	5
girls	0	1	1	
Developmental disorders				
boys	5	15	20	24
girls	2	2	4	
Psychotic disorders				
boys	3	6	9	12
girls	1	2	3	
Others				
boys	4	10	14	22
girls	2	6	8	
Totals	37(23%)	127(77%)	164(100%)	

period of both inpatient and daypatient care has been added up in each child's case. Thus multiple admissions are considered as a single treatment process, and any period of daypatient treatment has been added on to the period of inpatient care. This is because daypatient treatment in these cases has usually been a continuation or extension of the same treatment programme. Children treated only as day-patients are not included in this table. While in most groups the mean stay was between 4 and 5 months, the variations were wide, ranging from about one month (occasionally even less) to over a year.

The particularly long mean stay of girls with conduct disorders was due largely to difficulty in finding suitable residential schools to which to discharge girls requiring further help in such a setting. The figure is

Table 9.7 Mean period of inpatient/daypatient care

	Boys	*Girls*	*Both sexes*
Conduct disorders	4m 7d ($n = 47$)	6m 14d ($n = 15$)	4m 24d ($n = 62$)
Neurotic disorders	4m 7d ($n = 16$)	4m 18d ($n = 16$)	4m 12d ($n = 32$)
Developmental disorders	4m 19d ($n = 18$)	1m 5d ($n = 3$)	4m 5d ($n = 21$)
Psychoses	6m 13d ($n = 9$)	4m 5d ($n = 3$)	6m 1d ($n = 12$)

inflated by the very long stays of a small number of girls who had to wait inordinate lengths of time for boarding-school places. It probably does not represent a special treatment need in this group. On the other hand, the psychotic children did tend to stay longer, though their numbers are small and, again, the mean length of stay is inflated by a few who stayed a very long time. The short mean stay of the girls with developmental disorders is of little significance, since there were only three girls in the inpatient group and two of these were admitted for assessment only.

Table 9.8 shows the mean duration of treatment of the inpatients in

Table 9.8 Mean periods of inpatient/daypatient care – 'treatment' cases only

	Boys	*Girls*	*Both sexes*
Conduct disorders	5m 3d ($n = 35$)	7m 5d ($n = 14$)	5m 21d ($n = 49$)
Neurotic disorders	4m 10d ($n = 15$)	5m 26d ($n = 12$)	5m 6d ($n = 27$)
Developmental disorders	5m 12d ($n = 14$)	32d ($n = 1$)	5m 3d ($n = 15$)
Psychoses	9m 9d ($n = 6$)	6m 29d ($n = 2$)	8m 21d ($n = 8$)

the group of 'treatment' cases. The few 'treatment' cases discharged prematurely against medical advice have been excluded, as well as the assessment cases. Again, the psychotic children appear as those receiving treatment for the longest period.

The 16 children who were treated only as daypatients are too few to justify detailed analysis. Table 9.9 shows the diagnoses. There were

Table 9.9 Children treated or assessed as daypatients only

	Boys	*Girls*	*Both sexes*
Conduct disorders	5	1	6
Neurotic disorders	0	1	1
Mixed neurotic and conduct disorders	1	0	1
Developmental disorders	2	1	3
Other groups	3	2	5
Totals	11	5	16

no psychotic children among the daypatients. Twelve were 'treatment' cases and four were admitted as daypatients only for assessment. The mean period of treatment was 6 months 5 days in the 'treatment' group and 1 month 2 days in the 'assessment' group. In almost all cases the children attended five days a week while they were daypatients, but sometimes with breaks for holidays, intercurrent illness and similar factors.

Age Range

The inpatient and daypatient sections of the Charles Burns Clinic normally admit only children up to age twelve. Under exceptional conditions older children are sometimes taken, but this is less common nowadays than it was during the first three years, since the pressure on places is greater.

Table 9.10 shows the ages of the 164 children at the time of their

Table 9.10 Age at first admission

	Below 4	*4+*	*5+*	*6+*	*7+*	*8+*	*9+*	*10+*	*11+*	*12+*	*13+*	*Total*
Boys	4	9	10	8	15	13	20	14	15	5	2	115
Girls	2	3	6	4	5	3	5	5	10	4	2	49
Total	6	12	16	12	20	16	25	19	25	9	4	164

admission. The only striking feature when age at admission is considered in relation to diagnosis is that only one neurotic child (out of 33) was first admitted below the age of seven, whereas 19 out of the 68 children with conduct disorders were below seven on first admission (Table 9.11).

The peak age period for first admission of neurotic disorders comes

Table 9.11 Age on first admission in two diagnostic groups

	Below 4	*4+*	*5+*	*6+*	*7+*	*8+*	*9+*	*10+*	*11+*	*12+*	*13+*	*Total*
Conduct disorders	2	5	4	8	10	6	13	9	9	2	—	68
Neurotic disorders	—	—	1	—	1	3	6	7	10	4	1	33

a little later than that for conduct disorders (Table 9.11). Much the commonest reason for admitting a neurotic child for treatment was school refusal, and presumably this only becomes severe enough to justify admission over the age of about seven or eight.

Discussion

The figures quoted in this chapter must be regarded cautiously. Admission policy depends on the number of inpatient and daypatient places available, the demands made by the community upon the unit, the length of the waiting list, the policy, opinions and state of morale of the staff of the unit and many other factors. Thus, the type of admission to a unit which has no waiting list and can take urgent cases in straight away is likely to be very different to those in a unit with a long waiting list. The waiting period for the Charles Burns Clinic has varied enormously and this has caused admission policy to vary. A further change of emphasis came with the appointment to the clinic, during the period under review, of a consultant with a special interest in children with developmental language disorders. The main results of this, however, were seen in the admission pattern after the period reviewed here.

All authorities seem to be agreed that admission policy must take into account the children already in the clinic, and that a balance between the different types of disorder shown by the children is necessary. In particular, too many aggressive, anti-social, limit-testing children cannot be dealt with satisfactorily at any one time. Yet this is much the biggest group of children on whose behalf applications for admission are received. This is reflected in the admissions to the Charles Burns Clinic in the three years reviewed. The development of effective techniques for helping these children is clearly a matter of central importance, and has been discussed in Chapter 3.

With these reservations, the pattern of work implied by the figures set out above is probably fairly typical of that of a regional child psychiatry unit serving a large area. The rather small number of children with psychosomatic disorders who were admitted may reflect a natural tendency for them to be admitted, when necessary, to the psychiatric ward in the children's hospital in the city.

It seems that treatment is usually a matter of months, though the figures conceal wide variations in length of stay. But only nine children received treatment in the clinic for a continuous period of more than a year. As a group, psychotic children seem to need the longest period of treatment. The differences between the groups are not striking and, where they exist, may be more a reflection of the facilities available to receive the children on discharge than anything else.

These figures for the Charles Burns Clinic are similar to those reported by Barker and Jamieson (1967) for a regional unit in Scotland (conduct disorders, 47 per cent; neurosis, 18 per cent; habit (or 'developmental') disorders, 13 per cent; psychosis, 11 per cent). This may simply reflect the fact that the same consultant was responsible for admission policy in each unit. Probably, however, the patterns of admissions in both units were closely related to the demands from the community. Indeed, during the period in question the admissions to the Charles Burns Clinic came predominantly from 'outside' clinics. The pattern of admissions to a regional adolescent unit (Berg and Griffiths, 1970) was a little different, the proportion of patients with conduct disorders being lower, while a bigger percentage suffered from school refusal.

Results

The results of treatment are difficult to assess. Undoubtedly the majority of the children treated improved markedly during their period in the clinic, the psychotic children being the main exception to this statement. But the testing time usually comes on discharge. Subsequent events are often decided, it seems on looking at the later progress of the children, by the continuing care that is provided for them and their families.

The children in the three-year cohort described here are the subject of a follow-up study which aims to assess the progress of all of them 3–4 years after discharge. To date, the follow-up of only the 1968 admissions is complete; this is referred to further in Chapter 11.

Staffing Levels

The establishment of staff at the Charles Burns Clinic was gradually increased during the period reviewed, and since. The present staff look after a total of 39 inpatients and daypatients; they also provide an outpatient service seeing between 300 and 400 new referrals per year. The clinic has heavy teaching commitments and an active programme of research.

The establishment of staff at the Charles Burns Clinic (1973)

Nursing staff	*Hours worked*	*Number of staff involved*
Day staff		
Nursing officer	Full-time	1
Senior nursing officer	Half-time	1
Sisters/Charge nurses	Full-time	5 (including 2 on secondment)
Staff nurses	Full-time	2
Enrolled nurse	Full-time	1
Nursery nurses	Full-time	3
Nurse-therapists (Nursing assistants)	Full-time	15
	Part-time (total 60 hours per week)	3
Night staff		
Sisters/Charge nurses	Full-time	2
Staff nurse	Part-time (34 hours)	1
State Enrolled Nurses	Full-time	2
Nursing assistants	Full-time	2

Medical staff	*Half-day sessions worked at CBC*	*Number of staff involved*
Consultant psychiatrists	21	4
Consultant paediatrician	2	1
Senior registrar psychiatrists	14	2
Registrar psychiatrist	11	1
Clinical assistants	10	4
Clinical psychologists		
Senior	15	2
Basic	10	1
Social workers		
Principal	8	1
Senior	8	1
Basic	15	2
Occupational therapists	20	2
Teachers	40	4
Child psychotherapist	5	1
Speech therapist	10	1

Summary

This review of the work of a newly-established regional inpatient clinic for emotionally disturbed children, shows that the greatest demand is for the treatment of children with conduct disorders. Neurotic children were the second biggest group treated. The mean periods of treatment were between five and six months for most groups, with longer periods for psychotic children. In addition some children were admitted for shorter periods of assessment.

CHAPTER TEN

The Child Psychiatric Nurse: Training for Residential Care

S. Brown, I. Kolvin, D. McI. Scott and E. G. Tweddle

Psychiatric Service Needs

In 1968 Ackral *et al.* estimated that the psychiatric bed needs for children and adolescents in the United Kingdom were approximately 4,000. As it is accepted that the nurse: child ratio in child units needs to be in the vicinity of 1:1 in order to keep step with residential facilities, some 4,000 nurses need eventually to be found. This ratio appears high but, as Haldane *et al.* (1965) point out, such an overall staff: patient ratio allows at best a ratio of 1:3 by day and 1:6 by night. The evidence from Wardle's 1970 survey was that there were at that time over 1,100 day and inpatients being cared for in psychiatric units by over 800 nursing staff of which only 38 per cent were registered, and of these only a few had any special qualifications in the care of children. Despite the fact that some five hospitals have initiated training schemes, there still remains a serious shortage of trained staff which will inevitably limit the expansion of residential psychiatric services and reduce the quality of nursing care.

Ackral *et al.* expressed the view that the most urgent need was initially to train senior or experienced staff who would set the pattern and be guides and mentors to junior and untrained staff. They organised an experimental course in Newcastle, which was supported by the Nuffield Provincial Hospitals Trust under the aegis of the Department of Adult Education, University of Newcastle. More recently the

Association for the Psychiatric Study of Adolescents (1972) has underlined the view that the establishment of post-registration courses is a desirable and urgent matter, and further recommended that a properly trained and experienced nurse tutor should be available to each course.

Yet, since the majority of child psychiatric units are still in their infancy, there is no general pool of suitably qualified nurses to act as clinical instructors and tutors. There are, indeed, few trained nurses. These must therefore be closely involved in training and teaching. Some believe that only the nurse already trained in the adult psychiatric field is a suitable candidate for work in child psychiatry, while others feel these are too set in their ways, having learned inappropriate techniques. The same contradictory beliefs are held about nurses with paediatric, subnormality and also general training. Such personal views are dependent on the training and preconception of their proponents. The truth, in fact, is that we do not know. Experience leads us to believe that none of these preconceptions has so far proved to have any general validity. Previous training provides a solid nursing foundation and a reservoir of experience. Such previous experience is insufficient for work in a child psychiatric setting. These nurses lack an appreciation of the deeper emotional needs of children and must be capable of modifying personal attitudes and reactions. However, recent recommendations (Briggs, 1972) envisage an opportunity for the trainee nurse to choose between the child and adult fields for her mandatory psychiatric experiences. In future this may well be seized upon by a number of nurses, especially those interested in paediatrics. The prospect of entering child psychiatry will not always, therefore, be seen as unfamiliar and daunting.

A debate has raged over the last five years about whether the nursing profession is the most appropriate one to care for psychiatrically disturbed children (Berg, 1970). We do not want to enter this debate, except to comment with Stevens (1969, pp. 802, 803) that we are convinced that there exist serious psychiatric problems of childhood which patently call for nursing assessment, decision and action. In the authoritative USA working party report, *Nursing in Child Psychiatry* (Chisholm, 1968), the view is expressed that successful clinical nursing practice with a perceptive assessment of psychological, social and physical needs can only be based on a sound theoretical rationale.

Many units, from expedience, must rely on the intuition, experience or in-service training of their staff, but intuitive flair has little more than local value unless it can be conceptualised into principles which can then be made generally available. Even worse, many units have staff with no previous child experience, who on a rotation basis accept a care-taking or custodial role. Ackral *et al.* (1968) consider that the solution lies in providing comprehensive theoretical and practical further training. Acquisition of nursing skills through trial-and-error management of patients appears foolhardy and retrogressive when an increasing body of knowledge about the theory and practice of modern methods of management and therapy is being developed.

Unlike Stroh (1968) we would not support an emphasis on in-service training alone. This, we feel, leads to the perpetuation of traditional practices which often can become outmoded. In order to avoid parochial thinking, courses need to be open to wider academic influences. They can achieve this if located in a college or university setting or if brought under the wing of a national nursing body which will control standards. Inevitably some hospital units will have both.

As has already been mentioned, a case has been made (Berg, 1970) for the development of a new group of hospital assistants working as child social therapists who would be trained in the tradition of social-workers. We agree with Haldane, Lindsay and Smith (1971) that residential child-care training alone would insufficiently prepare such staff to care and manage children with psychosomatic, organic or rare but serious disorders such as anorexia nervosa or schizophrenia. Nor would such staff have the necessary expertise to cope with pharmaco-therapy or relevant technical and diagnostic nursing procedures. Some of the more complex cases require expert nursing techniques which are only available in the hospital setting.

Qualities of the Child Psychiatric Nurse

The basic question to be posed is whether the child psychiatric nurse is a different breed from other nurses. This may be true, but opinions differ as to the most appropriate personal characteristics. Wardle (1970), who undertook a survey of child psychiatric departments, comments on the remarkable uniformity of unit directors' views concerning qualities required in nursing staff. Those most frequently mentioned were: adequate intelligence, adaptability and versatility, consistency and stability, a liking for children, patience and tolerance, warm-heartedness and motherliness, an ability to relate with sensitivity, empathy and skills in child care. The multi-disciplinary Joint

Board of Clinical Nursing Studies (1973) laid stress on the capacity for warmth and affection while being aware of the dangers of over-possessiveness, the need for staff to understand and take into account the individual differences of patients and the need for toleration of parents. On the other hand, senior nurses in the United States (Chisholm, 1968) offered the view that child psychiatric nurses tended, after training, to differ from other nurses in their greater awareness of dynamic and social factors and of the need for direct intervention in child and family disturbances.

Three essential characteristics which are seldom acknowledged but which we recognise from our practical experience are an ability to tolerate anxiety, a sense of humour and a greater degree of physical fitness than is necessary in adult work. Some authorities (Haldane, Smith *et al.*, 1971) actually list undesirable qualities which are mainly extremes of attitudes or traits, such as indulgent sentimentality, self-righteousness, severe self-doubting or brash over-confidence, extreme passivity or marked authoritarianism; but these are merely opinions and not the fruits of research. What is necessary is some operational research undertaken by vocational psychologists to ascertain the features most predictive of the successful nurse. For instance, research in another context (Truax and Carkhuff, 1969) has indicated that important features for psychotherapeutic success include non-possessive warmth, correct empathy and genuineness. Such divergent views advanced by medical directors, senior psychiatric nurses and general research suggest that techniques of student selection may be a particularly rewarding area for research. Attention must be paid not only to delineating the salient characteristics of the successful psychiatric nurse, but also to seeking objective ways of uncovering these characteristics in potential candidates and testing preconceived notions of the desirability of previous training. We are not, however, seeking to establish a stereotype. Haldane, Smith *et al.* (1971) point out that within a pool of trained staff not all individuals will possess the same capacities and skills, nor will one individual respond most appropriately to all situations. Within the total staff the range of qualities and therapeutic skills needed should be available for all clinical contingencies. In short, it is likely that there is no one ideal type of personality for work with children and adolescents.

Selection Procedure at the Nuffield Child Psychiatry Unit, Newcastle

Though we consider the interview to be the cornerstone of selection, nevertheless full background details are required to be submitted on application. Additionally, all applicants are given opportunities of viewing the unit and meeting the staff. This allows them to absorb the atmosphere of the unit and permits staff to meet candidates in a more relaxed and informal setting.

All candidates are subjected to a searching personal interview. Following this they are invited to complete intelligence and personality tests, for research but not for selection purposes. An analysis of these research findings has recently been undertaken. The mean scores of the selected nurses were very close to population norms for neuroticism and extraversion. By comparison, candidates rejected tended to have higher neuroticism scores and to be more introverted than accepted candidates. On the group intelligence test used (Otis, 1937) the mean scores of accepted candidates lay towards the upper end of the normal range though candidates' mean scores proved to be marginally higher. Those with the lowest scores on IQ testing tended to have an objective history of poor scholastic pre-registration attainments. It must be emphasised that the reliability of a short (30 minute) group IQ test given immediately after a searching interview is open to question. This may have led to a slight underestimation of the general intelligence of all candidates.

Correlation coefficients were calculated between psychological measures, age, and performance in written examinations and practical assessments at the end of the course. The only significant correlation was a negative one between age and performance in written examinations. It seems that younger nurses produce better written papers but practical work does not show a similar age difference. There was also a complete absence of correlation between intelligence and performance in written and practical examinations. It thus appears that there is little value to be obtained from the continuing use of intelligence tests in selection. Since, however, the small number of candidates with lowest IQ scores showed greater study difficulties before registration, probably more attention should be paid to previous scholastic history than to IQ results for selection purposes. However, some kind of intellectual screen may still be necessary if nurses are accepted for post-registration courses when they have not yet completed the full general training (State Enrolled Nurses).

Provided places are available for them, candidates have been rejected only on interview evidence of personality or emotional difficulties.

The general overall impression, based on test results and a review of personalities and work efficiency of the nurses, is of an absence of common denominators either for success or failure. The only exception is that the younger nurses have tended to cope better with written examinations. Though the older student tends to have some academic difficulties, she clearly brings her maturity and experience to bear on practical situations. This does not mean to say that problems of rigidity of attitude, degrees of obsessionality, neurotic conflicts and poor academic motivation have not been encountered. Candidates who have looked less promising at selection did in fact show slow progress initially, but subsequently, with academic supervision and practical direction, showed dramatic improvement and maturation by the end of the course. Of the students who showed high promise at interview, two subsequently did not do so well.

In conclusion, though it seems desirable in the future to seek more sophisticated objective psychological selection techniques, at the moment careful selection using references, a study of the student's previous educational progress and careful interviewing appears a reasonably satisfactory way of selecting registered nurses for this field of work.

Roles and Skills and Course Objectives

John *et al.* (1963) describe seven main skills which the psychiatric nurse should possess – skills in the areas of basic nursing, technical nursing, occupational and recreational activities, communication both with patients and co-workers, human relationships, organisation and observation. The Joint Board (1973) describes skills related to maintaining the physical well-being of children (including child care and specific technical nursing skills), emotional well-being, social well-being, the application of individual and group sociotherapeutic techniques, co-ordination, co-operation and communication skills, management, administrative and teaching skills. It is to be noted that these different views, the first from the adult and the second from the child field, overlap to an appreciable extent.

The omission by John *et al.* of child care and parent surrogate skills is understandable, but there is no obvious explanation for the lack of reference to therapeutic skills. Over the last ten years the psychiatric nursing literature has increasingly described a developing use of therapeutic skills, both in the hospital and in the home. To quote the Government publication, *Psychiatric Nursing: Today and Tomorrow* (Department of Health and Social Security, 1968), 'Much psychiatric treatment today sees the patient as an active participant in treatment – not as a passive object for the exercise of medical skills. This means that the nurse – who is often beside the patient all day – is the key therapeutic figure.' This document advocates the introduction of the nurse to a variety of therapeutic ventures such as behaviour therapy, group therapy and therapeutic communities. Others, too, have underlined this point: 'We have no evidence to suggest that experienced nurses are less able to help patients who need continuing care than psychiatric social workers or doctors and they are sometimes helpful when other members of the staff have achieved nothing. They only are available throughout the 24 hours' (Watson *et al.*, 1970).

It is now also widely agreed that the general psychiatric nurse must develop a major role in the community. Hospital patients often develop an over-dependence on nurses and this can be reduced by earlier discharge and after-care in the community. Not only have psychiatrists and psychiatric nurses been attracted to the idea of extending the nurse's role to domiciliary and community work, but also a leading social worker has added his support to this new development (Hunter, 1960, 1962, 1970).

In child psychiatry parallel developments have been described in the nursing literature. A changing and developing role has clearly been indicated over the span of time even by a single author. In 1944 Szurek wrote that he viewed the nurse as a daily supervisor with child-care functions. In 1956 he reported that he then recognised an important therapeutic role. Such a role was facilitated by the greater number of therapeutic encounters between the nurse and the child patient during the day and the fact that the nurse acted as a collaborative therapist on the team. Then in 1966 in an American Nursing Association publication (Chisholm, 1968) there is a discussion of the appropriateness of the psychiatric nurse specialist functioning as a therapist, though some do not entirely agree with this (American Nurses Association, 1967; Churchill, 1967).

It is our view that the question is not whether psychotherapy is a suitable undertaking for child psychiatric nurses, but rather which nurses are suitable for psychotherapeutic training. Such training must inevitably evolve, otherwise highly trained nurses become dissatisfied with their limited role in the multi-disciplinary team. We anticipate that over the next decade there will be much discussion concerning the depth of therapy which the nurse is capable of undertaking. This, to a considerable extent, will be determined by the philosophy of each treatment centre.

The next role which merits consideration is the domiciliary one. For instance, Hunter (1970) has written convincingly about psychiatric nursing in the domiciliary situation in relation to general psychiatry, and much of what he has written has direct relevance to child psychiatry. He does not view all trained nurses as being suitable at the present time for this type of work. He feels that the experience of a patient's environment adds an additional useful dimension to the nurse's understanding and management of the patient. Often families can be given practical assistance with management of the patient. They can also be provided with support, advice and supervision, especially with regard to medication and with recognition of side-effects of medication. In certain cases, the nurse can undertake a preventive role. Hunter also stresses the significance of the relationship between the nurse and the patient.

Already one child psychiatric department has reported the introduction of the nurse to the preliminary home visit prior to admission (Haldane, Lindsay and Smith, 1971) but we feel that this should be extended to the after-care service. Hospital staff could contribute to the follow-up care as a graduated exercise leading towards final discharge. Clearly, such individual continuity of care on a one-to-one basis could not be that nurse's only function, as the exercise would then become uneconomic (Simms, 1966). Total care, as practised by the nurse, would have to take into account emotional factors within the patient and also family, cultural, physical and pharmacological factors. Such a programme would be doomed to failure unless there were a free flow of communication within the multi-disciplinary team (psychiatrists, social workers, psychologists) and extending beyond it to the general practitioner.

Then there are the additional roles of the specialist nurse in child psychiatry which one can only list:

As a consultant to other bodies and disciplines.

A leadership role for the junior and less well-trained staff.

A supervisory role in relation to the less trained staff.
An administrative role. Most authorities are not very happy with this being the only role for a senior nurse, since direct nursing care of children is the distinctive characteristic of child psychiatric nursing. Without it, nursing becomes either completely technical or rigidly administrative (Reiter, 1966).

Training

Child psychiatry is a dynamic and developing subject. Since the implementation of the National Health Service Act there has been an appreciable increase in the body of knowledge in the fields of medicine and the behavioural sciences which has radically influenced our approach to the management of the disturbed child. To keep abreast of these developments nurses who are already qualified need further training and a preparation for the kind of role change we foresee as essential for this type of work.

It is probably true to say that the traditional supervisory, domestic and care-taking role of the child psychiatric nurse is now insufficient and we should accept nothing less than skilled professional management of children, whether individually or in groups. In this way nurses will cease to be psychiatric auxiliaries to other professionals and become specialists in their own right, with professional standing comparable with that of other specialists in child psychiatry.

The broad objective is to create a nursing specialist or consultant capable of maintaining a humane individual approach (Simms, 1966), operating from a sound theoretical frame of reference and capable of functioning not only as a nurse practitioner but as a consultant to professional colleagues and the general public (Royal College of Nursing, 1970).

The main aim of our course is to provide a practical and theoretical basis for the recognition and understanding of emotional disturbance in children and their families and to plan nursing care and treatment on a day or residential basis. In order to achieve such objectives the student has to acquire certain skills, knowledge and attitudes, as suggested by the Joint Board of Clinical Nursing Studies (1973). The objectives of our course were classed as primary and secondary. There is no significance in the order in which they have been listed.

Primary Objectives of Training

1. To help the student to acquire basic information about physical, emotional and cognitive aspects of human development.
2. To provide basic sociological knowledge: this includes an understanding of the dynamics of human behaviour and of relationships, both individually within families and within social settings, of role theory and communications theory, and of attitudes and attitude change.
3. To provide a working knowledge of some personality theories and their relevance to child psychiatric practice.
4. To provide an account of the aetiology of child psychiatric disorders.
5. To provide an understanding of the personal emotional needs of individual children and young people.
6. To familiarise the student with the range of psychological disorders they are likely to meet in any child or adolescent setting, that is in the family, in school, in social care, in establishments for sick, psychiatrically disturbed or handicapped children, and so on.
7. To provide an appreciation of the multidisciplinary nature of the diagnostic assessment process in child psychiatry.
8. To help the nurse improve skills of communication.
9. To provide a working knowledge of the principles and techniques of a variety of treatment methods: psychotherapy, either individually or in groups, case work and family therapy, play therapy, behaviour therapy and drug therapy. To these must be added principles of residential treatment and the nurse's individual and collaborative role in such activities.
10. To provide an appreciation of the importance of relationships among staff and relationships between staff and patients occurring in the special ambience of a psychiatry department. The nurse must become aware of a number of functions which, taken together, are unique to the child–nurse relationship: intimacy of contact in physical caring, her presence in a variety of social and nurturing situations, her inevitable involvement in the child's daily crises calling for skilful intervention and effort at resolution.
11. To provide an understanding of the philosophical assumptions underlying decisions about policy and practical management

and the effects of such policies on staff and patient treatment practices. Examples are the open versus the closed door issue, concepts of tight and loose structure for child management, and implications of technological advances.

12. To provide some knowledge and understanding of the functions of the other disciplines working in this area and an appreciation of their need for a degree of overlapping.
13. To help the nurse to develop skills of recording, observation and interpretation.

Secondary Objectives of Training

1. To help the nurse to gain a working knowledge of the principles of nursing care of the physically ill child.
2. To familiarise the student with the main features of adult mental disorders.
3. To provide an understanding of the principles of administration including selection, supervision, counselling, deployment of staff and an introduction to the evaluation of nursing management.
4. To provide a knowledge of hospital and community resources.
5. To provide elementary teaching skills.
6. To provide some knowledge of the importance of research.

The Nuffield Unit Training Scheme

(a) *Background*

No training scheme can be divorced from the orientation, activities, organisation and administration of the department in which it is located. The administration and staff of the unit must accept responsibilities in the training exercise which it has accepted. In this exercise there are two essentials: the first is a nucleus of senior staff and the second is staff continuity (Hallman, 1960). Indeed it is disastrous to train junior staff without prior training of senior staff as conflicts about theory and practice quickly develop. This is doubly essential because child and adolescent units are invariably small and most senior personnel have to accept training roles and functions. Some senior staff are able to function adequately by virtue of their experience alone. However, challenging questions about establishment policy cannot easily be answered nor can new ideas be readily assimilated when theoretical knowledge is inadequate. With regard to continuity, the practice of rotating trained nursing staff from child units to adult psychiatric or general hospital settings is now unanimously condemned as it both complicates the running of the unit and prevents the development of special skills, as well as militating against continuity of care for the individual patient.

The philosophy and activity of the department has previously been described (Ackral, *et al.*, 1968) and only salient features merit comment here. The clinical work of the department consists of the psychological diagnosis, care and treatment of disturbed children. The department's treatment approach is eclectic with a major emphasis on psychodynamic principles. Students do, however, have the opportunity to gain experience of behaviour modification and pharmacotherapy. The facilities for both day and inpatients are integrated to provide a service for children usually below 16 years of age. The children are divided into three groups, one for the nursery range and two for the older children of varied ages. Each group has its own nucleus of permanent nursing staff, each under the supervision of a nursing sister. Every nurse takes an individual responsibility for one or two children, and gives general attention to the rest in her group. Careful observations of children's behaviour are recorded daily by the nursing staff and the salient features are included in the monthly progress report.

The school has been organised on a horizontal basis into three broad age bands – nursery-infant, junior and secondary. While most children attend the school group most appropriate to their age, some attend according to ability. The size of classes is determined by many factors, including the age and accessibility of the children and the range and severity of the disorders. Similar grouping principles are applied to occupational therapy situations. During play periods and after school hours, spontaneous regroupings of the children facilitates the emergence of free unstructured play activities.

(b) *Design of the course*

Some consider that, apart from time devoted to studies and instruction, the nurse should have full nursing responsibilities; others feel she should be supernumerary. We believe that supernumerary status prevents full involvement in the therapeutic relationship and the

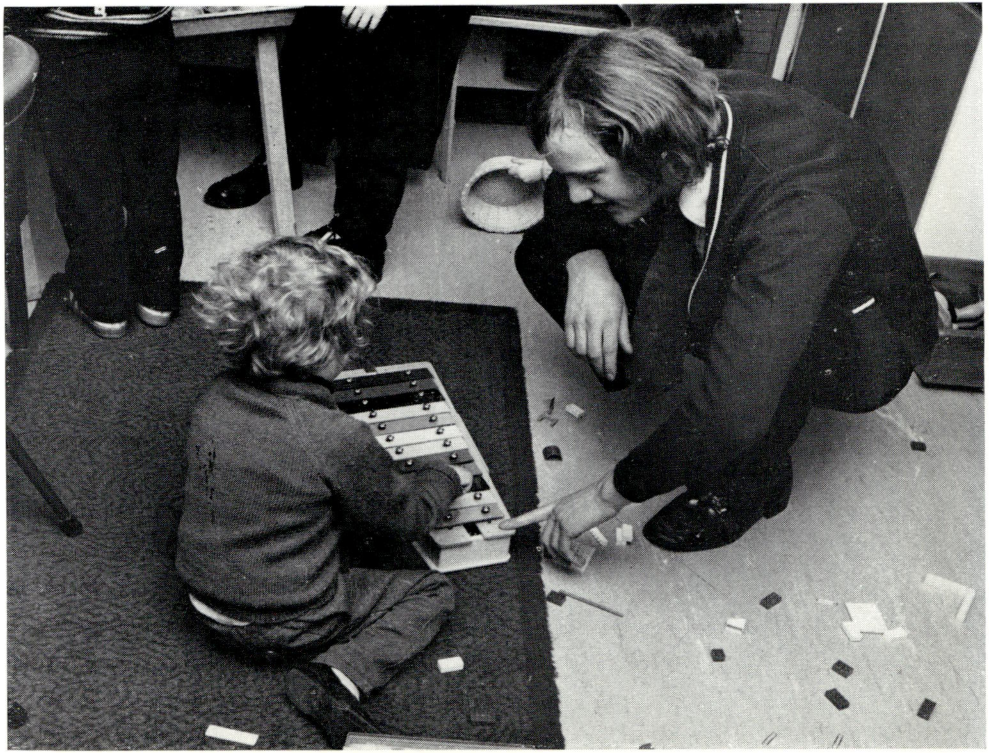

Fig. 10.1

At the Nuffield Child Psychiatry Unit

acceptance of clinical responsibility for patients but, at the same time, student status needs to be respected so that post-graduate nurses are not just used as 'a pair of hands'.

Another issue is the length of the course. Experience led us to decide that twelve months was a necessary minimum for the acquisition of a new set of skills, acquiring adequate knowledge and suitable modification of attitudes. The nurses attending the course are allowed considerable time during the academic year for educational purposes. One full day a week is devoted to lectures and tutorials. All students initially attend individual or small group seminars with both their academic and practical tutors, and are given one to two hours for private study. They join each nursing group for their weekly meetings to discuss the organisation of group activities, the handling of children on an individual or group basis and interpersonal relationships. They attend one or two interdisciplinary conferences a week. They also observe the work of teachers and occupational therapists. We estimate that on the average the equivalent of one-and-a-half days and, on occasions, up to two days a week during academic terms are devoted to formal and semi-formal teaching sessions. The Joint Board of Clinical Studies has suggested that students should be rotated between child and adolescent units, perhaps in four-month modules. From our experience we believe the first two of these blocks should be in the same setting, since anything less than eight months is inadequate for the continuity of experience of care of children and personal supervision by tutors.

Student Supervision

Personal counsellors. Our students vary in their background experience and a number need to make major attitude adjustments. Because we recognise this as a potential source of stress we have arranged for personal counselling to be available within the unit.

Academic tutors. The academic tutor organises the course schedule, conducting seminars, allocating case student projects and setting essays, organising educational visits, and arranging terminal tests and final examinations.

Practical tutors. The practical tutors are drawn from the senior nursing staff and their main function is to promote clinical competence through daily supervision and direction and weekly small group tutorials.

Induction Period

This is a crucial exercise for many reasons. Some nurses have to make major adjustments to becoming students again, but all have to be introduced to the nature of post-graduate education. New recruits to child psychiatry have to be familiarised with a multi-disciplinary staff, their teachers, the resources and organisation of the departments and the disordered patients cared for in the department. They also have to develop relationships with their colleagues within the department and their peers on the course. For such reasons we have now organised a three-week induction period as part of the course.

Course Content

From a survey of the literature Haldane (1965) comments that the content of such post-registered courses varies little and usually includes formal lectures, seminars and case conferences, educational visits, and practical work consisting of practical supervision, written child studies, learning a creative skill (for example, a handicraft such as can be used in relation to an individual child) and training in counselling and psychotherapy of various kinds. The Nuffield course follows this pattern but, additionally, it is designed to build on previous knowledge and skills deriving from basic nurse training and experience. Though adjustments for individual experience are possible, most students have preferred to undergo the full course of lectures and seminars. In view of the above we have assumed the minimum of knowledge in all nurses but have allowed the course to be flexible so as to make good any specific deficiencies with a particular kind of basic training.

Lectures and Seminars

(i) *Child development.* This provides an account of the normal and abnormal physical, emotional and cognitive development over all stages of childhood and adolescence. It includes knowledge of the developing parent–child relationships and interactions and provides an introduction to the major theories of personality development. It deals with the roles and functions of the psychologist in diagnosis and treatment and gives an account of normal and special education. The importance of individual and group play in child development is stressed.

Breakdown

Lectures	23 hours
Seminars	9 hours
Educational visits, observations and films	10 hours

(day nursery, mental subnormality hospitals, training centres)

(ii) *Aetiological and dynamic factors in child psychiatry.* This provides an account of the psychosocial and biological origins of behaviour with particular emphasis on psychological defence mechanisms, crisis theory, cycles of deprivation, family dynamics, and so on.

Breakdown

Lectures	10 hours
Seminars	5 hours
Films	1 hour

(iii) *Social and environmental factors.* This is designed to cover social and environmental factors operating both in the community and within institutions. Visits are paid to community homes and community assessment centres.

Breakdown

Lectures	4 hours
Seminars	2 hours
Visits	5 hours

(iv) *Child psychiatry – symptoms, disorders and assessment.* This section covers the identification, classification, diagnosis and treatment of psychiatric disturbances in childhood. It lays emphasis on the nature and importance of multidisciplinary assessments.

Breakdown

Lectures	21 hours
Seminars	10 hours
Demonstrations	9 hours
Films	3 hours

(v) *Principles of therapy and management.* This section covers the theory and practice of individual, group and family therapy. Particular attention is devoted to such themes as crisis intervention, principles of residential therapy (Rogers, 1965), the nature and place of social casework and counselling, communication theory, the theory and practice of behaviour modification (operant conditioning), the principles of pharmacotherapy in childhood, and also the place of the supporting therapies – occupational therapy, play therapy, drama therapy, speech therapy, etc. Finally, it covers the principles of child psychiatric nursing, child–nurse relationships and the development of a therapeutic milieu.

Breakdown

Lectures	27 hours
Seminars	45 hours
Films	1 hour
Projects	10 hours
Visits to schools for maladjusted children	2 hours

Experience – a direct involvement, both individually and in groups, with children of different ages undergoing various therapies is arranged. Experience is also provided in the co-operative planning of general therapeutic and nursing care and opportunities are made available for observing and participating in behaviour therapy.

(vi) *Observation, recording and interpretation.* This covers the skill of behaviour observation and recording in various settings and interpretations of data.

Breakdown

Lectures	2 hours
Seminars	3 hours

(vii) *Relevant medical and other disorders.* This comprises the nature and treatment of paediatric disorders with psychiatric components such as epilepsy, appetite and eliminative disorders, asthma, eczema, ulcerative colitis and deafness. Adult psychoses, neuroses and character disorders are also covered.

Breakdown

Lectures	10 hours
Seminars	10 hours
Visits	12 hours

(viii) *Principles of social administration.* This includes an account of hospital and community resources.

Breakdown

Lectures	6 hours
Seminars	3 hours

(ix) *Principles of teaching and place of research.* These topics are covered generally in other seminars.

Academic Terms

It has been found useful to relate the theoretical programme to the academic terms but not the academic year. The course heavily relies on university staff for lectures and tutorials and such staff are more likely to be available during academic terms. Furthermore, it is administratively more convenient if the holidays of the student nurse can coincide with school holidays. Finally, starting at Easter rather than in September gives students the summer to settle more adequately into their practical work and consolidate in a more leisurely way what they have already learned before embarking on the next two academic terms.

Supervision

Clinical supervision aims at helping the student apply theoretical knowledge to the practical nursing situation and attempts to modify those attitudes which may adversely influence handling.

Evaluation of the Newcastle Course

Some Statistics of Students Attending the Course

So far, five courses have been run, attended by 36 nurses. Only two students have not stayed the course. Eleven of the students were male and 25 female (a ratio of 1:2·3). This high female/male ratio probably results from the unit's situation within a children's hospital. There was a fair spread of ages, with 50 per cent of the students being under

30 years of age, about 30 per cent between 30 and 40, and about 20 per cent over 40 years. Forty-four per cent of the nurses were doubly trained and a further 11 per cent were trebly trained. Table 10.1 indicates that there is a wide dispersal of students at the end of each course and a wide variety of chosen field of work. Most have continued to work with children in child or adolescent psychiatry; others have opted for special responsibilities for children in subnormality institutions or for work in paediatric wards.

Table 10.1 Dispersal of nurses

Chosen fields	*Students remaining in Newcastle*	*Students outside Newcastle*	*Total*
Child and adolescent psychiatry	7	7	14
Schools (maladjusted, etc.)	—	2	2
Paediatrics	2	1	3
Academic tutor	1	—	1
Subnormality	3	4	7
General psychiatry	1	1	2
Further training (general nursing or psychiatry)	2	1	3
Others (married, left nursing, etc.)	1	1	2
Left course	1	1	2
Totals	18	18	36

The students completing the courses up to 1972 have progressed reasonably well in terms of careers. Their subsequently achieved status in nursing (whether or not still in nursing) is indicated in Table 10.2. Understandably, higher nursing grades have been achieved by nurses completing the course in its first year.

Table 10.2 Status of previous students in hospital service

Salmon grading	*Year 1969*	*1970*	*1971*	*1972*	*Total*
7 or higher	3	1	1	1	6
6	2	2	2	4	10
5	—	1	4	2	7
Totals	5	4	7	7	23

Assessment of Students

Initially, only a final written and oral examination at the end of the course was used. Subsequently it was decided to supplement this with continuous assessment of the student's practical work which took into account attitudes and attitude change during the course.

Students take three written papers of which there are five sections: child development, social and family factors in child psychiatry, psychiatric disorders in children and adolescence, organisation and administration, and therapy in child psychiatry. The oral examination accounts for 25 per cent of the marks, continuous assessment for 30 per cent, and the written examination for 45 per cent. Candidates need 50 per cent in each section and an overall 50 per cent to pass.

The course is supervised by an Examination Moderating Board which is composed of members from both the Hospital and the University and supplemented by an external assessor. The Board meets once or twice annually, controls standards and supervises the examination.

Feedback from the Students

Frank evaluations of the course have been regularly sought from students in terms of presentation, content and overall value. Their comments varied from year to year but we offer some recurring themes which are of general interest.

(i) Early in the course students prefer seminars to be closely linked with material presented in formal lectures. This aids the assimilation of the large amount of factual information needing to be covered. The students reject the currently fashionable proposal that they glean basic knowledge through private studies.

(ii) Routine visits to a variety of institutions are of little educational value unless combined with informed discussion of the philosophy and practices of the setting concerned.

(iii) A detailed timetable of the lectures, seminars and visits should be available at the beginning of the term. This helps the students to plan their reading.

(iv) There is a dearth of good instructional film material in the child psychiatry field.

(v) The students have made persistent requests for:
more pure study time
more revision seminars
more multidisciplinary meetings and conferences.

(vi) They have argued for greater therapeutic opportunities and administrative responsibility.

(vii) They prefer frequent progress reports to be given on a frank and individual basis by a nurse tutor rather than in a seminar or group setting where frankness is often muted.

(viii) They have made many valuable comments, both about organisation of the course and the organisation of the day and residential unit. For instance, they have pointed out that if lectures and seminars in administrative subjects are given early they can quickly gain a grasp of the organisation and administration of the department and the ramifications of the work. Some of their comments have led to the abolition of certain tedious or unnecessary nursing chores.

Scope and Prospects

It has been our experience that suitable recruits are available, given reasonable post-graduate training facilities and career prospects. Indeed, as has been shown, prospects in face of the current shortage of trained nurses are good, not only in child psychiatry but in wider fields such as paediatric units, subnormality units, special schools and children's homes. Unfortunately, the career structure in child psychiatry is a rather truncated one with units unlikely to be able to negotiate a status beyond a Salmon 7 (deputy matron). Advancement beyond this level will usually necessitate a move into general nursing administration. In these circumstances, post-registered courses should not only prepare students to work as clinical nurses but also give them an introduction to some of the problems faced by the nursing administrator or tutor.

A word must be said about the economic viability of such courses, since each department can train only a small number of nurses at one time. While we recognise the essentially specific aspects of child psychiatric nursing care, we feel that much of the advanced course's content is basic to a wide variety of professional disciplines in fields concerned with emotionally disturbed children. We would therefore argue for the establishment of a generic form of training which would provide core experience for other health workers such as occupational therapists, residential care workers, teachers in special units and so forth (Royal College of Psychiatrists, 1971). Clearly some specific professional training would additionally have to be provided for each of the different groups. This would lead to considerable financial economies and economic use of lecturer-time in a field where resources are short.

We must thank Professor Sir Martin Roth for continued encouragement and toleration of experimental educational programmes in his department, Mr E. Hughes, Director of the Department of Adult Education, for his personal breadth of vision which has allowed the course to flourish, and the senior members of the nursing staff of the Newcastle University Hospitals for their essential practical help and encouragement.

CHAPTER ELEVEN

The Results of Inpatient Care

Philip Barker

The results of the treatment in hospital of children with psychiatric disorders are difficult to assess for a number of reasons. One is that the aims of treatment vary from child to child. Another is that it is impossible ever to know precisely what the prognosis would have been without inpatient care. It is also impossible to determine the contributions to change made by, on the one hand, inpatient care itself, and, on the other hand, other treatment given to child or family before, during or after the period of inpatient care. Yet another complication is that the nature of inpatient care varies from unit to unit, as the contributions to this book show, and even from time to time in the same unit.

Measuring change in the condition of children is also difficult. Sometimes, moreover, it is a change in the family group as a whole that is more important than change in a particular child. As with hospital admission in general, a frequent reason for admission is the severity of the illness or disorder. Just as patients ill enough to require care in general hospitals are admitted regardless of whether or not they are likely to be cured, or even have their condition alleviated, in the same way disturbed children are sometimes admitted for help in hospital primarily because of the severity of their symptoms. Relief for the community rather than radical cure of the child's disorder may be the main aim of treatment.

The aims of inpatient care can include any of the following:

(a) Assessment and investigation.
(b) The short-term treatment or alleviation of severe or acute emotional disorders.
(c) The provision of short-term relief for the family or the wider community.
(d) The provision of short-term relief for the child facing environmental stress.
(e) Help with particular problems such as depression, acute or severe neurotic anxiety, anti-social behaviour, psychosomatic symptoms or educational problems (especially when these are related to emotional disturbance).
(f) An attempt to bring about a substantial change in the course of the child's personality growth and development.
(g) The treatment of serious psychotic disorders (see Chapter 6).

Short-term treatment may be expected to have short-term results; it is less likely to result in a change in the child's long-term development than is a longer period of treatment. Long-term results, however, are going to be affected also by the many other experiences and treatments that may follow the period of inpatient care, as well as by the process of maturation. In particular, the changing social situation of a child can have profound effects on him, regardless of the treatment he receives. The following case-history illustrates this.

Neville was first admitted to the Charles Burns Clinic at the age of nine, the main problems being soiling and a behaviour disorder. His family was an unstable and troubled one, and there was great disharmony between the parents. Neville himself did well in hospital and after four months was discharged home. He no longer soiled and his behaviour was much improved.

Neville at first did well at home after his stay in the clinic. Unfortunately the parents' marital difficulties worsened, and this led to Neville's mother leaving home. The father, a night-shift worker, attempted to look after the children on his own, with help and support from a social worker from the social services department. He managed quite well with the other three children, but Neville relapsed. His soiling recurred and he began truanting and wandering off. At the request of the social worker who had been called in he was readmitted, now aged ten. The hope was that without Neville the father could manage to care adequately for the other children.

This worked out quite well. Neville's symptoms again improved rapidly and he did not present any serious behaviour problems in the clinic. The father also managed to look after the other three children. After due consideration of the home situation it was decided that on his discharge Neville should be admitted to the care of the local authority and placed in a children's home, from which he could conveniently visit his own home. A place was also found for him in a school near the children's home.

After discharge all went well at first, but after about three months complaints were received from the school that Neville was displaying aggressive behaviour with which the staff could not cope. His outbursts of aggression were said to follow teasing by other children. In one attack he threw a chair at a teacher and in another he ripped a teacher's dress. He was also said to disrupt seriously the work of the open-plan school, in which he could never be confined to the area where he was supposed to be. This led to Neville's exclusion from the school, though his adjustment in the children's home remained good.

Was Neville's inpatient treatment a success? On each occasion it seemed to be at the time. Unfortunately the situation was complicated on the first occasion by the parents' subsequent separation, and on the second by Neville's position in an open-plan, permissive school which apparently provided him with too few controls and too little structure at a stage when he lacked internal controls. It could have been argued that the inpatient care would have been a lasting success if the parents' marriage had not broken up.

Perhaps the clinic staff should have worked harder on the marital problem, though it is questionable whether the marriage was capable of repair. On the second occasion, perhaps a more suitable school should have been selected. Yet there was no other more suitable school available in the area of the children's home, which itself did meet Neville's needs very well. It can certainly be said that inpatient treatment is no panacea for children such as Neville, even in the short term. But it can be useful as one of a range of facilities including social-work services, residential care and special schools.

The difficulties in assessing the longer-term results of inpatient care are illustrated by the following two cases.

Mandy was admitted to the Charles Burns Clinic in 1968 at the age of seven. She was one of eight children. The first four were the children of her mother's husband, but currently her mother lived with the father of the last four children, to whom she was not married. Mandy was the second of this man's four children. He himself was a sick man, unable to work and requiring frequent hospital treatment.

Mandy was admitted because of her violent screaming attacks, jealousy of her sister and reluctance to go to school. She was, indeed, quite beyond the control of her weak, indulgent mother over whom she had gained a demanding ascendancy.

Mandy tested out the clinic's limits thoroughly after admission but eventually settled down and her behaviour improved greatly. She was able to work through some personal anxieties in her psychotherapeutic sessions with her doctor.

Within a few weeks of discharge Mandy's behaviour again became difficult. She had been sent, at her request, to a different school, but she began to complain about this. At home she again began to display tantrums whenever her mother attempted to deny her anything she wanted. This always led to her mother giving in. Mandy soon decided she disliked her school and refused to go, so her mother arranged for her to go to another. Again Mandy, after a brief 'honeymoon' period, refused to go.

By this time Mandy's behaviour was again very disturbed and so she was readmitted to the clinic. This time she spent six months as an inpatient followed by six months as a daypatient. Once again she 'tested out' the clinic very thoroughly. At one stage she took to running away home. Eventually she seemed well enough for discharge, and this time a place was found for her in a day school for maladjusted children. Predictably, Mandy found it not entirely to her liking, stopped attending regularly and demanded a change of school which, again predictably, her mother tried to arrange. By now, however, this was more difficult as Mandy's reputation was known to the local schools. Throughout this time Mandy remained an outpatient of the clinic, as indeed she is at the time of writing.

Next, a place was found for Mandy in a residential school for maladjusted children. Here things went well for a few terms. Then Mandy began to find fault with the school and at the beginning of term refused to return. She was by this time aged twelve.

All attempts to persuade Mandy to return to school failed and instead she got her mother to apply for her admission to every secondary school in the area. None would take her, however. It was now agreed by the various professional people trying to help the family that a care order should be sought from the juvenile court on the grounds of Mandy's failure to attend school. This was duly obtained and Mandy was found a place in a children's home from which she could visit her home and also go (as a boarder) to the residential school for maladjusted children to which she had refused to return.

Mandy and her mother were furiously indignant about these procedures. Much negative feeling was expressed towards the writer (and others) and an appeal against the care order was threatened by the family. Quite quickly, however, Mandy came to accept the situation and settled down in school and in her new way of life which allowed her frequent, but controlled, access to home at weekends and during school holidays. It seemed as if she was, at one level, relieved that at last some limits had been set. Her mother, who undoubtedly loved her children and cared for them well in material ways, had been like a chair which always collapsed when sat on. She could never stand up to her wilful, demanding daughter.

Mandy received a total of 18 months treatment in the clinic, 12 months as an inpatient and six as a daypatient. Yet at the time when the follow-up study of 1968 admissions was being carried out she was refusing to return to her residential school. Hardly a successful result! But the large amount of psychiatric effort which had been expended had probably not been wasted. At least the dynamics of the family were quite well understood (a brother was by now also under treatment as an outpatient), and useful relationships with Mandy, her mother and one of her brothers had been established. It was in the context of all the previous work with the family that a halt to Mandy's demanding manipulation of her mother could finally be called. How far this process could have been gone through without Mandy being admitted to hospital is not clear; nor is it clear whether earlier court action would have been helpful. At last, however, real progress seemed to be occurring in Mandy's treatment and rehabilitation.

Neil was admitted to the Charles Burns Clinic, also in 1968, at the age of nine. He was an illegitimate child abandoned by his mother and living in a children's home. His first five years had been spent in a residential nursery. He was referred because of his violently aggressive and destructive behaviour in the children's home where he lived. He had physically attacked staff, would not share anything with other children and occasionally soiled and smeared faeces.

Following admission Neil proved a very difficult and aggressive boy who taxed the resources of the clinic fully. Medication and consistent handling were followed by some improvement in Neil's behaviour and cessation of his soiling. After 3½ months' inpatient care Neil was returned to the children's home where his adjustment now seemed better. Close outpatient support and treatment for Neil and his house-parents was planned. Unfortunately these house-parents left a few months later.

Their successors proved quite unable to cope with Neil and said that he must be removed, or they would go. Neil was therefore removed to another children's home.

Things went no better at the next home. Indeed, further difficulties appeared and these led to Neil being sent eventually to an approved school, the status of which later changed to that of a community school. It was fortunate that this school was an unusually enlightened, progressive and therapeutic one. Neil was able to remain for a prolonged period at this school and to receive expert help with his problems. The result was that at follow-up in 1972 he was making excellent progress, both as regards the symptoms he formerly had and also in the matter of his personality development generally.

Thus Neil showed a better result at follow-up than did Mandy, but his progress had very little to do with the treatment he had had 4½ years previously at the Charles Burns Clinic. Mandy, looked at by any sort of objective criteria at the time of follow-up, had done less well despite more treatment. Yet in her case the clinic had been a major and significant part of her childhood experiences. Without it her precarious adjustment in her family and the community in which she lived might well have broken down long since. With its help a series of crises in Mandy's development and in the life of the family (crises not mentioned in the brief history above) have been met and, in some measure at least, overcome. Mandy has, in consequence, achieved a level of maturity which did not at one stage seem attainable. Neil, too, has done well, but because of treatment carried out during the years which followed his inpatient stay.

The above considerations suggest that long-term follow-up studies of child psychiatric inpatients should be treated with reserve. Inpatient care might be compared with one instrument in an orchestra, the music of which should be judged with and without that instrument. Consideration of inpatient treatment on its own is liable to lead to results as fallacious as judging the potential of a double-bass simply on what it can achieve played as a solo instrument.

Despite these reservations, follow-up studies are of interest and some examples are worth examining. One of the earliest follow-up studies is that of Potter and Klein (1937). These authors followed up 175 children who had been treated in the New York State Psychiatric Institute and Hospital. The follow-up contact was made at least a year after discharge. Adjustment was classed as 'satisfactory' or 'unsatisfactory'. Sixty-four children had 'organic reactions', and of these the adjustment of only ten was classified as satisfactory; six of the group were dead at follow-up. Results were even worse in the 14 'schizophrenic reaction' group: only one of these was classed as satisfactory. The 'situational reaction' group did best. Here 55 were satisfactory and 42 unsatisfactory. The different sub-categories are shown in Table 11.1. The psychoneurotic cases thus seemed to do best of all, an experience common to most child psychiatry units.

Table 11.1 Social Adjustment of 'Situational Reaction Group' at Follow-up (Potter and Klein, 1937)

	Personality and habit problems	*Conduct disorders*	*Psychoneurosis*	*Total*
Satisfactory	14	26	15	55
Unsatisfactory	11	25	6	42
Totals	25	51	21	97

Benjamin and Weatherly (1947) described a follow-up study of 44 children treated in the children's psychiatric ward of the Illinois Psychiatric Institute. Each had been discharged for at least five months, but the mean time to follow-up was not stated. The average inpatient stay had been 9·3 months; only five children stayed five months or less. Twenty-seven were boys, 17 girls. About half showed antisocial behaviour, the other half 'neurotic behaviour'. Of the 44 children, 11 (25 per cent) showed 'great improvement', 6 (14 per cent) 'improvement', 14 (32 per cent) 'little improvement' and 9 (20 per cent) 'no improvement'. In four cases the outcome is listed as 'unknown'. In view of the multiple factors which affect outcome it is open to question how much significance figures of this sort have.

Barker and Milligan (1947), in one of the earliest British reports, described seven years' work at St James Hospital, Portsmouth, to which children were first admitted in 1940. The children were not treated in a separate children's unit though many of them were housed in 'a special wing of the female convalescent villa'. The length of stay was up to three years. Behaviour disorders were common. 'A secure background to the lives' of the children was a central part of the treatment. Some 80 per cent recovered or were much improved and 'all the children were followed up', though for how long is not stated. It would seem that this service was seen as valuable by the community it served, for the authors state that when it became known that they were offering such a service for children they were inundated with requests to arrange admissions. This unit was the forerunner of the present Wessex Unit for Children and Parents (see Appendix B).

McTaggart (1965) described an eight-bedded child psychiatric unit in the University of Alberta Hospital, a general teaching hospital. Opened in 1960, the unit admitted about 85 new cases per year, with an average stay of only 25 days. Milieu therapy was supplemented by occupational therapy, educational help, group sessions and, where appropriate, individual psychotherapy. It was considered important to have a family available for the child. The author believed that such short-term treatment could be of value as a therapeutic experience, as well as helping in diagnosis and prognosis. He gives follow-up data on 93 patients, the mean interval after discharge being 2·3 years. According to parents' reports 67 per cent of the children were in an improved state, 23 per cent were unchanged and 10 per cent were worse. The male: female ratio in this unit, as in most others, was about 2:1.

Davids *et al.* (1968) described a follow-up of 27 male patients who had been treated at one of the units of the Emma Pendleton Bradley Hospital, a neuropsychiatric unit for children, in Rhode Island. The ten cases of 'childhood schizophrenia' were compared with seventeen diagnosed as 'passive–aggressive personality'. The mean age on admission was 7·2 years, and at follow-up 15·2 years. Rather less than half of the subjects were making a 'favourable adjustment' at follow-up. Although there were significant differences in the symptoms of the two groups at the time of admission, there were few differences between the groups when variables present during treatment were compared, particularly the amount and type of treatment given. There were also no significant differences in the measures of adjustment used at follow-up. These authors considered that their findings indicated that outcome depended more on the symptoms and behaviour the children brought with them when coming for treatment, than on the treatment given.

Levy (1969) reported a long-term follow-up of former patients of the Menninger Clinic's Children's Hospital (formerly called Southard School). One hundred (85 per cent) of the 113 patients discharged between 1945 and 1960 were traced. All contact was by telephone or letter. At follow-up the ex-patients' ages ranged from 17 to 41 years, and they had been discharged 8 to 23 years previously.

The diagnoses of the total group of 113 patients were:

Chronic brain syndrome	12
Psychosis (usually schizophrenic reaction)	27
Neurosis (usually 'severe')	21
Personality disorder	13
Neurotic behaviour disorder (usually 'severe')	24
Emotional maladjustment	16
	113

Thirty-four were leading lives that appeared ordinary, 24 had a more marginal adjustment, 7 were 'more actively peculiar', 6 had been seriously ill after discharge but had subsequently improved. Eleven were chronically ill but currently out of hospital, 10 were in psychiatric institutions, 3 in penal establishments and 5 dead. About 60 were self-supporting. In all, 37 patients had required subsequent inpatient treatment. Among diagnostic groups the 'schizophrenic' or 'psychotic' children tended not to do so well. At the time of discharge, it was thought by the staff that 55 patients had been helped. The follow-up study however suggested that 50 of these had been helped. Several other patients thought not to have been helped seemed, or claimed, to have been helped at follow-up. This study was conducted entirely by means of letters and telephone calls, the latter usually lasting between 30 minutes and 2 hours. The author comments on the 'compelling data' that can be obtained in these ways, particularly by telephone. The paper is an unusually interesting one in that it gives an indication of the life pattern that followed residential treatment. It is not surprising that patients who were discharged to the care of 'relatively well adjusted families' did much better than those whose families were very disturbed.

Treffert (1969) described follow-up data relating to the unit at Winnebayo State Hospital. The figures related to children who had been discharged at least one year previously. Unfortunately Treffert's figures are based chiefly on patients' and parents' reported opinions on the results of treatment, rather than on any more objective assessment. Nevertheless, 65 per cent of former patients were either in a regular school setting or had graduated from high school; from the meagre clinical data given, however, it is hard to be sure whether or not this is a good result.

Even more uncertain is the significance of the view of 80 per cent of the patients (and also 80 per cent of their parents) that they had improved while in hospital. It is perhaps of more interest that 58 per cent of patients felt there was little or no stigma attached to having been in hospital. Indeed, 16 per cent felt that 'the known fact of hospitalisation' helped to have people accept them.

The type of problem dealt with in this unit is indicated by the following diagnostic breakdown of six years' admissions:

Schizophrenia	40
Childhood schizophrenia	33
Adjustment reaction	297
Chronic brain syndrome	53
Mental deficiency	22

Warren (1965b), discussing a follow-up study of adolescent psychiatric inpatients, points out that 'diverse further factors' affect the ultimate outcome. He emphasises the need for detailed description of the syndromes followed up. He reported in this paper follow-up data on 157 patients (94 boys and 63 girls), the clinical features of which had been described in an earlier paper (Warren, 1965a). The age range was 11 to 19½, most being in 'the middle of this range'. This is an important study because of the considerable amount of clinical detail given (though only some of the subjects' ages fall in the range with which the present book is chiefly concerned). In summary, about two-thirds of the patients with neurotic disorders did well. Just over half of those with mixed neurotic and conduct disorders did well, while this only applied to just under half of those with conduct disorders. Only a quarter of the children with psychotic disorders and of those with 'other' disorders did well. Younger patients tended to do better than older ones.

Because of the complexity of the matter there is much to be said for follow-up studies of particular diagnostic groups. An example is the report of Berg (1970) on a group of school phobic adolescents treated in an inpatient unit. Twenty-one out of a total of 23 discharged school phobic patients were followed up on average 13 months after discharge. The mean period of inpatient treatment had been 9 months. Of the 21 subjects, 16 were attending school, technical college or work satisfactorily (though some of these had other adjustment problems) and 5 were not. These results are similar to those of some other studies of children with school refusal.

The children admitted to the Charles Burns Clinic in 1968–70, and reviewed in Chapter 9, are being systematically followed up 3–4 years after discharge. At present data for the 1968 admissions only are available. During this year 32 *inpatients* were admitted for *treatment* (as distinct from those for whom admission was primarily for assessment purposes). One of the 32 was classified as having no psychiatric disorder. This was the sister of a boy with a conduct disorder; she was admitted with her brother at the same time as the mother was herself admitted to hospital for psychiatric treatment.

The father was dead, and this plan was thought better than separating the siblings. This girl, classified as an admission for 'treatment' because her admission was part of a family treatment plan, remained well at follow-up 3 years 8 months later. Two other children, both girls who had been admitted because of neurotic school refusal, could not be traced; one of these had only been in the unit 18 days when she was discharged by her parents.

The outcome in the remaining cases is summarised in Tables 11.2, 11.3 and 11.4. Age is shown to the nearest half-year and duration of inpatient treatment to the nearest half-month. Wherever possible an interview with child and parents, or parent-substitutes, was carried out either by the author or by another member of the psychiatric staff of the clinic.* These children were assessed using a standard form devised for the purpose, together with a routine clinical assessment. In the other cases reports were obtained from professional people such as psychiatrists in local child guidance clinics, psychologists, social workers and head teachers of schools. In some cases several reports were available.

Children were rated as 'improved' only if there was clear, unequivocal evidence of substantial improvement in the signs and symptoms originally present, without the substitution of other serious symptoms. All the evidence available – the interview with the patient, parents' account, school report and any other reports – in each case was considered. If there was any suggestion of deterioration the outcome was judged to be 'worse'. Children who were marginally better or substantially the same were rated as showing 'no change'.

Most of the children had improved. This applied to 10 out of the 12 children with conduct disorders and 6 out of the 9 neurotic children. The numbers are, however, too small for any general conclusions to be drawn. It is of interest, though, that 10 of the children with conduct

* I am grateful to Dr C. Zacharias for undertaking some of this work.

Table 11.2 Charles Burns Clinic 1968 admissions – Follow-up Data

Case No., sex and age on admission	*Duration of treatment (months)*	*Length of follow-up (years–months)*	*Method of follow-up*	*Result I = improved NC = no change W = worse*	*Remarks*
CONDUCT DISORDERS					
1. M(9)	3½	4– 6	Report	I	At community school
2. M(8½)	15	2–10	Report	I	At residential special school
3. M(7)	5½	3– 8	Interview	I	In foster home
4. M(10½)	2	4– 0	Report	I	At day school for maladjusted children
5. M(10)	2½	4– 2	Interview	I	Had been at residential school for maladjusted children
6. M(5½)	3½	4– 1	Interview	NC	Recent relapse
7. M(1)	6½	3– 2	Interview	I	At residential school for maladjusted children
8. M(9½)	7½	3–11	Report	I	At residential special school
9. M(5)	2½	3– 0	Interview	I	In children's home Had been re-referred
10. F(12)	6	4– 4	Report	I	—
11. F(10½)	2½	4– 3	Interview	I	Epileptic girl, subsequent neurosurgery Now at residential special school
12. F(8)	4½	4– 2	Interview	NC	Fluctuating course Residential school for maladjusted children

Table 11.3 Charles Burns Clinic 1968 admissions – Follow-up Data

Case No., sex and age on admission	*Duration of treatment (months)*	*Length of follow-up (years–months)*	*Method of follow-up*	*Result I = improved NC = no change W = worse*	*Remarks*
NEUROTIC DISORDERS					
13. M(12)	2	3–11	Interview	I	Symptom-free
14. M(12)	8	3– 9	Interview	I	Symptom-free Had been at residential school for maladjusted children
15. M(11)	7½	3– 5	Report	W	Subsequent mental hospital and community school care
16. M(10)	3	4– 6	Interview	I	—
17. M(10)	4	3– 6	Report	W	Relapsed. Now in community school
18. F(10)	2½	3– 7	Interview	I	Very well
19. F(12)	5	3–10	Interview	I	Still lacks self-confidence
20. F(12)	6½	3– 6	Report	NC	Needed further inpatient care. Current difficulty over going to work
21. F(9½)	5	2–11	Interview	I	Symptom-free

disorders received further help, usually in a special school. Only three continued to live full-time with their natural parents, and one of these attended a day school for maladjusted children. Thus ten children were placed in a special school or home situation, and in all instances but one this was done on the recommendation of the Charles Burns Clinic staff.

Seven out of the 9 children with neurotic disorders were discharged to live at home full-time and attend an ordinary school, but two of these (cases 17 and 20) subsequently relapsed and proved to have long-standing personality problems which still persist. The other two had particularly disturbed families and were discharged to attend residen-

Table 11.4 Charles Burns Clinic 1968 admissions – Follow-up Data

Case No., sex and age on admission	*Duration of treatment (months)*	*Length of follow-up (years–months)*	*Method of follow-up*	*Result I = improved NC = no change W = worse*	*Remarks*
MIXED NEUROTIC AND CONDUCT DISORDER					
22. M(10½)	2	4– 2	Interview	I	Still receiving outpatient treatment at CBC
PSYCHOSIS					
23. M(7)	11½	2–10	Interview	I	At day special school
24. M(9½)	6½	3– 7	Report	NC	At residential special school
25. F(5)	13	3–10	Report	W	In subnormality hospital
OTHERS					
26. F(12)	2	3–10	Report	I	Anorexia nervosa – transferred to another hospital for further treatment
27. M(6)	7	3– 6	Report	I	Emotional dwarfism – subsequently taken into care
28. M(8½)	2	4– 0	Interview	I	Encopresis. Very well. Mother died during follow-up period
29. M(4½)	6	3– 8	Interview	NC	Developmental language disorder. At residential special school

tial schools for maladjusted children; one of them did very well (case 14) but one relapsed and has required further treatment (case 15).

Twenty-one out of the 29 disturbed children followed up had improved, but it is clear from the tables that most of the children had further special help. Even those in whom this is not mentioned normally had continued outpatient support. Inpatient care was thus often a passport to further help rather than a complete treatment in itself. This is probably inevitable in a short- to medium-term unit, and may well be the best way for a unit of this sort to operate. The child is given 'primary' treatment, which is often urgently needed, and when some progress has been made is passed on for further help in some other appropriate setting.

These children were probably a particularly severely disturbed group. They were the first year's admissions to a new unit, and some had been long awaiting the unit's opening. Almost all had severe disorders on admission; the school refusers had been out of school for periods of up to two years. The outcome 3–4 years later may therefore be judged fairly satisfactory.

The three children rated 'worse' include two neurotic children who at the time of follow-up had recently relapsed, and one autistic child who had been placed in a mental subnormality hospital.

The 'no change' group included two children with conduct disorders; these had both recently relapsed and were receiving further help from the clinic. One neurotic child had required further inpatient treatment in an adolescent unit and was currently having difficulty in attending her work, on account of neurotic symptoms. The other two children showing 'no change' were a boy with late onset psychosis (case 24) and one with severe receptive developmental language disorder who showed no response to treatment (case 29).

Conclusions

The outcome of the residential psychiatric treatment of children depends on a variety of factors, most of which are difficult to measure precisely. Follow-up studies, to be of value, should take into account the nature, severity and background of the presenting disorder in each case, and also the various other family, social, biological and educational factors operating during and after inpatient care.

It seems inherently implausible that a period of several months' residence in a hospital unit, especially one designed for the treatment of emotional disorders, will have *no* effect on the developing personality of a child. The task of the staff of such a unit, therefore, is to integrate appropriate experiences for the child in hospital with a wider and longer-term treatment plan. This plan will always take into account the family, as well as other social, educational and biological factors.

It is clear, from comparing inpatient facilities with prevalence rates for emotional disorders in the community, that only a tiny proportion of disturbed children are admitted for inpatient care. Those that are admitted are presumably some of the more severely disturbed and most reports suggest that a majority of them make satisfactory progress subsequently. There are indications that neurotic children do better, on the whole, than those with conduct disorders. Psychotic children, and those with evidence of severe biological disabilities, do less well.

In the final analysis the treatment of disturbed children in hospital, like the treatment of other categories of patient, is a response to human need. It may be as worthwhile to admit the incurably psychotic child to enable the family to go on holiday as it is to admit a child with a more hopeful prognosis. Yet it is almost certain that residential psychiatric treatment of children has much more to offer than relief for those who have to care for severely disturbed children.

The children admitted have usually suffered much emotional trauma and damage, and without help the future outlook for many of them is, from the evidence available, bleak. Inpatient care offers hope as well as help, and inpatient units also provide unique opportunities to observe and study disturbed children and their response to different modes of treatment.

CHAPTER TWELVE

The Future

Philip Barker

Hospital units for the inpatient treatment of children are now an established and developing part of the psychiatric services in Great Britain and other Western countries. It is possible to regret not only that they have been found necessary, but also that the need for them seems to be increasing. Yet it may be better to treat emotional disorders in childhood than to leave them until adult life, as has perhaps happened in the past. Many adults with psychiatric disorders, personality problems and records of antisocial behaviour have shown evidence of psychiatric disorder in childhood; and the follow-up study of Robins (1966) shows how grim the adult prognosis of children with conduct disorders can be.

The question is thus not so much whether psychiatric units for children will increase in number and scope, but in what way they will develop. Children's units tended at first to be modified adult psychiatric wards. Indeed, children used often to be treated with adults in the same wards. This happens much less frequently nowadays, certainly in Great Britain. And as more children's and adolescent units have opened a body of knowledge and expertise in the running of them has been acquired by their staffs. Some of this has been put on record in the present book.

The development of particular units has naturally depended upon local circumstances, including the other facilities available and, above all, the personality and interests of the staff, especially the director. The development of an adolescent unit has been described by Allchin (1969). His description has some parallels in the development of units generally. Allchin sees adolescent units as facing two of the key problems both of institutions generally and of adolescence, namely authority and communication. These matters are also very important issues in children's units. In order to have a significant and helpful effect on the developing personalities of their patients, units must come to terms with both of them. It is no exaggeration to say that most disturbed children have, as central features of their disorders, difficulties with authority figures (usually including their parents) and problems of communication.

As Allchin points out, the younger the children the less amount of democratic authority it is possible for them to have in a unit. Children's needs for dependable adults to whom to relate, and a secure background for their lives, must never be forgotten. Children generally, but disturbed children in particular, must learn to communicate their feelings, wishes and needs in a non-pathological way (rather than through their symptoms and disturbed behaviour). Whatever their age they need to take some degree of responsibility for themselves, both individually and as groups, and a psychiatric treatment unit should help them to do this. This is something which institutions, including those for mentally sick adults, have in the past often failed to do. Yet the sort of therapeutic community described by Jones (1952) for adults is not suitable for children. They cannot be expected to take responsibility for themselves as adults should. They are still at a dependent stage of development, though in any one unit there are bound to be a number of children at different stages in the process of growing up.

The future development of units for children will certainly see continuing efforts to overcome these dual problems of communication and authority. As Allchin says, there is a limit to the rate of progress possible 'within the context of the administrative setting of a national service, with its inevitable rigidities'. It is for this reason, Allchin suggests, that small, independent units, often schools, have pioneered developments in this area. But hospital units as a whole are probably moving in the direction which Allchin describes for the unit of which he is writing. This is, broadly, towards a community in which communication is as free as possible and authority is shared as appropriate among all members of the community.

Developments in Nursing

The central importance of nurses in children's psychiatric units has been repeatedly stressed in this book. The development of training schemes for nurses, discussed in Chapter 10, is therefore a major advance. Moreover, the syllabus for the post-registration training of nurses in this field, recently published by the Joint Board of Clinical Nursing Studies (1973) is both comprehensive and forward-looking. Once courses based on this syllabus get under way it should be possible to build up a body of highly expert nurses to work in this very special field.

When special training for registered nurses is established it will be necessary to devise schemes for the training of other nurses. The post-registration courses should provide highly expert senior staff, but it is unrealistic to expect all the nurses to have this training. Yet all staff should be adequately trained, and there will be a need for nurses trained in the practical, day-to-day care and treatment of the children to work under the supervision and guidance of the senior staff. This is the most logical step and it is already under discussion among those concerned with the problem.

Administrative Changes

The changes currently taking place in the structure of the National Health Service are bound to affect children's psychiatric units in Great Britain. It is too early to say precisely how units will be affected, but the unification into one organisation of the hospital, general practitioner and public health services offers great possibilities. While it has always been possible to establish links, and to work with other agencies and services whatever the administrative set-up, the new arrangements should facilitate closer collaboration between hospital units and other community facilities. The limitations of admitting a disturbed child to hospital, if work is not done in the community to prepare for his return, are obvious.

It may be that the years ahead will see hospital psychiatric units for children and adolescents developing as an integral part of the community's psychiatric services. This would be a logical step and might lead to earlier intervention and the treatment of families before individual children in them had got as disturbed as they often are when referred nowadays.

More Emphasis on Day Care

This book has not looked closely at daypatient treatment, but day care is likely to be a developing feature of child psychiatric services. More than a decade ago Connell (1961) pointed out some of the advantages of daypatient treatment, and nowadays many inpatient units take also some daypatients. This is certainly the trend at the Charles Burns Clinic, where there are nowadays usually more daypatients than the ten for which we nominally have places, this being compensated for by a smaller number of inpatients. When the second three years' admissions are reviewed the proportion of daypatients will certainly be much higher than it was in the first three years.

The literature on day treatment is limited, but Chazin (1969) has pointed out that in many cases continued daily contact with the home and family has advantages. Chazin describes a type of day treatment milieu similar to that found in many residential units. Marshall and Stewart (1969) also provide an interesting discussion of the merits of daypatient treatment, which can be carried out in association with an inpatient service. It is not, however, clear whether day treatment units should ideally be separate from inpatient units; at present very few are.

Involvement of Families

From the start, children's units have involved their patients' families in treatment more than is usual in adult psychiatric hospitals. Close involvement of families, or at least mothers, has always been a characteristic of the child-guidance movement, and this tradition has tended to be carried on by inpatient units. It often consists, however, of no more than the traditional 'casework interviews' of child-guidance clinics, though sometimes group therapy is also offered to parents. Yet the inpatient or daypatient treatment setting offers much greater scope for the involvement of parents in therapy. Bruggan (1971) has described their involvement in the admission process, in the assessment of progress and in discharge, and this is surely an advance on the situation in which the hospital staff decide when the child is ready for discharge (or admission) and inform the parents. The process could perhaps be carried even further and the parents, with the child patient, be closely involved in much other decision-taking involving their child in the unit.

Such greater participation by families in the inpatient treatment process would present difficulties, but would also be helped by the closer links with community agencies which the new administrative arrangements will make possible. Inpatient, or daypatient, care might thus become a means whereby the care and treatment of a child are taken over from the family only to the minimum extent necessary. At present we tend either to leave the child at home or to take over his care completely by admitting him, with all the implications of failure which this may have for the parents. The radical alterations in family dynamics which admission can cause have been discussed recently by Copus and Walker (1972), who recommend a flexible use of inpatient, daypatient and outpatient treatment.

Sometimes participation by the family in treatment might extend to their entry into hospital with the child. This, however, would often involve providing special accommodation, as well as, in many cases, a rather drastic review of the treatment arrangements. It is an area in which experiment is probably due, however.

Treatment Methods

There will be a continuing need to review and develop treatment methods. This book has looked at methods currently in use, and these will no doubt be modified in the light of experience and new theoretical knowledge. The psychotic child provides a continuing challenge, and at present the results of the treatment of children with psychotic disorders are on the whole disappointing. The hyperaggressive, acting-out child is also one who normally taxes the resources of an inpatient unit to the full, though the importance of providing effective treatment has been well brought out in Chapter 3.

Behaviour therapy techniques promise to be of real value as part of the treatment programme. Their use has been referred to elsewhere in the book, and Lehrer *et al.* (1972) have provided a useful account of how operant techniques can be used in a hospital unit for adolescents. This paper well shows how operant techniques and more traditional methods can be integrated in a consistent treatment plan. These techniques can also be used by, and with, families and may be very suitable for use as part of a programme involving the whole family and the home setting as well as the hospital.

Conclusions

Residential psychiatric treatment for children now has an established place in the hospital service. The various contributions to this book illustrate its present scope and some of the ways in which units run. Now that the usefulness of these units is generally accepted, the way is open for their further development. There is a need for the evaluation of treatment methods at present used in inpatients' units and for the development of new ones. The general paucity of academic posts and units has affected this aspect of child psychiatry as it has all others. Staff training is another important area for future development.

The place of inpatient care in the community's mental health services generally will also change; it is to be hoped that inpatient, day-patient, outpatient and whole-family treatment will become integral parts of the mental health services in each district of the reorganised National Health Service.

Appendix A Admission Procedure at Charles Burns Clinic

1. Admissions of children to the clinical groups to be kept under review by a panel consisting of the nursing officer (or deputy), one of the senior registrars (in his absence, the other senior registrar), one of the clinical psychologists and a member of the teaching staff. This panel should meet at least once weekly and review patients on the waiting list with a view to allocating a time for their admission. Its members should maintain contact with the language unit staff so as to be informed of the number of inpatient places needed by this group. The panel will take into account the length of time a child has been on the waiting list, the nature of the child's disorder and its urgency and the balance of the different groups, and of the children in the clinic as a whole.
2. As soon as possible after a child is placed on the waiting list the admission panel will decide the group into which the child will ultimately be admitted. This will enable the social-worker concerned with the group to make preliminary contact with the family while the child is awaiting a place.
3. The charge nurse or deputy of each clinical group will inform the admission panel as soon as the probable date for any discharge is known, using the relevant form. If possible, discharges will normally be planned two to three weeks ahead, so that the presence of places to admit children into can be anticipated by the admission panel.
4. Once the approximate admission date is known a nurse-therapist

will be allocated, probably at the next meeting of the group. At this time arrangements will usually be made for the social worker and nurse-therapist to visit the family at home as a preliminary to admission.

5. Once a firm admission date has been agreed by the group (the admission panel only giving a date from which a place will be available) a letter confirming the arrangements should be sent to the parents by the doctor concerned with the case, outlining the proposed arrangements for a preliminary visit and for admission. The nurse-therapist will then fill in seven copies of the admission slip – for school, OT, nursing office, staff-room, receptionist (two copies) and sister's office. Admission should be arranged for a time when the nurse-therapist will be on duty; it should also be convenient to the social worker and doctor concerned. Once a firm date has been agreed the doctor should write to the GP informing him of it, and should also make out a case summary (on the form provided): there should be a copy each for OT, school and nursing group.
6. On arrival the child should be met by his nurse-therapist and the parents by the charge nurse (or deputy) concerned. The nurse-therapist will normally show the child his room and bed, and introduce him to other staff and children. The charge nurse will be available to answer parents' queries about visiting, pocket-money, telephone calls, clothes, etc.
7. If either the social worker or doctor wishes to see the parents (for example to obtain additional history), he should do so *after* the charge nurse has finished seeing them. Similarly, if the receptionist requires to obtain additional information for the front sheet (which, however, will normally have been filled in previously), she should do so after they have seen the social worker or doctor, by mutual arrangement.
8. The child should be seen by his doctor on the day of admission and a physical examination should normally be done that day. If necessary it can be supplemented later.
9. Emergency admissions should, if at all possible, be handled by the admission panel, or those members of it who are available. If necessary they should consult with the consultant staff should difficulties arise.

The admission procedure may need to be modified in the case of emergencies.

Appendix B Residential Psychiatric Units in the United Kingdom

The information given here was obtained by circulating all known children's and adolescent units in the UK during the summer of 1972. The information was checked and brought up to date, as far as possible, in September 1973. Only units taking patients below the age of 15 are included.

England and Wales

BECKENHAM, KENT
Adolescent Unit, The Bethlem Royal Hospital, Monks Orchard Road, Beckenham, Kent

Consultant psychiatrists	Dr W. Warren, Dr P. H. Connell
Number of beds	17 male, 16 female (33 total)
Daypatient places	nil
Age-range	12–16½ approx.
Other information	Length of stay not usually more than one year

BEVERLEY, YORKSHIRE
Adolescent Unit (West End) Broadgate Hospital, Waltington, Beverley, Yorkshire, HU17 8RN

Consultant psychiatrist	Dr V. L. Doughty
Number of beds	12
Daypatient places	Up to 5
Age-range	12–16 years

BIRMINGHAM

Psychiatric Unit, Children's Hospital, Birmingham, B17 8SD

Consultant psychiatrist	Dr J. E. Varley
Number of beds	10
Daypatient places	5
Age-range	0–15 years

Adolescent Unit, Hollymoor Hospital, Northfield, Birmingham, B31 5EX

Consultant psychiatrist	Dr E. M. Irwin
Number of beds	10 male, 10 female (20 total)
Daypatient places	5
Age-range	12–16 years
Other information	Median length of stay 100 days

Charles Burns Clinic, Queensbridge Road, Moseley, Birmingham, B13 8QD

Consultant psychiatrists	Dr P. Barker, Dr G. K. R. Jamieson, Dr E. M. D. O'Brien, Dr H. M. N. Rees
Number of beds	29
Daypatient places	10 (sometimes increased at the expense of inpatient numbers)
Age-range	Up to 12 years

BRISTOL

Psychiatric Unit, Ward 8, Royal Hospital for Sick Children, St Michael's Hill, Bristol

Consultant psychiatrists	Professor D. Russel-Davis, Dr Lumsden Walker, Dr Martin Gay, Dr Hugh Coulstine
Number of beds	6
Daypatient places	6
Age-range	2–14 years
Other information	Primarily short-term and diagnostic (up to three months)

BROADSTAIRS, KENT

Lanthorne Hospital, Lanthorne Road, Broadstairs, Kent

Consultant psychiatrist	Dr K. M. Fraser
Number of beds	25
Daypatient places	Up to 5
Age-range	4–15 years
Other information	Specialises in psychosomatic disorders. Maximum stay one year. Usual length approx. two school terms

CAERLEON, MONMOUTHSHIRE

Polland's Well Children's Unit, St Cadoc's Hospital, Caerleon

Consultant psychiatrist	Dr V. A. Wills
Number of beds	6 male, 6 female (12 total)
Daypatient places	6
Age-range	Up to 12–13 years

CANTERBURY, KENT

Beech House, St Augustine's Hospital, Chartham, Canterbury, Kent

Consultant psychiatrist	Dr G. C. Turle
Number of beds	23 male
Daypatient places	nil
Age-range	12–16 years

CARDIFF, S. WALES

Young People's Unit, Vehindre Road, Whitchurch, Cardiff, CF4 7JG

Consultant psychiatrist	Dr H. V. R. Jones
Number of beds	8 male, 8 female (16 total)
Daypatient places	nil
Age-range	13–17 years

CARMARTHEN, S.W. WALES

Adolescent Unit, St David's Hospital, Carmarthen, S.W. Wales

Consultant psychiatrist	Dr Evan Davies
Number of beds	6 male, 9 female (15 total)
Daypatient places	nil
Age-range	12–18 years
Other information	Psychotic adolescents not admitted. Optimum length of stay 3–4 months

CARSHALTON, SURREY

Ward C8, Queen Mary's Hospital, Carshalton, Surrey

Consultant psychiatrist	Dr G. Crosse
Number of beds	16
Daypatient places	8
Age-range	2–15 approx.
Other information	Unit attached to Queen Mary's Hospital Day School

CHANDLERS FORD, HANTS

Leigh House, Adolescent Psychiatric Unit, Hursley Road, Chandlers Ford, Hants

Consultant psychiatrists	Dr W. H. Allchin, Dr L. Rosenberg
Number of beds	15 male, 15 female (30 total)
Daypatient places	nil
Age-range	12–18+
Other information	Specialises in long-term analytical psychotherapy where indicated – serious neurotic disorders or borderline psychosis. Average stay one year. Admission for up to 2–3 years acceptable

CHESTER

The Adolescent Unit, Maple Ward, Moston Hospital, Liverpool Road, Chester

Consultant psychiatrist	Dr J. D. Richardson
Number of beds	8 male (or 10), 10 female (or 8) (18 total)
Daypatient places	7
Age-range	12–16+

COLCHESTER, ESSEX
Children's Unit, Royal Eastern Counties Hospital, Turner Road, Colchester, Essex

Consultant psychiatrist	Dr B. M. Crocket
Number of beds	12
Daypatient places	Up to 6
Age-range	Normally up to 13 years, sometimes up to 15
Other information	Length of stay up to one year. Average four months

DERBY
The Grange, Etwall Road, Mickleover, Derby

Consultant psychiatrist	Dr D. J. Salfield
Number of beds	10
Daypatient places	4
Age-range	Up to puberty

DENBIGHSHIRE
Gwynfa Residential Clinic, Old Colwyn, Denbighshire

Consultant psychiatrists	Dr E. Simmons, Dr G. M. Nicholl, Dr J. Pryce
Number of beds	25
Daypatient places	On demand
Age-range	4–16 years

EPSOM, SURREY
Adolescent Unit, Long Grove Hospital, Epsom, Surrey

Consultant psychiatrists	Dr P. Johnson, Dr A. B. Monro
Number of beds	18 male, 18 female (36 total)
Daypatient places	nil
Age-range	11–17 years
Other information	Length of stay approx. 8–10 months. No drug addicts or mentally subnormal patients

EXETER
Dryden Clinic, Dryden Road, Exeter

Consultant psychiatrists	Dr C. J. Wardle, Dr P. M. Jackson
Number of beds	18 children, 12 adolescents
Daypatient places	10
Age-range	Children 6–14; Adolescents 14–17
Other information	Unit specialises in emotional problems of older children and adolescents who have conduct disorders

FAREHAM, HANTS
Meon House Young People's Unit, Knowle Hospital, Fareham, Hants

Consultant psychiatrist	Dr A. Harbott
Number of beds	10 male, 10 female (20 total)
Daypatient places	nil
Age-range	12–18 years
Other information	Organised as intensive therapeutic community. Length of stay about six months

HAYWARDS HEATH, SUSSEX

Colwood Hospital, Hurstwood Lane, Haywards Heath, Sussex

Consultant psychiatrists	Dr M. D. A. Heller, Dr M. G. E. Morgan
Number of beds	15 male, 15 female (30 total)
Daypatient places	nil
Age-range	12–16/17 years
Other information	Known serious drug-takers, very dull children and severely aggressive acting-out children not admitted

HENLEY-ON-THAMES, OXFORDSHIRE

Smith Hospital, Henley-on-Thames, Oxfordshire

Consultant psychiatrists	Dr G. O'Gorman, Dr J. Aitken
Number of beds	About 28
Daypatient places	About 22 (total 50)
Age-range	0–12 years
Other information	Severely disturbed and autistic children. Length of stay up to twelve years

HOVE, SUSSEX

Children's Unit, Lady Chichester Hospital, Hove, Sussex, BN3 4A6

Consultant psychiatrist	Dr J. Ross
Number of beds	10
Daypatient places	nil
Age-range	0–12 years
Other information	Average length of stay five months

HULL

The Child Psychiatric Unit, Baynard House, De la Pole Hospital, Willerby, Hull, Yorkshire, HV10 6ED

Consultant psychiatrist	Dr P. J. Beynon
Number of beds	15
Daypatient places	6
Age-range	4–14 years (mainly 5–13)

ILFORD, ESSEX

Adolescent Unit, Brookside School, Goodmayes Hospital, Goodmayes, Ilford, Essex

Consultant psychiatrist	Not yet appointed
Number of beds	20 total
Daypatient places	15
Age-range	12–18 years
Other information	Unit not fully operational when list went to press

ILKLEY, YORKSHIRE

Kanner Children's Unit, High Royds, Menston, Ilkley, Yorkshire

Consultant psychiatrist	Dr Ian Berg
Number of beds	12
Daypatient places	Occasional daypatients only
Age-range	0–11 years
Other information	Admits especially childhood psychosis, brain damage, very severe personality disorders, wetting, soiling. Typical length of stay approx. five months

High Lands Adolescent Unit, Scalebor Park Hospital, Burley-in-Wharfedale, Ilkley, Yorkshire, LS29 7AJ

Consultant psychiatrist	Dr I. Berg
Number of beds	10 male, 10 female (20 total)
Daypatient places	6
Age-range	11–16 inclusive

IPSWICH

'Hightrees' Adolescent Unit, The Ipswich Hospital, Foxhall Wing, Ipswich

Consultant psychiatrist	Dr J. G. Howells
Number of beds	6 male, 4 female (10 total)
Daypatient places	nil
Age-range	14½–19 years

LANCASTER

Children's Unit, Lancaster Moor Hospital, Lancaster

Consultant psychiatrists	Dr T. W. Rogers, Dr D. Ross
Number of beds	14, mainly boys
Daypatient places	Average 4
Age-range	5–12+
Other information	Length of stay usually 6–20 weeks

LEICESTER

Oakham House, 493 Gipsy Lane, Leicester, LE5 OTD

Consultant psychiatrists	Dr K. D. Hopkirk, Dr S. M. W. Pittock
Number of beds	15 female
Daypatient places	9
Age-range	11+–16+
Other information	Medium term stay 3–5 months.

LINCOLN

Lawn Hospital Inpatient Psychiatry Unit for Children, Union Board, Lincoln

Consultant psychiatrists	Dr J. S. Edmondson, Dr P. I. G. Wateling
Number of beds	12
Daypatient places	2
Age-range	0–12

LIVERPOOL

Department of Psychological Medicine, W Ward, Alder Hey Children's Hospital, West Derby, Liverpool, 12

Consultant psychiatrists	Dr J. G. Neville, Dr Dewi Jones
Number of beds	12
Daypatient places	Up to 4 nominal
Age-range	0–15 years

Royal Liverpool Children's Hospital, Heswall, Cheshire

Consultant psychiatrist	Dr P. Pinkerton
Number of beds	25 male, 25 female (50 total)
Daypatient places	10
Age-range	2–15 years
Other information	Unit deals with psychosomatic disorders. Gross behaviour disturbances not admitted. Length of stay three months–several years. Small children admitted with mothers

LONDON

Children's Department, The Maudsley Hospital, Denmark Hill, London, SE5

Consultant psychiatrists	Dr W. Warren, Dr L. A. Hersov
Number of beds	25
Daypatient places	6
Age-range	Children 1–12 years
Other information	Length of stay: few 1–2 months, majority 3–15 months, few 8 months–2 years. Average 6 months

Department of Child and Adolescent Psychiatry, Guy's Hospital, London, SE1 (Hector Cameron Ward)

Consultant psychiatrist	Dr G. F. Vaughan
Number of beds	7
Daypatient places	4
Age-range	Up to 15 years

Psychiatric Part of Children's Unit, Whipps Cross Hospital, Whipps Cross Road, Leytonstone, London, E11

Consultant psychiatrist	Dr W. R. Little
Number of beds	8 male, 4 female (total 12 + 1 for toddler and mother)
Daypatient places	6
Age-range	5–12 (5–13 for school refusers)

MACCLESFIELD

The Young People's Unit, Victoria Road, Macclesfield, Cheshire

Consultant psychiatrist	Dr P. G. Wells
Number of beds	10 male, 10 female (20 total)
Daypatient places	Variable
Age-range	12–17 years
Other information	Admission based on therapeutic agreement preferably with whole family

MANCHESTER

Child Psychiatric Unit, Booth Hall Hospital, Charlestown Road, Blackley, Manchester, M9 2AA

Consultant psychiatrists	Dr T. R. Malloy, Dr S. A. Leslie, Dr J. Erulkar
Number of beds	22
Daypatient places	As required, usually 3–6
Age-range	0–12 years
Other information	Regarded as short stay by Regional Board; long stay determined by needs of case

MIDDLESBROUGH

Department of Child and Family Psychiatry, 'Brynteg', 26a Belle Vue Grove, Middlesbrough, Teesside (St Luke's Hospital)

Consultant psychiatrists	Dr G. L. Davies, Dr A. G. Chisholm
Number of beds	8 male, 4 female (total 12 + 1 mother)
Daypatient places	8
Age-range	Inpatients – up to 11, day patients – up to 15

MORPETH

Stannington Children's Hospital, Stannington, Morpeth, Northumberland

Consultant psychiatrist	Dr S. T. Morton
Number of beds	10 male, 10 female (20 total)
Daypatient places	nil
Age-range	5–15 years
Other information	Usual length of stay 8–11 months. Specialises in adolescent development disorders, psychosomatic disorders and psychiatric problems in long-stay paediatric disorders.

NEWCASTLE-ON-TYNE

Nuffield Child Psychiatry Unit, Hospital for Sick Children, Great North Road, Newcastle-on-Tyne, NE2 3AX

Consultant psychiatrists	Dr I. Kolvin, Dr S. T. Morton, Dr M. D. Rowbotham
Number of beds	20 ($\frac{2}{3}$ male, $\frac{1}{3}$ female)
Daypatient places	22
Age-range	0–12/13 years

NOTTINGHAM

Children's Unit, St Ann's Hospital, Porchester Road, Nottingham

Consultant psychiatrist	Dr E. Arkle
Number of beds	20
Daypatient places	10
Age-range	3–11 years
Other information	Special interest in children under 5 and epileptic children with conduct disorders or hyperkinetic disorders

Adolescent Unit, St Ann's Hospital, Porchester Road, Nottingham

Consultant psychiatrist	Dr E. Arkle
Number of beds	10 male, 6 female (16 total)
Daypatient places	10
Age-range	11–school-leaving age

NUNEATON

Bramcote Hospital, near Nuneaton, Warwickshire

Consultant psychiatrist	Dr J. Warner
Number of beds	6
Daypatient places	nil
Age-range	0–15 years
Other information	Six beds in a medium-stay paediatric unit chiefly for cases of school refusal, encopresis, severe enuresis, mild behaviour problems

OXFORD

Highfield Adolescent Unit, Warneford Hospital, Headington, Oxford

Consultant psychiatrists	Dr W. L. Parry-Jones, Dr J. B. McWhinnie
Number of beds	8 male, 8 female (16 total)
Daypatient places	Occasional daypatients only
Age-range	14–18 years
Other information	Short to medium-stay with emphasis on family therapy

The Park Hospital for Children, Old Road, Headington, Oxford

Consultant psychiatrists	Dr D. C. Taylor, Dr J. Lindsay, Dr C. Ounsted
Number of beds	33 + 3 mothers
Daypatient places	Variable
Age-range	7 weeks–15+ years

PORTSMOUTH

Wessex Unit for Children and Parents, Milton Ford, Locksway Road, Portsmouth, PO4 8LD

Consultant psychiatrists	Dr C. Haffner, Dr D. Thornber
Number of beds	42
Daypatient places	30 (full time equivalent)
Age-range	0–school-leaving age
Other information	Facilities for admitting parents, mainly mothers

RICHMOND, SURREY

Families Unit, The Cassel Hospital for Functional Nervous Disorders, Ham Common, Richmond, Surrey

Consultant psychiatrist	Dr A. R. Wilson
Number of beds	30
Daypatient places	nil
Age-range	0–15 years
Other information	For the psychotherapy of neurosis occurring in family settings. Children are admitted usually with one or more parents for whom treatment is also available

ST ALBANS, HERTS

Adolescent Unit, Hill End Hospital, St Albans, Herts

Consultant psychiatrist	Dr P. Bruggen
Number of beds	11 (half male, half female)
Daypatient places	Indefinite
Age-range	Up to 16 years

High Wick Hospital, Highfield Lane, St Albans, Herts

Consultant psychiatrists	Dr G. Stroh, Dr S. Tischler
Number of beds	18
Daypatient places	nil
Age-range	3–13 years
Other information	Treats autistic and other psychotic children and children with severe behaviour disorders

SHEFFIELD
Child Psychiatry Annexe (Shirle Hill), Nether Edge Hospital, Sheffield, S11 9EL

Consultant psychiatrists	Dr F. G. Thorpe, Dr K. Dawson-Butterworth
Number of beds	16
Daypatient places	4
Age-range	3–14 (pre-adolescent children)

SLEAFORD, LINCOLNSHIRE
The Adolescent Unit, Rauceby Hospital, Sleaford, Lincolnshire

Consultant psychiatrists	Dr A. H. Lorimer, Dr A. N. Varma
Number of beds	15 male
Daypatient places	5
Age-range	12–16 years
Other information	Duration of stay three months to one year. Average 4½ months

SOUTHPORT, LANCS
Child Psychiatric Unit, Hawkeshead Hospital, Southport, Lancs

Consultant psychiatrist	Dr J. M. Naylor
Number of beds	12 male, 6 female (18 total)
Daypatient places	Variable, total number of patients rarely exceeds 18
Age-range	0–12+ boys, 0–14+ girls
Other information	Usual length of stay three months. Day patients longer

STOCKTON-ON-TEES, TEESSIDE
Forensic Psychiatry Centre, Winterton Hospital, Sedgefield, Stockton-on-Tees, Teesside, TS21 3EJ

Consultant psychiatrist	Dr D. G. A. Westbury
Number of beds	18 male
Daypatient places	Variable
Age-range	13–17 years
Other information	Only for current offenders

STRATFORD-ON-AVON
Children's Recovery Hospital, Stratford-on-Avon, Warwicks

Consultant psychiatrists	Dr P. J. Crowley, Dr P. H. Wotton-McTurk
Number of beds	16
Daypatient places	10
Age-range	3–11 years
Other information	Usual length of stay about three months

SUTTON, SURREY
Children's Unit, Belmont Hospital, Brighton Road, Sutton, Surrey

Consultant psychiatrist	Dr M. J. Shepperd (locum)
Number of beds	12
Daypatient places	Occasionally 1 or 2
Age-range	3–7 years
Other information	Non-communicating children. Period of treatment six months–one year

TAUNTON

Merrifield Children's Unit, Norton Fitzwarren, Taunton, Somerset

Consultant psychiatrists	Dr A. H. Bakker, Dr M. F. Bethell
Number of beds	24 male, 12 female (36 total)
Daypatient places	Up to 4
Age-range	4½–13 with some up to 15
Other information	High percentage of non-communicating children

WARWICK

Adolescent Unit (Agnes Jones Ward), Central Hospital, Warwick

Consultant psychiatrist	Dr P. J. Crowley
Number of beds	17 female
Daypatient places	Variable
Age-range	13–19 years

WIRRAL, CHESHIRE

Pensby Children's Wing, Irby Road, Heswell, Wirral, Cheshire

Consultant psychiatrists	Dr D. M. Zausmer, Dr M. Rogers, Dr J. L. Lanceley
Number of beds	16
Daypatient places	4
Age-range	4–12 years
Other information	Unit specialises in treatment of psychosomatic disorders. Usual length of stay about six months. Unit houses an active pre-school playgroup

WROUGHTON, SWINDON

West Stowell Clinic, Burderop Hospital, Wroughton, near Swindon, Wilts

Consultant psychiatrist	Dr Male
Number of beds	20
Daypatient places	Up to 4–5
Age-range	3–11 years
Other information	Chiefly psychotic children. Relatively long-stay in conditions simulating intensive child care. Average stay 2–3 years

YORK

Children's Unit, Fairfield Hospital, Skelton Road, York

Consultant psychiatrist	Dr C. H. Neville-Smith
Number of beds	12
Daypatient places	Up to 4
Age-range	5 to puberty (roughly 12½)
Other information	Average length of stay three months

Southfield Adolescent Unit, 31 Shipton Road, York, YO3 6RE

Consultant psychiatrist	Dr D. J. Galbraith
Number of beds	6 male, 8 female + 1 either sex (15 total)
Daypatient places	2–3 maximum
Age-range	12–18 years
Other information	Usual stay up to 4–8 months

Mental subnormality hospitals with special units for emotionally disturbed children

Cranage Hall Hospital, Cranage, Crewe, Cheshire, CW4 8EG

Consultant psychiatrists	Dr G. C. Kanjilal, Dr P. N. Sarkar
Number of beds	70 male, 60 female (130 total)
Daypatient places	2
Age-range	3–15 years

Harperbury Hospital, Harper Lane, Shenley, Radlett, Herts, WD7 9HQ

Consultant psychiatrist	Dr D. M. Ricks
Number of beds	100
Daypatient places	nil
Age-range	Up to 16 years

Bryn-Y-Neuadd Hospital, Llanfairfechan, Caernarvonshire

Consultant psychiatrists	Dr G. M. Nicholl, Dr J. Price
Number of beds	50
Daypatient places	On demand
Age-range	0–16 years

Scotland

ABERDEEN

Ward 7, Royal Aberdeen Hospital for Sick Children, Cornhill Road, Aberdeen

Consultant psychiatrists	Dr I. M. Lowit, Dr J. Taunch
Number of beds	10
Daypatient places	6
Age-range	3–14+
Other information	Five-day ward. Average stay five months

BROXBURN, WEST LOTHIAN

Adolescent Unit, Bangour Village Hospital, Broxburn, West Lothian

Consultant psychiatrist	Dr B. E. A. Magill
Number of beds	8 male, 8 female (16 total)
Daypatient places	No definite number
Age-range	12–15 years
Other information	Length of stay averages 6–8 months

CUPAR, FIFE

Department of Child and Family Psychiatry, Playfield House, Stratheden Hospital, Cupar, Fife

Consultant psychiatrists	Dr J. D. Haldane, Dr S. F. Lindsay
Number of beds	30
Daypatient places	Variable
Age-range	Pre-school–18 years

DUMFRIES

Department of Child Psychiatry, Ladyfield, Glencaple Road, Dumfries, DG1 4TE

Consultant psychiatrists	Dr J. Currah, Dr J. C. Powell
Number of beds	55
Daypatient places	Up to 10
Age-range	Up to 12
Other information	Department comprises three separate units, each catering for particular types of child

DUNDEE

Liff House Children's Unit, Royal Dundee Liff Hospital, Dundee

Consultant psychiatrists	Dr I. C. Menzies, Dr H. S. Mathewson
Number of beds	16
Daypatient places	4
Age-range	Up to 12

EDINBURGH

Forteviot House, Royal Hospital for Sick Children, 14/16 Hope Terrace, Edinburgh, EH9 2AR

Consultant psychiatrists	Dr S. Wolff, Dr J. Blachford Rogers
Number of beds	24
Daypatient places	Usually about 3, inpatient numbers being reduced by the numbers of day patients attending
Age-range	Up to school-leaving age
Other information	Usual length of stay three months

GLASGOW

Department of Child and Family Psychiatry, Royal Hospital for Sick Children, Yorkhill, Glasgow, G3 8SJ

Consultant psychiatrists	Dr F. H. Stone, Dr I. F. Sutherland, Dr D. S. James
Number of beds	16 plus 4 parent-and-child rooms
Daypatient places	16
Age-range	0–12 years

Woodcroft House, Woodilee Hospital, Lenzie, Glasgow

Consultant psychiatrists	Dr G. E. Swinney, Dr T. S. Bedi
Number of beds	20 male
Daypatient places	nil
Age-range	12–15 years

Northern Ireland

BELFAST

Child Psychiatry Unit, Lissue Hospital, Ballinderry Road, Lisburn, near Belfast

Consultant psychiatrist	Dr W. M. Nelson
Number of beds	20
Daypatient places	5
Age-range	0–13 years
Other information	Medium-stay diagnostic and treatment unit

References

ABERCROMBIE, M. L. J. (1972) 'Parent–staff communications in a children's unit.' *Proceedings of the Royal Society of Medicine*, **65**, 335–338.

ACHENBACH, T. M. (1966) 'The classification of children's psychiatric symptoms: a factor analytic study.' *Psychological Monographs*, **80**, 1–37.

ACKERSON, L. (1931) *Children's Behaviour Problems*. Chicago: University of Chicago Press.

ACKRAL, N., KOLVIN, I. and SCOTT, D. MCI. (1968) 'A post-registration course in child psychiatry for nurses.' *Nursing Times*, Occasional Paper, 5 April 1968.

AHNSJO, S. (1969) 'Residential care of children.' In *Modern Perspectives in International Child Psychiatry*. Edited by Howells, J. G. Edinburgh: Oliver and Boyd.

AICHORN, A. (1935) *Wayward Youth*. New York: Viking Press.

ALLCHIN, W. H. (1969) 'A living myth: the problem of communication within a community.' In *Adolescence: Psychological Perspectives*. New York: Basic Books.

ALT, H. (1960) *Residential Treatment for the Disturbed Child*. New York: International Universities Press.

AMERICAN NURSES ASSOCIATION (1967) Division of psychiatric nursing practice: statement of psychiatric nursing practice.

AMERICAN PSYCHIATRIC ASSOCIATION (1957) *Psychiatric Inpatient Treatment of Children*. (Principal Editor, J. Franklin Robinson). Washington.

ANTHONY, E. J. (1957) 'An experimental approach to the psychopathology of childhood: encopresis.' *British Journal of Medical Psychology*, **30**, 146–175.

ANTHONY, E. J. (1958) 'An experimental approach to the psychopathology of childhood: autism.' *British Journal of Medical Psychology*, **31**, 211–225.

ANTHONY, E. J. (1967) 'Psychoneurotic disorders of childhood.' In *Comprehensive Textbook of Psychiatry*. Edited by Freeman, A. M. and Kaplan, H. Baltimore: Williams Wilkins.

ASSOCIATION FOR THE PSYCHIATRIC STUDY OF ADOLESCENTS (1972) Memorandum on Nurse Training.

BAGLEY, C. (1971) *The Social Psychology of the Child with Epilepsy*. London: Routledge and Kegan Paul.

BARKER, E. G. W. and MILLIGAN, W. L. (1947) 'Inpatient treatment of the maladjusted child.' *British Medical Journal*, **1**, 805–807.

BARKER, P. (1968) 'The inpatient treatment of school refusal.' *British Journal of Medical Psychology*, **41**, 381–387.

BARKER, P. (1971a) *Basic Child Psychiatry*. London: Crosby Lockwood Staples.

BARKER, P. (1971b) 'Occupational therapy in a child psychiatry unit.' In *Occupational Therapy: Today–Tomorrow*. (Proceedings of the Fifth International Congress of the World Federation of Occupational Therapists). Edited by Binswanger, R. and Spindle, I. D. Basle: S. Karger.

BARKER, P. (1973) *Care Can Prevent: Child Care or Child Psychiatry*. London: National Children's Home.

BARKER, P. and JAMIESON, R. (1967) 'Two years' admissions to a regional child psychiatry unit.' *British Medical Journal*, **2**, 103–106.

BARKER, P. and MUIR, A. (1969) 'The role of occupational therapy in children's inpatient psychiatric units.' *American Journal of Occupational Therapy*, **23**, 431–436.

BARKER, P. and WARD, P. A. (1972) 'Milieu therapy in a child psychiatry unit: the effects of a change in mealtime arrangements.' *Nursing Times*, **68**, 1579–1581.

BARNES, E. (Editor) (1968) *Psychosocial Nursing*. London: Tavistock.

BARTAK, L. and RUTTER, M. (1971) In *Infantile Autism, Concepts, Characteristics and Treatment*. Edited by Rutter, M. Edinburgh and London: Churchill, Livingstone.

BENDER, L. (1937) 'Group activities on a children's ward as methods of psychotherapy.' *American Journal of Orthopsychiatry*, **7**, 1151–1173.

BENDER, L. (1947) 'Childhood schizophrenia: clinical study of 100 schizophrenic children.' *American Journal of Orthopsychiatry*, **17**, 40–57.

BENDER, L. (1961) 'Clinical research from inpatient services for children.' *Psychiatric Quarterly*, **35**, 88–120.

BENJAMIN, A. and WEATHERLY, H. E. (1947) 'Hospital ward treatment of emotionally disturbed children.' *American Journal of Orthopsychiatry*, **17**, 665–674.

BERES, D. (1956) 'Ego deviation and the concept of schizophrenia.' *Psychoanalytic Study of the Child*, **11**, 164–235.

BERG, I. (1970) 'Correspondence.' *British Journal of Psychiatry*, **116**, 239–240.

BERG, I. and GRIFFITHS, B. (1970) 'Two years' admissions to a regional adolescent psychiatry unit.' *Medical Officer*, **73**, 5–7.

BERRY, M. F. (1969) *Language Disorders of Children*. New York: Appleton-Century-Crofts.

BESKIND, H. (1962) 'Psychiatric inpatient treatment of adolescents: a review of clinical experience.' *Comprehensive Psychiatry*, **3**, 354–369.

BETHELL, M. F. (1968) 'Caring for children: developing a psychiatric unit for special groups.' *Nursing Times*, **64**, 457–459.

BETTELHEIM, B. (1950) *Love Is Not Enough*. Illinois: Free Press of Glencoe.

BETTELHEIM, B. (1966) 'Training the child care worker in a residential centre.' *American Journal of Orthopsychiatry*, **36**, 694–705.

BETTELHEIM, B. and SYLVESTER, E. (1952) 'A therapeutic milieu.' *American Journal of Orthopsychiatry*, **22**, 314–334.

BETZ, B. J. (1945) 'A children's psychiatric service.' *American Journal of Nursing*, **45**, 817–820.

BEUHLER, R. E., PATTERSON, G. R. and FURNESS, J. M. (1966) 'The reinforcement of behaviour in institutional settings.' *Behaviour Research and Therapy*, 157–167.

BIRCH, H. G. (1964) *Brain Damage in Children*. London: Bailliere, Tindall and Cox.

BOOKBINDER, L. J. (1962) 'Simple conditioning *v*. the dynamic approach to symptoms and symptom substitution: a reply to Yates.' *Psychological Reports*, **10**, 71–77.

BORGAONKAR, D. S., UNGER, W. M., MOORE, S. M. and CROFTON, T. A. 'XYY Syndrome, height and institutionalisation of juvenile delinquents.' *British Journal of Psychiatry*, **120**, 549–550.

BOWLBY, J. (1964) *Maternal Deprivation and Mental Health*. Geneva: World Health Organisation.

BRADLEY, C. (1936) 'A children's hospital for neurological and behaviour disorders.' *Journal of the American Medical Association*, **107**, 650–652.

BRIDGLAND, M. (1971) *Pioneer Work with Maladjusted Children*. London: Staples Press.

BRIGGS, A. (1972) *Report of the Committee on Nursing*. London: H.M.S.O.

BRITISH NATIONAL FORMULARY (1971) London: B.M.A. and Pharmaceutical Press.

BRITISH PAEDIATRIC ASSOCIATION (1959) 'Medical care of the adolescent.' *Lancet*, **1**, 825–826.

BROWN, G. D. and TYLER, V. O. (1968) 'Time out from reinforcement: a technique for dethroning the "duke" of an institutionalised group.' *Journal of Child Psychology and Psychiatry*, **9**, 203–211.

BROWN, S. L. (1972) 'Family group therapy.' In *Manual of Child Psychopathology*. Edited by Welman, B. New York: McGraw-Hill.

BRUGGAN, P. (1971) 'The reason for admission as the focus of work.' In *Proceedings of the Sixth Conference of the Association for the Psychiatric Study of Adolescents*.

CAMERON, K. (1949) 'A psychiatric inpatient department for children.' *Journal of Mental Science*, **95**, 560–566.

CAPLAN, H. L. (1970) 'Hysterical "conversion" symptoms in childhood.' M.Phil. dissertation: University of London.

CHAPEL, J. L. (1967) 'Treatment of a case of school phobia by reciprocal inhibition.' *Canadian Psychiatric Association Journal*, **21**, 25–28.

CHAUDHARY, N. A. and TRUELOVE, S. C. (1961) 'Human colonic motility: a comparative study of normal subjects, patients with ulcerative colitis, and patients with the irritable colon syndrome (effects of emotions).' *Gastroenterology*, **40**, 27–36.

CHAZIN, R. (1969) 'Day treatment of emotionally disturbed children.' *Child Welfare*, **48**, 212–218.

CHESS, S. (1969) *An Introduction to Child Psychiatry* (2nd edition). New York: Grune and Stratton.

CHISHOLM, M. M. (1968) *Nursing in Child Psychiatry: Working Conference*. Massachusetts: Boston University School of Nursing.

CHURCHILL, J. (1967) 'An issue: nurses and psychotherapy.' *Perspectives in Psychiatric Care*, **5**, 160–162.

CHRIST, A. E. and WAGONER, N. N. (1966) 'Iatrogenic factors in child residential treatment.' In *Current Psychiatric Therapies*. Edited by Masserman, J. H. London: Grune and Stratton.

CLANCY, H., ENTSCH, M. and RENDLE-SHORT, J. (1969) 'Infantile Autism: the correction of feeding abnormalities.' *Development Medicine and Child Neurology*, **11**, 569–578.

CLANCY, H. and MCBRIDE, G. (1969) 'The autistic process and its treatment.' *Journal of Child Psychology and Psychiatry*, **10**, 233–244.

CLARKE, A. D. B. (1968) 'Learning and human development.' *British Journal of Psychiatry*, **114**, 1061–1077.

COHEN, R. L. (1964) 'The influence of child guidance practices on children's in-patient units.' *Journal of the American Academy of Child Psychiatry*, **3**, 151–160.

CONNELL, P. H. (1961) 'The day patient approach in child psychiatry.' *Journal of Mental Science*, **107**, 969–977.

COOLIDGE, J. C., HAHN, P. B. and PECK, A. L. (1957) 'School phobia: neurotic crisis or way of life.' *American Journal of Orthopsychiatry*, **27**, 296–306.

COOLIDGE, J. C., WILLER, M. L., TESSMAN, E. and WALDFOGEL, S. (1962) 'Patterns of aggression in school phobia.' *Psychoanalytic Study of the Child*, **17**, 319–334.

COPUS, P. E. and WALKER, W. L. (1972) 'The psychiatric ward in a children's hospital: a review of the first two years.' *British Journal of Psychiatry*, **121**, 323–326.

CREAK, M. (1964) 'Schizophrenic syndrome in childhood: a further progress report of a working party.' *Developmental Medicine and Child Neurology*, **4**, 530–535.

CREAK, M. (1971) 'Gaps in medical education.' *Proceedings of the Royal Society of Medicine*, **65**, 106–107.

CRYSTAL, D. (1972) 'The case of linguistics: a prognosis.' *British Journal of Disorders of Communication*, **1**, 3–16.

CUNNINGHAM, M. A., PILLAI, V. and ROGERS, W. J. B. (1968) 'Haloperidol in the treatment of children with severe behaviour disorders.' *British Journal of Psychiatry*, **114**, 845–854.

CURRAN, F. J. (1939) 'Organisation of a ward for adolescents in Bellevue Psychiatric Hospital.' *American Journal of Psychiatry*, **95**, 1365–1388.

DALTON, K. (1960) 'Effect of menstruation on schoolgirls' weekly work.' *British Medical Journal*, **1**, 326–328.

DAVIDS, A., RYAN, R. and SALVATORE, P. D. (1968) 'Effectiveness of residential treatment for psychotic and other disturbed children.' *American Journal of Orthopsychiatry*, **38**, 469–475.

DAVIDSON, S. (1961) 'School phobia as a manifestation of family disturbance'. *Journal of Child Psychology and Psychiatry*, **1**, 270–278.

DE HIRSCH, K. (1970) 'A review of language development.' *Developmental Medicine and Child Neurology*, **12**, 87–97.

DEPARTMENT OF HEALTH AND SOCIAL SECURITY (1968) 'Psychiatric Nursing Today and Tomorrow.' (Report of the joint sub-committee of the Standing Mental Health and the Standing Advisory Committee.) London: H.M.S.O.

DES LAURIERS, A. M. (1962) *The Experience of Reality in Childhood Schizophrenia.* New York: International Universities Press.

DESPERT, J. L. (1938) 'Schizophrenia in children.' *Psychiatric Quarterly*, **12**, 366–371.

DESPERT, J. L. and SHERWIN, A. C. (1958) 'Further examination of diagnostic criteria of psychosis in infancy and early childhood.' *American Journal of Psychiatry*, **114**, 784–790.

DOCKAR-DRYSDALE, B. (1968) 'Residential treatment of "frozen" children.' In *Therapy in Child Care* (collected papers). London: Longman Green.

EASTMAN, R. D. and JARCAR, J. (1971) 'Epilepsy and forate deficiency.' *British Medical Journal*, **4**, 361–362.

EISENBERG, L. (1957) 'The course of childhood schizophrenia.' *Archives of Neurology and Psychiatry*, **78**, 69–83.

EISENBERG, L. (1958) 'School phobia: diagnosis, genesis and clinical management.' *The Paediatric Clinics of North America*, **5**, 645–666.

EISENBERG, L. (1967) 'Psychotic disorders in childhood.' In *Biologic Basis of Paediatric Practice*. Edited by Cooke, R. E. New York: McGraw-Hill.

EVANS, J. (1970) 'Conflicts, crises and tensions in a residential unit.' In *Proceedings of the Fifth Conference of the Association for the Psychiatric Study of Adolescents.*

EVANS, I. M. (1970) 'A modular teaching unit for research and therapy with children.' *Journal of Child Psychology and Psychiatry*, **11**, 63–67.

EYSENCK, H. J. (1959) 'Learning theory and behaviour therapy.' *The Journal of Mental Science*, **105**, 61–75.

FALCONER, M. A. (1972) 'Place of surgery for temporal lobe epilepsy in children.' *British Medical Journal*, **2**, 631–635.

FEDERAL SECURITY AGENCY (1952) *Residential Treatment Centres for Emotionally Disturbed Children:* a listing.

FLANAGAN, J. C. (1954) 'The critical incident technique.' *Psychological Bulletin*, **51**, 327–328.

FLECK, S. (1972) 'Some basic aspects of family pathology.' In *Manual of Child Psychopathology*. Edited by Wolman, B. New York: McGraw-Hill.

FRENCH, E. L. (1963) 'Residential treatment for emotionally disturbed young people.' *Mental Hospitals*, **14**, 386–389.

FREUD, A. (1948) *The Ego and the Mechanism of Defence*. London: The Hogarth Press.

FREUD, A. (1966) *Normality and Pathology in Childhood.* London: The Hogarth Press.

FREUD, A. (1970) 'The symptomatology of childhood.' *The Psychoanalytic Study of the Child*, **25**, 19–41. New York: International Universities Press.

FREUD, S. (1925) *Negation*. London: Hogarth Press.

FRICK, W. B. (1964) 'School phobia: a critical review of the literature.' *Merrill Palmer Quarterly*, **10**, 361–373.

FRY, D. B. and WHETNALL, E. (1954) 'The auditory approach in the training of deaf children.' *Lancet*, **1**, 583–587.

GAIR, D. S. and SALOMON, A. D. (1962) 'Diagnostic aspects of psychiatric hospitalisation of children.' *American Journal of Orthopsychiatry*, **32**, 445–460.

GARVEY, W. P. and HEGRENES, J. R. (1966) 'Densensitization techniques in the treatment of school phobia.' *American Journal of Orthopsychiatry*, **36**, 147–152.

GIBBENS, T. C. N. (1961) 'Trends in juvenile delinquency.' *World Health Organisation Public Health Papers No. 5.*

GILBERTSON, R. J. L. and SUTTON, H. (1943) 'A children's psychiatric service.' *American Journal of Nursing*, **43**, 570–572.

GINOTT, H. G. (1961) *Group Psychotherapy with Children.* New York: McGraw-Hill.

GOODRICH, D. W. and BOOMER, D. S. (1958) 'Some concepts about therapeutic intervention with hyperaggressive children.' *Social Casework*, **39**, 207–211 and 286–292.

GOLD, S. (1965) 'Diagnosis and management of hysterical contractures in children.' *British Medical Journal*, **1**, 21–23.

GREENWOOD, E. D. (1955) 'The role of psychotherapy in residential treatment.' *American Journal of Orthopsychiatry*, **25**, 692–698.

GROUP FOR THE ADVANCEMENT OF PSYCHIATRY (1966) 'Psychopathological disorders in childhood: theoretical considerations and a proposed classification.' *Volume 6, Report No. 62.*

HALDANE, J. D. (1963) 'The functions, selection and training of the nurse in a residential psychiatric unit for children.' *International Journal of Nursing Studies*, **1**, 27–36.

HALDANE, J. D., CRUNLEY, R., SMITH, J. D. and STEPHEN, D. (1965) 'Psychiatric nursing of children and adults: some comparisons and contrasts.' *International Journal of Nursing Studies*, **2**, 23–31.

HALDANE, J. D., LINDSAY, S. F. and SMITH, J. D. (1971) 'Nursing in child, adolescent and family psychiatry.' *International Journal of Nursing Studies*, **8**, 91–102.

HALDANE, J. D., SMITH, J. D., MCINNES, J. and HENDERSON, J. (1971) 'The training of nurses in child, adolescent and family psychiatry.' *Nursing Times:* Occasional Paper.

HALLMAN, N. (1965) 'Nursing education for child care.' In *Report on a Seminar convened by the Regional Office for Europe of the World Health Organisation.* Copenhagen: W.H.O. (Regional Office for Europe).

HARRINGTON, J. A. and LETEMENDIA, F. J. J. (1958) 'Persistent psychiatric disorders after head injuries in children.' *Journal of Mental Science*, **104**, 1205–1218.

HARTMANN, E., GLASSER, B. A., GREENBLATT, M., SOLOMON, M. H. and LEVINSON, D. J. (1968) *Adolescents in a Mental Hospital.* New York: Grune and Stratton.

HELFER, R. E. and KEMPE, C. H. (Editors) (1968) *The Battered Child.* University of Chicago Press.

HENDRICKSON, W. J. and HOLMES, D. J. (1959) 'Control of behaviour as a crucial factor in intensive psychiatric treatment in an all adolescent ward.' *American Journal of Psychiatry*, **115**, 969–973.

HERBERT, G. W. and WEDELL, K. (1970) 'Communication handicaps of children with specific language deficiency.' Paper read at Annual Conference of British Psychological Society.

HERMELIN, B. I. and O'CONNOR, N. (1970) *Psychological Experiments With Autistic Children.* Oxford: Pergammon Press.

HERSOV, L. A. (1960a) 'Persistent non-attendance at school.' *Journal of Child Psychology and Psychiatry*, **1**, 130–136.

HERSOV, L. A. (1960b) 'Refusal to go to school.' *Journal of Child Psychology and Psychiatry*, **1**, 137–145.

HERSOV, L. A. (1972) 'School refusal.' *British Medical Journal*, **3**, 102–104.

HEWITT, L. E. and JENKINS, R. L. (1946) *Fundamental Patterns of Maladjustment: The Dynamics of Their Origin*. Springfield: State of Illinois.

HUNTER, P. (1960) 'The changing function of professional staff in the mental hospital.' *A.P.S.W. Ventures in Professional Co-operation:* London.

HUNTER, P. (1962) 'After care for the mentally ill as a British hospital provides it.' *Nursing Outlook*, **10**, 604–606.

HUNTER, P. (1970) 'The role of the psychiatric nurse and some thoughts on training.' Presented as Evidence to the Committee on Nursing.

HUTT, S. S., HUTT, C., OUNSTED, C. and LEE, D. (1965) 'A behavioural and electro-encaphalographic study of autistic children.' *Journal of Psychiatric Research*, **3**, 181–197.

HYLTON, L. F. (1964) *The Residential Treatment Center*. New York: Child Welfare League of America.

INGRAM, T. T. S. (1972) 'The classification of speech and language disorders in young children.' In *The Child with Delayed Speech*. Edited by Rutter, M. and Martin, J. A. M. London: Heinemann.

JOHN, A. L., LEITE-RIBEIRO, M. O. and BUCKLE, D. (1963) 'The nurse in mental health practice: report on a technical conference.' (Public Health Papers, No. 22). Geneva: World Health Organisation.

JOHNSON, A. M., FALSTEIN, E. I., SZUREK, S. A. and SVENDSEN, M. (1941) 'School phobia.' *American Journal of Orthopsychiatry*, **11**, 702–711.

JOINT BOARD OF CLINICAL NURSING STUDIES (1973) Outline Curriculum in Child and Adolescent Psychiatric Nursing for Registered Nurses (Course No. 600) London.

JONES, M. (1952) *Social Psychiatry*. London: Tavistock.

JONES, M. (1962) *Social Psychiatry in Practice*. Harmondsworth: Penguin Books.

JONES, R. S. (1966) 'Assessment of respiratory function in the asthmatic child.' *British Medical Journal*, **2**, 972–978.

KAHAN, V. L. (1971) *Mental Illness in Childhood: A Study of Residential Treatment*. London: Tavistock.

KANNER, L. (1943) 'Autistic disturbance of affective contact.' *Nervous Child*, **2**, 217–250.

KANNER, L. (1957) *Child Psychiatry*. 3rd Edition. Springfield, Illinois: Charles C. Thomas.

KANNER, L. (1958) 'The 33rd Maudsley lecture: trends in child psychiatry.' *Journal of Mental Science*, **105**, 581–593.

KENNEDY, W. A. (1965) 'School phobia. Rapid treatment of fifty cases.' *Journal o Abnormal Psychology*, **70**, 285–289.

KESSLER, J. W. (1972) 'Neurosis in childhood.' In *Manual of Child Psychopathology*. Edited by Wolman, B. New York: McGraw-Hill.

KING, R. D., RAYNES, N. V. and TIZARD, J. (1971) *Patterns of Residential Care*. London: Routledge and Kegan Paul.

KLEIN, M. (1924) 'The role of the school in the libidinal development of the child.' *International Journal of Psychoanalysis*, **5**, 312–331.

KLOPP, H. I. (1932) 'The children's institute of the Allentown State Hospital.' *American Journal of Psychiatry*, **88**, 1108–1118.

KOLVIN, I. and ASSOCIATES (1971) 'Studies in the childhood psychoses.' *British Journal of Psychiatry*, **118**, 381–419.

KRUG, O. (1952) 'The application of the principles of child psychotherapy in residential treatment.' *American Journal of Psychiatry*, **108**, 695–700.

KRUG, O., HAYWARD, H. and CRUMPACKER, B. (1952) 'Intensive residential treatment of a nine-year-old girl with an aggressive behaviour disorder, petit mal epilepsy and enuresis.' *American Journal of Orthopsychiatry*, **22**, 405–427.

LAURENCE, D. R. (1973) *Clinical Pharmacology*. 4th Edition. London: J. & A. Churchill.

LAZARUS, A. A. and ABRAMOWITZ, A. (1965) 'The use of "emotive imagery" in the treatment of children's phobias.' In *Case Studies in Behaviour Modification*. Edited by Ullmann, L. P. and Krasner, L. New York: Holt, Rinehart and Winston.

LAZARUS, A. A., DAWSON, G. C. and POLEFKA, D. A. (1965) 'Classical and operant factors in the treatment of a school phobia.' *Journal of Abnormal Psychology*, **70**, 225–229.

LEHRER, P., SCHIFF, L. and KRIS, A. (1972) 'Operant conditioning in a comprehensive treatment program for adolescents.' In *Residential Treatment of Emotionally Disturbed Children*. Edited by Weber, G. H. and Haberlein, B. J. New York: Behavioural Publications.

LENNEBERG, E. H. (1967) *Biological Foundation of Language*. New York: Wiley.

LEVENTHAL, T. and SILLS, M. (1964) 'Self-image in school phobia.' *American Journal of Orthopsychiatry*, **34**, 685–695.

LEVENTHAL, T., WEINBERGER, G., STANDER, R. J. and STEARNS, R. P. (1967) 'Therapeutic strategies with school phobia.' *American Journal of Orthopsychiatry*, **37**, 64–70.

LEVY, E. Z. (1969) 'Long-term follow-up of former inpatients at the Children's Hospital of the Menninger Clinic.' *American Journal of Psychiatry*, **125**, 1633–1639.

LOVAAS, O. I. (1966) 'A programme for the establishing of speech in psychotic children.' In *Early Childhood Autism*. Edited by Wing, J. K. Oxford: Pergammon.

LOURIE, N. V. and SCHULMAN, R. (1952) 'The role of the residential staff in residential treatment.' *American Journal of Orthopsychiatry*, **22**, 798–808.

MACKEITH, R. C. and RUTTER, M. (1972) 'A note on the prevalence of language disorders in young children.' In *The Child with Delayed Speech*. Edited by Rutter, M. and Martin, J. A. M. (Clinics in Developmental Medicine, No. 43) London: Heinemann.

MACKINNON, I. L., MACKINNON, P. C. B. and THOMPSON, A. D. (1959) 'Lethal hazards of the luteal phase of the menstrual cycle.' *British Medical Journal*, **1**, 1015–1017.

MCREYNOLDS, L. (1966) 'Operant conditioning for investigation of speech sound discrimination in aphasic children.' *Journal of Speech and Hearing Research*, **9**, 519–528.

MCTAGGART, A. N. (1965) 'The psychiatric care of children in a teaching hospital.' *Canadian Medical Association Journal*, **10**, 332–337.

MAHLER, M. S. (1952) 'On child psychosis and schizophrenia: autistic and symbiotic and infantile psychoses.' *Psychoanalytic Study of the Child*, **7**, 286–305.

MAHLER, M. S. (1965) 'On early infantile psychosis: the symbiotic and autistic syndromes.' *Journal of the American Academy of Child Psychiatry*, **4**, 554–568.

MAPSTONE, E. (1969) *Children in Care* (Concern No. 3). London: National Children's Bureau.

MARKS, I. M. (1969) *Fears and Phobias*. London: Heinemann.

MARSHALL, K. A. and STEWART, M. F. (1969) 'Day treatment as a complementary adjunct to residential treatment.' *Child Welfare*, **48**, 40–44.

MILHAM, S. (1971) 'Some problems posed by the residential care of adolescents.' In *Proceedings of the Sixth Conference of the Association for the Psychiatric Study of Adolescents*.

MILLER, D. (1964) *Growth to Freedom: The Psychological Treatment of Delinquent Youth*. London: Tavistock Publications.

MINISTRY OF HEALTH (1964) 'Inpatient accommodation for mentally ill and seriously maladjusted children and adolescents.' (Circular H.M. (64) 4). London: H.M.S.O.

MOIR, A. T. B., HALLIDAY, J. and WILLIAMS, R. (1971) 'Lack of effect of folic acid on the mental state and fit frequency of drug treatment.' *Lancet*, **2**, 798–800.

NEILL, A. S. (1962) *Summerhill*. London: Victor Gollancz.

NELSON, R. O. and EVANS, I. M. (1968) 'The combination of learning principles and of speech therapy techniques in the treatment of non-communicating children.' *Journal of Child Psychology and Psychiatry*, **9**, 111–124.

NEUBAUER, C. (1970) 'Mental deterioration in epilepsy due to folate deficiency.' *British Medical Journal*, **2**, 759–761.

NOSHPITZ, J. D. (1962) 'Notes on the theory of residential treatment.' *Journal of the American Academy of Child Psychiatry*, **1**, 284–296.

O'CONNOR, N. (1956) 'The evidence of the permanently disturbed effects of mother–child separation.' *Acta Psychologica*, **12**, 174–191.

ORNITZ, E. M. and RITVO, E. R. (1968a) 'Perceptual inconstancy in early infantile autism.' *Archives of General Psychiatry*, **18**, 76–98.

ORNITZ, E. M. and RITVO, E. R. (1968b) 'Neurophysiologic mechanisms underlying perceptual inconstancy in autistic and schizophrenic children.' *Archives of General Psychiatry*, **19**, 22–27.

OTIS, A. S. (1937) *Otis Quick Scoring Mental Ability Tests: Manual of Directions for Gamma Test*. Yonkers-on-Hudson, New York: World Books.

PATTERSON, G. R. (1964) 'An empirical approach to the classification of disturbed children.' *Journal of Clinical Psychology*, **20**, 326–337.

PESHKIN, M. M. (1930) 'Asthma in children refractory to treatment – a plea for a "Home" as a restorative measure.' *American Journal of Diseases of Children*, **39**, 774–781.

PETERSON, D. R. (1961) 'Behaviour problems of middle childhood.' *Journal of Consulting Psychology*, **25**, 205–209.

PINKERTON, P. (1958) 'Psychogenic megacolon in children: the implications of bowel negativism.' *Archives of Disease in Childhood*, **33**, 371–380.

PINKERTON, P. (1965) 'The psychosomatic approach in child psychiatry.' In *Modern Perspectives in Child Psychiatry*, 306–335. Edited by Howells, J. G. Edinburgh: Oliver and Boyd.

PINKERTON, P. (1967) 'Correlating physiological with psychodynamic data in the study and management of childhood asthma.' *Journal of Psychosomatic Research*, **11**, 11–25.

PINKERTON, P. (1969) 'Managing the psychological aspects of cystic fibrosis. *Arizona Medicine*, **26**, 348–351.

PINKERTON, P. (1970) 'The influence of sociopathology in childhood asthma.' *Psychotherapy and Psychosomatics*, **18**, 231–238.

PINKERTON, P. (1971a) 'Childhood asthma.' *British Journal of Hospital Medicine*, **6**, 331–338.

PINKERTON, P. (1971b) 'Re-appraisal of "parentectomy" in childhood asthma.' *The Medical Officer*, **125**, 63–65.

PINKERTON, P. (1972a) 'Psychosomatic aspects of asthma.' *The Practitioner*, **208**, 430–436.

PINKERTON, P. (1972b) 'The psychosomatic approach in paediatrics – an exercise in interdisciplinary liaison.' *Nursing Times*, **68**, 311–316.

PINKERTON, P. (1972c) 'Depression *v.* denial in childhood asthma: equipotent fatal hazards.' *Proceedings of the 4th Union European Pedopsychiatrists Congress*, Stockholm, 1971, 187–192.

POLLACK, M. and GOLDFARB, W. (1957) 'Patterns of orientation in children in residential treatment for severe behaviour disorders.' *American Journal of Orthopsychiatry*, **27**, 538–552.

POND, D. A. (1961) 'Psychiatric aspects of epileptic and brain damaged children.' *British Medical Journal*, **2**, 1377–1382 and 1454–1459.

POTTER, H. W. (1934a) 'A service for children in a psychiatric hospital.' *Psychiatric Quarterly*, **8**, 16–31.

POTTER, H. W. (1934b) 'The treatment of problem children in a psychiatric hospital.' *American Journal of Psychiatry*, **91**, 869–880.

POTTER, H. W. and KLEIN, H. R. (1957) 'An evaluation of the treatment of problem children as determined by a follow-up study.' *American Journal of Psychiatry*, **74**, 681–689.

PREMACK, D. (1971) 'Language in chimpanzee?' *Science*, **172**, 808–822.

QUAY, H. C. (1964) 'Dimensions of personality in delinquent boys as inferred from the factor analysis of case history data.' *Child Development*, **35**, 479–484.

REDL, F. (1959a) 'Life space interview techniques.' *American Journal of Orthopsychiatry*, **29**, 1–18.

REDL, F. (1959b) 'The concept of a "therapeutic milieu".' *American Journal of Orthopsychiatry*, **29**, 721–736.

REDL, F. and WINEMAN, D. (1951) *Children Who Hate*. Glencoe: The Free Press.

REDL, F. and WINEMAN, D. (1952) *Controls From Within*. Glencoe: The Free Press.

REES, H. M. N. and MORLEY, R. (To be published) 'Epidemiology of children in care.'

REES, H. M. N. and TAYLOR, J. (To be published) 'A teaching diagnostic programme for non-communicating children.'

REID REPORT (1969) *People with Epilepsy*. (Report of a Joint Subcommittee of the Standing Medical Advisory Committee on the Health and Welfare of Handicapped Persons.) London: H.M.S.O.

REID, J. H. and HAGAN, H. R. (1952) *Residential Treatment of Emotionally Disturbed Children*. New York: Child Welfare League of America.

REIDY, J. J. (1960) 'Community pressures and a state hospital program for children.' *American Journal of Psychiatry*, **117**, 336–341.

REITER, F. (1966) 'The clinical nursing approach.' *Nursing Forum*, **5**, 39–44.

REYNOLDS, E. H. (1967) 'Effect of folic acid on the mental state and fit frequency of drug treated epileptic patients.' *Lancet*, **1**, 1086–1088.

RIMLAND, B. (1964) *Infantile Autism*. New York: Appleton-Century-Crofts.

RINSLEY, D. M. (1963) 'Psychiatric hospital treatment – with special reference to children.' *Archives of General Psychiatry*, **9**, 489–496.

RIOCH, D. M. and STANTON, A. H. (1953) 'Milieu therapy.' *Psychiatry*, **16**, 65–72.

ROBINS, L. N. (1966) *Deviant Children Grown Up*. Baltimore: Williams and Wilkins.

ROBINS, L. N. and O'NEAL, P. L. (1969) 'The strategy of follow-up studies with special reference to children.' In *Modern Perspectives in International Child Psychiatry*. Edited by Howells, J. G. Edinburgh: Oliver and Boyd.

ROBINSON, J. F. (1947) 'Resident psychiatric treatment of children.' *American Journal of Orthopsychiatry*, **17**, 484–487.

ROBINSON, J. F. (1957) *Psychiatric Inpatient Treatment of Children*. Washington: American Psychiatric Association.

ROBINSON, J. F., MAXWELL, A. and DOMINGUEZ, K. E. (1947) 'Residential psychiatric treatment with children.' *American Journal of Orthopsychiatry*, **17**, 458–467.

RODDY, L. R. (1960) 'Children's unit, Eastern State Hospital.' *Virginia Medical Monthly*, **87**, 402–403.

ROGERS, J. B. (1954) 'A children's psychiatric unit in a mental hospital.' *British Medical Journal*, **2**, 1544–1546.

ROGERS, J. W. B. (1965) 'Children's inpatient units.' In *Modern Perspectives in Child Psychiatry*. Edited by Howells, J. G. Edinburgh: Oliver and Boyd.

ROSE, J. A. and SONIS, M. (1959) 'The use of separation as a diagnostic measure in the parent–child emotional crisis.' *American Journal of Psychiatry*, **116**, 409–415.

ROSENFELD, S. (1972) 'Reflections on borderline and atypical cases: borderline functioning in a traumatised child.' Paper given at the Twentieth Anniversary of the Hampstead Clinic, London.

ROSS, A. O. (1972) *Behaviour Therapy in Psychopathological Disorders of Childhood*. Edited by Quay, H. C. and Werry, J. S. New York: John Wiley and Sons.

ROYAL COLLEGE OF NURSING (1970) Document: Post certificate training and education of psychiatric nurses. London.

ROYAL COLLEGE OF PSYCHIATRISTS (1971) Memorandum of evidence to the committee on nursing. London.

ROYAL COLLEGE OF PSYCHIATRISTS (1973) Memorandum on training in child and adolescent psychiatry. London.

ROYAL MEDICO-PSYCHOLOGICAL ASSOCIATION (1957) 'Inpatient accommodation for child and adolescent psychiatric patients.' London.

ROYAL MEDICO-PSYCHOLOGICAL ASSOCIATION (1970) Report on an investigation into recruitment and training for nursing staff of inpatient units for children and adolescents. London.

RUBINFINE, D. L. (1962) 'Maternal stimulation.' *Psychoanalytic Study of the Child*, **7**, 286–305.

RUSSELL-DAVIS, D. (1972) *An Introduction to Psychopathology* (3rd Edition). Oxford University Press.

RUTTER, M. (1966) 'Prognosis: psychotic children in adolescence and early adult life.' In *Early Childhood Autism: Clinical, Educational and Social Aspects.* Edited by Wing, J. K. Oxford: Pergammon Press.

RUTTER, M. (1967) 'Psychotic disorders in early childhood.' In *Recent Developments in Schizophrenia.* Edited by Coppen, A. S. and Walk, A. London: Royal Medico-Psychological Association.

RUTTER, M. (1971) 'Parent–child separation: psychological effects on the children.' *Journal of Child Psychology and Psychiatry*, **12**, 233–260.

RUTTER, M. (1972) *Maternal Deprivation Re-assessed.* Harmondsworth: Penguin Books.

RUTTER, M. L., GRAHAM, P. and YULE, W. (1970) *A Neuropsychiatric Study in Childhood.* (Clinics in Developmental Medicine 35/36) London: Heinemann.

RUTTER, M., LEBOVICI, S., EISENBERG, L., SNEZNEVSKIJ, A. V., SADOUN, R., BROOKE, E. and LIN, T–Y. (1969). 'A tri-axial classification of mental disorders in childhood. An international study.' *Journal of Child Psychology and Psychiatry*, **10**, 41–61.

RUTTER, M. L. and LOCKYER, L. (1967) 'A 5 to 15 year follow-up of infantile psychosis.' *British Journal of Psychiatry*, **113**, 1169–1182.

RUTTER, M. TIZARD, J. and WHITMORE, K. (1970) *Education, Health and Behaviour.* London: Longman.

SANDS, D. E. (1953) 'A special mental hospital unit for the treatment of psychosis and neurosis in juveniles.' *Journal of Mental Science*, **99**, 123–129.

SCHRAGER, J. (1954) 'A focus for supervision of residential staff in a treatment institution.' *Bulletin of the Menninger Clinic*, **18**, 64–71.

SCOTTISH HOME AND HEALTH DEPARTMENT (1962) *Medical Services for Child Guidance.* Edinburgh: H.M.S.O.

SHAW, C. R. (1966) *The Psychiatric Disorders of Childhood.* New York: Appleton-Century-Crofts.

SHAW, C. R. and LUCAS, A. R. (1970) *The Psychiatric Disorders of Childhood* (2nd Edition). New York: Appleton-Century-Crofts.

SHEIMO, S. L., PAYNTER, J. and SZUREV, S. A. (1949) 'Problems of staff interaction with spontaneous group formations on a children's psychiatric ward.' *American Journal of Orthopsychiatry*, **19**, 599–611.

SIMMS, L. L. (1966) 'The clinical nursing specialist: an approach to nursing practice in the hospital.' *Journal of the American Medical Association*, **198**, 675–677.

SIMPSON, L. S. (1957) 'Hormones and behaviour pattern.' *British Medical Journal*, **2**, 839–843.

SKINNER, B. F. (1953) *Science and Human Behaviour.* New York: Macmillan.

SKYNNER, A. C. R. (1969) 'A group-analytic approach to conjoint family therapy.' *Journal of Child Psychology and Psychiatry*, **10**, 81–106.

SLAVSON, S. R. (1943) *An Introduction to Group Therapy.* New York: Harvard University Press.

SLAVSON, S. R. (1947) *The Practice of Group Therapy.* New York: International Universities Press.

SLAVSON, S. R. (1955) 'Criteria for selection and rejection of patients for various types of group therapy.' *International Journal of Group Psychotherapy*, **5**, 3–30.

SLOBIN, D. (1971) *The Orthogenesis of Grammar.* New York: Academic Press.

SPEIGEL, H. (1967) 'Is symptom removal dangerous?' *American Journal of Psychiatry,* **10**, 1279–1282.

SPERLING, M. (1961) 'Analytic first aid to school phobias.' *Psychoanalytic Quarterly,* **30**, 504–518.

SPERLING, M. (1967) 'School phobias: classification, dynamics and treatment.' *Psychoanalytic Study of the Child,* **22**, 375–402.

STAYTON, D. J., HOGAN, R. and AINSWORTH, M. (1971) 'Infant obedience and maternal behaviour: the origins of socialization reconsidered.' *Child Development,* **4**, 1057–1069.

STEVENS, R. A. (1969) 'Psychiatric nursing.' Course outline: University of Cincinnati.

STRATAS, N. E. and SCHMIDT, K. J. (1960) 'A children's unit in a state hospital.' *American Journal of Psychiatry,* **117**, 34–36.

STROH, G. (1960) 'Training scheme in a residential unit for severely disturbed children.' *Special Education,* **49**, 32–34.

STROH, G. (1962) 'Psychosis in childhood.' *Public Health,* **77**, 21–27.

STROH, G. (1968) 'The function of inservice training in the management of disturbed children.' *Journal of Child Psychology and Psychiatry,* **9**, 189–203.

STROH, G. and BUICK, D. (1964) 'Perceptual development and childhood psychosis.' *British Journal of Medical Psychology,* **37**, 291–299.

SUESS, J. F. and HOSHINO, A. Y. (1961) 'Therapeutic developmental management of an adolescent residential treatment service in a state hospital.' *American Journal of Psychiatry,* **117**, 891–895.

SUTTON, H. A. (1947) 'Some nursing aspects of a children's psychiatric ward.' *American Journal of Orthopsychiatry,* **17**, 675–683.

SZUREK, S. A. (1944) 'Child therapy procedures.' *Psychiatry,* **7**, 9–14.

SZUREK, S. A. (1947) 'Diagnosis of staff interaction in hospital psychiatric treatment of children.' *American Journal of Orthopsychiatry,* **17**, 652–664.

SZUREK, S. A. (1951) 'The family and the staff in hospital psychiatric therapy of children.' *American Journal of Orthopsychiatry,* **21**, 597–611.

SZUREK, S. A. (1956) 'Elements of psychotherapeutics with the schizophrenic child and his parents.' *Psychiatry,* **19**, 1–9.

THOMAS, A., CHESS, S. and BIRCH, G. (1968) *Temperament and Behaviour Disorders in Children.* New York: New York University Press.

TISCHLER, S. (1965) 'Observations based on psychotherapy with the parents of psychotic children.' In *Proceedings of the Sixth International Congress of Psychotherapy.* Basle: S. Kargar.

TISCHLER, S. (1971) 'Clinical work with the parents of psychotic children.' *Journal of Neurology, Neurosurgery and Psychiatry,* **74**, 225–249.

TIZARD, J. (1966) 'Mental subnormality and child psychiatry.' *Journal of Child Psychology and Psychiatry,* **7**, 1–16.

TREFFERT, D. A. (1968) 'Children and adolescents: hospital treatment programs.' *Hospital and Community Psychiatry,* **19**, 237–240.

TREFFERT, D. A. (1969) 'Child-adolescent unit in a psychiatric hospital.' *Archives of General Psychiatry,* **21**, 745–752.

TRUAX, C. B. and CARKHUFF, R. R. (1967) *Towards Effective Counselling.* Chicago: Aldine Publishing Co.

TURLE, G. C. (1960) 'On opening an adolescent unit.' *Journal of Mental Science*, **106**, 1320–1326.

WARDLE, C. J. (1961) 'Two generations of broken homes in the genesis of conduct and behaviour disorders in childhood.' *British Medical Journal*, **2**, 349–354.

WARDLE, C. J. (1962) 'Social factors in the major functional psychosis in society.' In *Society: Problems and Methods of Study*. Edited by Welford, A. T. London: Routledge and Kegan Paul.

WARDLE, C. J. (1967) 'Behaviour disorder in children with epilepsy.' *Journal of British Epilepsy Association* (Spring issue), 10–12.

WARDLE, C. J. (1969) 'Difficult children: problems in providing inpatient care.' Unpublished.

WARDLE, C. J. (1970) 'Report on investigation into recruitment and training for nursing staff of inpatient units for children and adolescents.' Report submitted to the Royal Medico-Psychological Association, London.

WARDLE, C. J. (1971) Evidence to Asa Briggs Committee.

WARREN, W. (1948) 'Acute neurotic breakdown in children with refusal to go to school.' *Archives of Disease in Childhood*, **23**, 266–272.

WARREN, W. (1952) 'Inpatient treatment of adolescents with psychological illness.' *Lancet*, **1**, 147–150.

WARREN, W. (1953) 'Treatment of youths with behaviour disorders in a psychiatric hospital.' *British Journal of Delinquency*, **3**, 234–247.

WARREN, W. (1965a) 'A study of adolescent psychiatric inpatients and the outcome six or more years later. I. Clinical histories and hospital findings.' *Journal of Child Psychology and Psychiatry*, **6**, 1–17.

WARREN, W. (1965b) 'A study of adolescent psychiatric inpatients and the outcome six or more years later. II. The follow-up study.' *Journal of Child Psychology and Psychiatry*, **6**, 141–160.

WARREN, W. (1970) 'You can never plan the future by the past.' *Journal of Child Psychology and Psychiatry*, **11**, 241–257.

WATSON, J. P., BENNET, D. H. and ISAACS, A. D. (1970) 'Psychiatric units in general hospitals.' *Lancet*, **1**, 511–514.

WEDDELL, D. (1961) 'Family centred nursing.' *International Nursing Review*, **8**, 20–25.

WEINER, H., THALLER, M., REISER, M. F. and MIRSKY, I. A. (1957) 'Aetiology of duodenal ulcer.' *Psychosomatic Medicine*, **19**, 1–10.

WEISS, M. and CAIN, B. (1964) 'The residential treatment of children and adolescents with school phobia.' *American Journal of Orthopsychiatry*, **34**, 103–112.

WEISS, M. and BURKE, G. B. (1967) 'A five–ten year follow-up of hospitalised school phobic children and adolescents.' *American Journal of Orthopsychiatry*, **37**, 294–295.

WENAR, C., RUTTENBERG, B. A., DRATMAN, M. L. and WOLF, E. G. (1967) 'Changing autistic behaviour (the effectiveness of 3 milieus).' *Archives of General Psychiatry*, **17**, 26–35.

WEST, D. J. (1967) *The Young Offender*. London: Penguin Books.

WILLS, W. D. (1960) *Throw Away The Rod*. London: Gollancz.

WING, L. (1969) 'The handicaps of autistic children: a comparative study.' *Journal of Child Psychology and Psychiatry*, **10**, 1–40.

WINNICOTT, D. W. (1953) 'Symptom tolerance in paediatrics.' *Proceedings of the Royal Society of Medicine*, **46**, 675–684.

WOLFF, H. H. (1971) 'The therapeutic and developmental functions of psychotherapy.' *British Journal of Medical Psychology*, **44**, 117–130.

YARROW, L. J. (1961) 'Maternal deprivation: towards an empirical and conceptual re-evaluation.' *Psychological Bulletin*, **58**, 459–490.

YATES, A. J. (1958) 'Symptoms and symptom substitution.' *Psychological Review*, **65**, 371–374.

YATES, A. J. (1962) 'A comment on Bookbinder's critique of symptoms and symptom substitution.' *Psychological Reports*, **11**, 102.

INDEX